OSTEOPOROSIS
A Guide for Clinicians

Pauline M. Camacho, MD, FACE
Associate Professor of Medicine
Division of Endocrinology and Metabolism
Loyola University Chicago Stritch School of Medicine
Director, Loyola University Osteoporosis and Metabolic
  Bone Disease Center
Maywood, Illinois

Paul D. Miller, MD
Distinguished Clinical Professor of Medicine
University of Colorado Health Sciences Center
Medical Director
Colorado Center for Bone Research
Lakewood, Colorado

Wolters Kluwer | Lippincott Williams & Wilkins
Health
Philadelphia · Baltimore · New York · London
Buenos Aires · Hong Kong · Sydney · Tokyo

Executive Editor: Charles Mitchell
Managing Editor: Sirkka Bertling
Developmental Editor: Grace R. Caputo, Dovetail Content Solutions
Project Manager: Fran Gunning
Senior Manufacturing Manager: Benjamin Rivera
Marketing Manager: Angela Panetta
Design Coordinator: Stephen Druding
Production Services: Nesbitt Graphics, Inc.
Printer: R. R. Donnelley, Crawfordsville

Library of Congress Cataloging-in-Publication Data

Camacho, Pauline M.
  Osteoporosis : a guide for clinicians / Pauline M. Camacho, Paul D. Miller.
    p. ; cm.
  Includes bibliographical references and index.
  ISBN-13: 978-0-7817-8619-5 (alk. paper)
  ISBN-10: 0-7817-8619-3 (alk. paper)
  1. Osteoporosis. 2. Osteoporosis—Treatment. I. Miller, Paul, 1943- II. Title.
  [DNLM: 1. Osteoporosis. WE 250 C172o 2007]
  RC931.O73C37 2007
  616.7'16—dc22

                                                                    2007000190

Care has been taken to confirm the accuracy of the information presented and to describe generally accepted practices. However, the authors, editors, and publisher are not responsible for errors or omissions or for any consequences from application of the information in this book and make no warranty, expressed or implied, with respect to the currency, completeness, or accuracy of the contents of the publication. Application of this information in a particular situation remains the professional responsibility of the practitioner.

The authors, editors, and publisher have exerted every effort to ensure that drug selection and dosage set forth in this text are in accordance with current recommendations and practice at the time of publication. However, in view of ongoing research, changes in government regulations, and the constant flow of information relating to drug therapy and drug reactions, the reader is urged to check the package insert for each drug for any change in indications and dosage and for added warnings and precautions. This is particularly important when the recommended agent is a new or infrequently employed drug.

Some drugs and medical devices presented in this publication have Food and Drug Administration (FDA) clearance for limited use in restricted settings. It is the responsibility of the health care provider to ascertain the FDA status of each drug or device planned for use in their clinical practice.

To purchase additional copies of this book, call our customer service department at (800) 638-3030 or fax orders to (301) 223-2320. International customers should call (301) 223-2300.

Visit Lippincott Williams & Wilkins on the Internet: at LWW.com. Lippincott Williams & Wilkins customer service representatives are available from 8:30 am to 6 pm, EST.

10 9 8 7 6 5 4 3 2 1

*This book is dedicated to our families.
You are our constant inspiration.
Thank you for being there for us.*

Preface

As the population ages, the prevalence of osteoporosis is increasing worldwide. Care of osteoporotic patients is in the hands of endocrinologists, rheumatologists, geriatricians, primary care physicians, and even physician assistants and nurse practitioners. The field of osteoporosis is evolving rapidly, with new agents, diagnostic methods, and management options being added every day. New data are being published monthly, and for clinicians busy in their practices it is challenging to find the luxury of time to learn these new developments.

Osteoporosis A Guide for Clinicians presents the disease in a comprehensive yet palatable and easily digestible form for busy clinicians, fellows, residents, and students. It delves into all aspects of the disease, from pathophysiology to diagnosis and management. Separate chapters have been devoted to vitamin D deficiency and workup and recognition of secondary causes of bone loss, because these are very important aspects in treating patients successfully. Two chapters focus on future agents on the horizon for osteoporosis and tailoring therapy to specific patient populations. We have also included real patient cases from our clinics and emphasized teaching points for each of the cases.

As an added bonus, we have annotated most of the references so that anyone interested in learning more about the studies mentioned in the text will have easy access to the research methodology, results, and conclusions. To our knowledge, this is the first osteoporosis book that has done this.

After reading *Osteoporosis*, the clinician should have a good understanding of the disorder and should feel comfortable treating it and implementing the appropriate workup and follow-up. We hope that this book will be a valuable tool in providing excellent osteoporosis care in clinics and will help individuals in teaching institutions in disseminating knowledge about the disease to their colleagues and trainees.

Acknowledgments

We would like to thank all of those who have helped make this book a reality: Charley Mitchell, the acquisitions editor at Lippincott Williams & Wilkins; Grace Caputo of Dovetail Content Solutions for her perseverance in keeping us on schedule; Alexandra Reiher, Elizabeth Dillard, Amanda Venti, Leslie Dalaza, and Monica Agarwal for annotating the references; Amit Dayal for his original illustrations; our secretaries, Charmaine Zawitaj, Colette Swain, and Abby Erickson; and most of all our families, who have inspired us and have always supported us in our academic pursuits.

Contents

Preface vii
Acknowledgments ix

1. Diagnosis 1
   Pauline M. Camacho

2. Pathogenesis 15
   Pauline M. Camacho

3. Assessment of Fracture Risk 25
   Paul D. Miller

4. Bone Densitometry: Using Dual-energy X-ray
   Absorptiometry for Monitoring 49
   Paul D. Miller

5. Biochemical Evaluation 63
   Pauline M. Camacho

6. Secondary Causes of Osteoporosis 81
   Pauline M. Camacho

7. Acquired Vitamin D Deficiency 115
   Pauline M. Camacho

8. Treatment Options 127
   Pauline M. Camacho

9. Tailoring Therapy to Individual Patients 149
   Paul D. Miller

10. Determining Success of Therapy and What to Do
    When Therapy Fails 177
    Paul D. Miller

11. Future Therapeutic Options 187
    Paul D. Miller

12. Case Studies 203
    Pauline M. Camacho and Paul D. Miller

Index 221

Diagnosis

Pauline M. Camacho

Aboyon, 1998

Burden of the Disease, 1
Clinical Picture, 1
Diagnosis, 3

Osteoporosis is a skeletal disorder characterized by compromised bone strength, which predisposes to increased risk of fractures [1,2]. Bone strength is a product of both bone density and bone quality. Bone density is expressed as grams of mineral per area or volume; bone quality refers to factors such as architecture, turnover, damage accumulation (e.g., micro-fractures), and mineralization [2]. Whereas bone density can be measured by various methods that are clinically available, bone quality is not readily quantifiable.

BURDEN OF THE DISEASE
Contrary to other common diseases that produce distinct symptoms, osteo-porosis can exist undetected for a long time before complications occur. It is estimated that this bone loss afflicts up to 28 million Americans; of these, 10 million have established osteoporosis [3]. Vertebral fractures are more common than breast cancer, stroke, and heart attack [3–5] (Fig. 1.1). A woman left untreated is predicted to have a 50% chance of suffering from an osteo-porotic fracture sometime in her life [6].

As the cost of healthcare in the United States and other countries continues to rise, it is becoming evident that the complications arising from this preventable and treatable disease account for an increasing chunk of our healthcare spending. With a cost of approximately $21,000 per hip fracture, the estimated total cost of treating hip fractures worldwide in the year 2050 will be $131.5 billion [7]. Thus, it is important that physicians and patients take measures to prevent and treat the disease.

CLINICAL PICTURE
Height Loss
Even without measuring bone mass using available technology, certain symptoms and signs should clue the physician to the presence of the disease. Perhaps the most common, yet the least noted during clinic visits, is

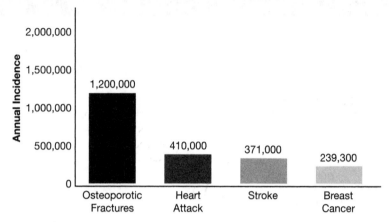

Figure 1.1. Osteoporotic fractures in women, compared with other diseases. Approximately 1.2 million osteoporosis-related fractures occur in women each year [3]. The incidence of osteoporosis-related fractures in women is greater than the annual combined incidence of heart attack [4], stroke [4], and breast cancer [5].

height loss. The majority of vertebral fractures are asymptomatic, with the only presenting symptom being height loss and dorsal kyphosis. Recent findings from the risedronate pivotal trials have shown that height loss of more than 2 cm over 3 years has a sensitivity of 35.5% for detecting new vertebral fractures, and specificity was 93.6% [8]. Furthermore, one study showed that height loss is highly predictive of low spine and hip bone mineral density (BMD) [9].

Dorsal Kyphosis
Dorsal kyphosis, or "dowager's hump," usually occurs as a result of multiple anterior wedge deformities in the thoracic and lumbar spine. It is important that clinicians explain to patients that this deformity is a result of osteoporotic fractures because even today, some patients still equate the "hump" with bad posture. Severe kyphosis also leads to impaired motion of respiratory muscles, leading to dyspnea and possibly restrictive lung disease.

Fragility Fractures
Fragility fractures are those that do not result from high trauma. These ostoeoporotic fractures usually result from falls. Other diseases that may cause low-trauma fractures include osteomalacia and metastatic bone disease.

In addition to vertebral fractures, common fracture locations include the wrist (Colles fractures), ankles, and hip, the fracture that carries the worst prognosis. Fractures in the pelvic bone do occur but are not typical of osteoporotic fractures. Occurrence of such should prompt an evaluation for osteomalacia or metastatic disease.

Acute compression fractures of the spine most commonly occur in the midthoracic region and present with sudden severe pain and tenderness. They usually occur while stooping or carrying a load, but sometimes occur with very little provocation. The pain usually requires multiple medications, such as analgesics and narcotics, for control and can last for weeks to months.

Patients with multiple compression fractures can suffer from chronic back pain, particularly in the lower back area. Hip fractures carry a mortality rate of up to 26%, most commonly due to associated complications such as infections and thromboembolic and cardiovascular events. Long-term disability and loss of independent function can occur in up to 50% of these patients [7,10–12].

DIAGNOSIS

Osteoporosis is most commonly diagnosed using bone densitometry. Various techniques are available to quantify bone mass (Table 1.1), but the most accurate and precise is the central dual-energy x-ray absorptiometry (DXA) scan.

Basic Principle

The basic principle of the DXA scan is that a beam of x-ray is generated and is allowed to pass through the area of interest, usually the spine or the hip. The density of the bone, which is usually determined by its calcium content, causes varying degrees of attenuation of the x-ray beam. As the beam passes through bone and soft tissue, two photoelectric peaks are quantified, and the device is able to subtract the contribution of soft tissue to the measured density. BMD is expressed as an area measurement in grams per square centimeter.

Bone Density and Fracture Risk

Fracture risk increases significantly with age (Fig. 1.2), and the incidence rises sharply after the menopausal years. Hip fractures occur about a decade later, with a sharp increase in incidence around age 70. A strong correlation exists between fracture risk and bone density, and it is said that this relationship is even stronger than that between cholesterol and heart disease (Fig. 1.3).

TABLE 1.1.   Bone Measurement Techniques

Technique	Precision (%)	Significant Change (%)
Spine DXA	1	3
Hip DXA	1.5	4
Q-CT	3	8
p-DXA	2	5
Ultrasound	4	11

DXA, dual-energy x-ray absorptiometry; Q-CT, quantitative computed tomography; p-DXA, peripheral dual-energy x-ray absortiometry

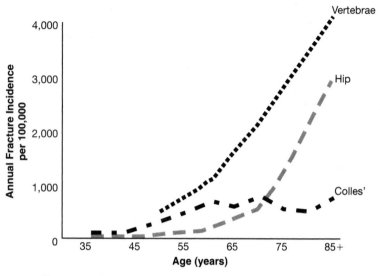

Figure 1.2. Fracture risk with aging in white women. (Adapted from Riggs BL, Melton LJ III. Involutional osteoporosis. N Engl J Med 1986;314:1676, with permission.)

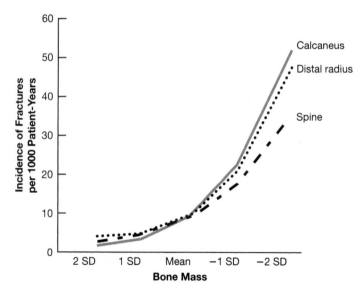

Figure 1.3. Fracture risk vs. bone density. There is an exponential relationship between decreasing bone mass and increasing incidence of fractures. (Adapted from Miller PD, Bonnick SL, Rosen CJ. Consensus of an international panel on the clinical utility of bone mass measurements in the detection of low bone mass in the adult population. Calcif Tissue Int 1996;58:207–214, with permission.)

T-Scores and Z-Scores

The T-score is the number of standard deviations that the BMD falls below or above the mean of a young control group. It is used for diagnosing osteoporosis. Z-scores compare the BMD with age- and sex-matched controls and give an idea of the age-appropriateness of bone loss.

World Health Organization Criteria

The World Health Organization (WHO) criteria are the widely accepted basis for osteoporosis diagnosis (Table 1.2). Based on an analysis of fracture incidence among white postmenopausal women, osteoporosis was defined as a T-score equal to or less than –2.5. T-scores above this cutoff but below –1.0 define osteopenia, or low bone mass. Normal BMD is 1 SD above or below the mean (T-score of –1 to +1). An individual who has a T-score of –2.5 or less and has suffered from an osteoporotic fracture is considered to have severe or established osteoporosis.

Use and Misuse of the World Health Organization Criteria

To fully appreciate the application of the WHO criteria, the original intent behind the creation of the criteria needs to be understood. These criteria were originally established to estimate the prevalence of osteoporosis and to estimate the economic burden of the disease worldwide. A cutoff T-score that roughly matched the estimates of fracture risk among women older than 50 years was chosen. A T-score of –2.5 represented approximately 30% of these women, corresponding to the lifetime fracture risk in the spine, hip, or forearm. In addition, approximately 16% of this population suffered from hip fractures and roughly the same percentage of women had T-scores in the femoral neck of –2.5 or less—thus, the osteoporosis T-score cutoff of –2.5. T-scores were used rather than absolute BMD to mitigate manufacturer- and machine-specific variabilities.

The T-score of –2.5, therefore, does not represent a threshold below which the fracture risk suddenly increases. Rather, fracture risk increases in a continuum, with lower T-scores clearly being associated with more fractures. In other words, a woman who has a T-score of –2.4 may not have significantly lower risk of fractures than a woman with a T-score of –2.6.

TABLE 1.2. **WHO Criteria for Assessing Disease Severity**

Diagnostic Classification	T-Score[a]
Normal	> –1.0
Osteopenia (low bone mass)	–1.0 to –2.5
Osteoporosis	≤ –2.5
Severe (established) osteoporosis	< –2.5 with fracture

WHO, World Health Organization.
[a]Bone mass T-score: the standard deviation in a patient's BMD, compared with the peak bone mass in a young adult of the same gender.

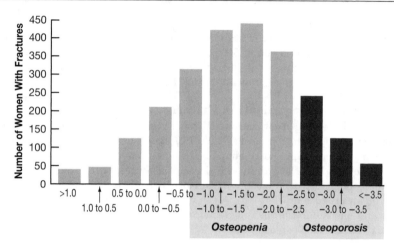

Figure 1.4. Fractures in women with normal or osteopenic T-scores. (Adapted from Siris ES, Chen YT, Abbott TA, et al. Bone mineral density thresholds for pharmacological intervention to prevent fractures. Arch Intern Med 2004;164:1108–1112, with permission.)

Perhaps the most common misuse of the WHO criteria is applying it to nonwhite postmenopausal populations. The fracture risk/T-score relationship used for these criteria was derived solely from a database of white, postmenopausal women. Thus, the criteria cannot be taken to mean or suggest the same fracture risk when the individual being measured is male, premenopausal, or nonwhite.

Another issue is that the WHO criteria do not apply to measurements obtained from peripheral sites. Several studies have shown this. Varney et al. [13] found that compared with central DXA results in the spine and proximal femur, a T-score of –1.9 or less using heel ultrasound (Hologic Sahara) gave the same prevalence of osteoporosis and osteopenia. Along the same lines, Pacheco et al. [14] found that a T-score threshold of –1.3 in the calcaneus as measured by DXA (Lunar Pixi) was the optimum threshold for diagnosing central osteoporosis. The National Osteoporosis Risk Assessment (NORA) study measured heel, phalanges, and forearm bone density and collected fracture data from 163,979 women [15]. In applying the WHO criteria, the prevalence of osteoporosis was found to be only 7.2% (T-score ≤–2.5), although the fracture rate among the whole population was 50% (Fig. 1.4). Thus, the T-scores obtained from peripheral sites do not have the same fracture implication as those obtained with central machines.

Diagnosis among Males
When considering the male population, two questions arise: (a) Is the definition of osteoporosis based on the WHO criteria applicable to males, even though it was derived from a female population? (b) What database shall we

compare males with? The International Society for Clinical Densitometry (ISCD) recommends using a uniform white male normative database for men, regardless of their race.

DXA manufacturers have begun to utilize the National Health and Nutrition Education Survey (NHANES) III database as the default database for their machines. This database allows for comparison of male BMD against a young male population. However, this database is limited in that it offers data only for hip BMD.

A male with a history of fragility fractures in the vertebrae, hip, or non-vertebral areas, with no other metabolic bone disorder, should be diagnosed with osteoporosis regardless of his T-score. When these fractures are not present, the use of a T-score cutoff of −2.5 against a young male population is the most widely accepted definition.

Diagnosis among the Nonwhite Population

As stated earlier, the database upon which the WHO criteria were based was comprised of white, postmenopausal women. What about nonwhite women? The NHANES III database, which includes proximal femur data from non-Hispanic blacks and Mexican Americans, provides a reference database for these large ethnic groups. This database is now the default database of most DXA machines in the United States, although other, smaller groups, such as Asians, are not represented in the database.

Diagnosing Osteoporosis Using Peripheral Devices

Peripheral devices are used widely in health fairs, some pharmacies, and physicians' offices. The biggest issue with using peripheral devices is that there is no standardized database, and each company has its set own reference population database. This leads to highly variant results.

In general, the T-scores obtained in peripheral sites correlate with lower scores in central sites. The probability of having a hip T-score (using central DXA) in the osteoporosis range when the heel T-score is less than −1.0 is 70%, whereas the probability of having a hip T-score less than −2.5 when the peripheral T-score is greater than −1.0 is less than 10%.

It is suggested that these results be interpreted in the light of a thorough risk factor assessment, and that in the absence of significant risk factors, a T-score of less than −1.0 should probably be followed by a central DXA measurement. If there are significant risk factors, such as prior fracture, a central DXA should be obtained regardless of the T-score from the peripheral device.

Common Misinterpretations of Dual-energy X-ray Absorptiometry Scan Results

It is highly advised that treating physicians review the DXA images to detect common artifacts that can affect BMD measurements (Figs. 1.5 to 1.9).

Spine Artifacts

Degenerative changes in the spine are exceedingly common among the elderly. These are seen as sclerotic changes in the facets and discs as well as os-

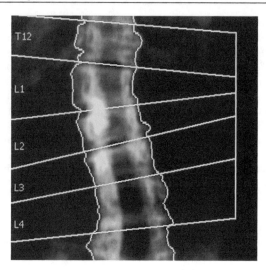

Figure 1.5. Anteroposterior lumbar spine dual-energy x-ray absorptiometry (DXA) scan showing degenerative changes in L1 and L2 and absence of bony structures in L1 to L5 due to laminectomy.

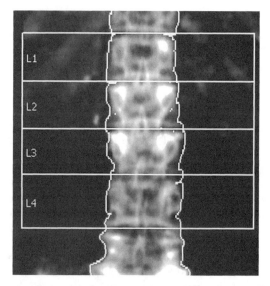

Figure 1.6. Anteroposterior spine dual-energy x-ray absorptiometry (DXA) scan showing sclerotic changes in the facets, which are most prominent in L1 to L3.

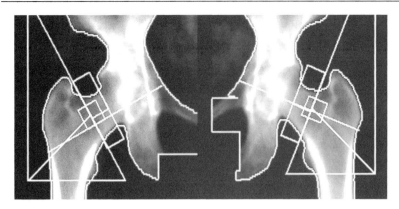

Figure 1.7. Properly positioned femoral neck markers and proper rotation of both hips. Note degree of prominence of internal trochanters.

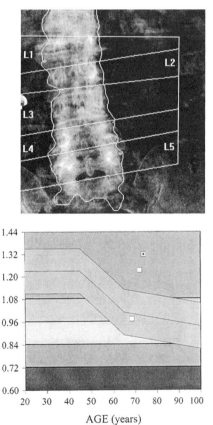

Figure 1.8. Multiple compression fractures in L1 to L4, resulting in elevated BMD and T-scores.   (*continued*)

Region	BMD (g/cm²)	Young-Adult (%)	(T)	Age-Matched (%)	(Z)
L1	1.310	116	+1.5	142	+3.2
L2	1.250	104	+0.4	126	+2.1
L3	1.304	109	+0.9	131	+2.6
L4	1.416	118	+1.8	142	+3.5
L2-L4	1.326	110	+1.0	133	+2.8

Figure 1.8. (*Continued*)

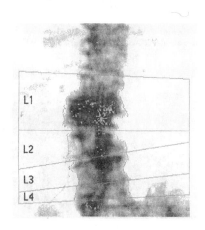

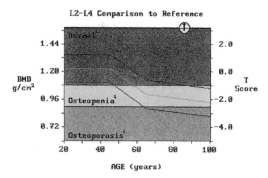

Region	BMD g/cm²	Young-Adult %	T-Score	Age-Matched %	Z-Score
L2-L4	1.648	137	3.7	171	5.7

Figure 1.9. Paget disease involvement of L1 and L2 and compression fractures in L3 and L4, leading to elevated bone mineral density.

teophyte formation. They elevate BMD and may lead to "falsely" normal BMD and T-scores in the spine.

Vertebrae with compression fractures are denser than normal vertebrae and would have higher T-scores. It would be a big mistake to withhold therapy for a patient who appears to have normal T-scores due to compression fractures.

Other artifacts in the spine that can lead to falsely elevated BMD include metal in clothing, metallic prosthesis from previous spine surgeries, Paget disease, inferior vena cava (IVC) filters, and severe atherosclerosis of the aorta.

Vertebral Markers
Unusually large and seemingly unphysiologic changes in BMD that are seen while patients are being monitored should prompt a thorough comparison of prior and current images. One possible mistake is improper positioning of L1 to L4 vertebral markers. With very few exceptions, the upper border of the ilium, or the iliac crest, should correspond with the lower border of L4.

Rotation of the Hip
The hip is more prone to technical differences due to difficulty with positioning of the hip of some elderly patients. Cushions are usually provided for placement under the legs to ensure proper internal rotation of the hip, although inconsistencies commonly arise. The degree of prominence of the internal trochanter can be used as a guide to compare the rotations of hip images.

Femoral Neck Marker
The width of the femoral marker must be kept consistent with each measurement, as significant differences in BMD will result when this is varied. Another common source of BMD technical differences arises from variable placement of the marker in the femoral neck.

REFERENCES
Annotations by Amanda Venti
1. **Kanis JA, Melton LJ III, Christiansen C,** et al. The diagnosis of osteoporosis. J Bone Miner Res 1994;9:1137–1141.
2. **NIH Consensus Development Panel on Osteoporosis prevention, diagnosis, and therapy.** JAMA 2001;285:785–795.

   Article summarizes the findings of a panel of 13 medical professionals representing a variety of subspecialities who were presented with data from 32 experts regarding prevention, diagnosis, and treatment of osteoporosis. The event, sponsored by the National Institute of Arthritis and Musculoskeletal and Skin Diseases and the National Institutes of Health Office of Medical Applications of Research, took place from March 27 to 29, 2000. A series of questions to be answered by the panel on the basis of the data presented was created beforehand. The material discussed included the results of a Medline search for January 1995 through December 1999. The panel concluded that osteoporosis affects all populations and age groups and has important physical, psychosocial, and financial consequences. The panel commented on risks for osteoporosis and fracture as well as factors determining who should be tested and treated. The group also drew conclusions regarding dietary supplementation and exercise, as well as the role of gonadal steroids in osteoporosis. The panel identified fracture prevention as the primary goal of therapy.

3. **National Osteoporosis Foundation.** 2003 Disease statistics (fast facts). Available at: http://www.nof.org.

4. **American Heart Association.** Heart disease and stroke statistics: 2003 update. Available at: http://www.americanheart.org.

5. **American Cancer Society.** Breast cancer facts & figures 2001–2002. Available at: http://www.cancer.org.

6. **Chrischilles EA, Butler CD, Davis CS,** et al. A model of lifetime osteoporosis impact. Arch Intern Med 1991;151:2026–2032.
   The objective of this study was to create a model for the impact of lifetime osteoporosis. The model was designed to predict the lifetime number of fractures in a cohort of 10,000 fifty-year-old white postmenopausal women, as well as the number of years of functional impairment they suffered secondary to fracture. Hip, vertebral, and Colles fractures were considered. According to this model, 54% of 50-year-old women will incur one of these fractures during the remainder of their lives, with 6.7% becoming dependent in their basic activities of daily living and 7.8% requiring nursing home care for approximately 7.6 years.

7. **Johnell O.** The socioeconomic burden of fractures: Today and in the 21st century. Am J Med 1997;103:20S–25S; discussion 5S–6S.
   This article discusses the cost-effectiveness of treating osteoporosis. The cost of hip fractures imposes a significant economic burden on society that could be reduced by treating the appropriate population preventively. The projected cost of hip fractures in the year 2050 is $131.5 billion. The paper states that models incorporating incidence, morbidity, mortality, costs of fractures, and efficacy of intervention can be used to quantify the potential benefit of treating osteoporosis. Cost-effectiveness is, of course, contingent upon the efficacy of treatment, patient compliance, age of the patient when treatment is initiated, and fracture risk. It is most beneficial to treat those at highest risk and to utilize the most effective interventions possible.

8. **Siminoski K, Jiang G, Adachi JD,** et al. Accuracy of height loss during prospective monitoring for detection of incident vertebral fractures. Osteoporos Int 2005; 16:403–410.
   This study included 985 postmenopausal women with osteoporosis in the placebo arms of the Vertebral Efficacy with Risedronate Therapy studies. The goal of the study was to determine the correlation between height loss and the development of new vertebral fractures, and whether height loss could be used in clinical practice to identify individuals with new fractures. The height of the participants was measured with a stadiometer each year for 3 years. The presence of new fractures was detected with quantitative and semiquantitative radiographic morphometry. The study concluded that height loss in cm = 0.95 × number of new vertebral fractures – 0.4 cm ($r = 0.33$). When height loss exceeded 4.0 cm, the odds ratio for the development of a new fracture went up to 20.6 (95% confidence interval, 9.3, 45.8). A height loss of more than 2.0 cm predicted a new vertebral fracture, with a sensitivity of 35.5% and a specificity of 93.6%.

9. **Moayyeri A, Ahmadi-Abhari S, Hossein-Nezhad A,** et al. Bone mineral density and estimated height loss based on patients' recalls. Osteoporos Int 2006;17:834–840.
   The study included a randomized clustered sampling of 457 individuals from all regions of Tehran, of both genders and all ages. These individuals were asked to recall their maximum height as measured previously. Each participant's current measured height was subtracted from his or her remembered maximum height. The results indicated a relationship between height loss (based on human memory) and bone mineral density (BMD). An estimated height reduction of greater than 5 cm correlated with lower L1 to L4 lumbar BMD, femoral neck BMD, and young adjusted T-scores. The investigators used a linear regression analysis to determine that height loss is a significant predictor of femoral neck T-score (standardized beta coefficient = –0.15; $p = 0.003$) and L1 to L4 lumbar T-score (beta = –0.078; $p = 0.048$). Height loss was a significant predictor for femoral neck T-score, even when age, gender, and weight were taken into consideration (beta = 10.078; $p = 0.043$). Height loss was a predictor of lumbar T-score only in participants younger than 50 years old.

10. **Cooper C, Atkinson EJ, Jacobsen SJ,** et al. Population-based study of survival after osteoporotic fractures. Am J Epidemiol 1993;137:1001–1005.

The study was based on a cohort of 335 residents of Rochester, Minnesota, diagnosed with vertebral fracture between 1985 and 1989. Of these, 76 died during 809 person-years of follow-up. Survival rates were much lower than expected, and at 5 years after diagnosis, survival was only 61%, in contrast to the predicted value of 76%. This corresponds to a relative survival of 0.81, 95% confidence interval 0.70 to 0.92. Findings were similar with reference to hip fractures with a 5-year survival equal to 0.82, 95% confidence interval 0.77 to 0.87. Five-year relative survival following distal forearm fracture was 1.00, with a 95% confidence interval 0.95 to 1.05.

11. **Davidson CW, Merrilees MJ, Wilkinson TJ,** et al. Hip fracture mortality and morbidity—can we do better? N Z Med J 2001;114:329–332.

This study examined the outcomes of all patients treated for a hip fracture at Christchurch Hospitals between May 1998 and April 1999. The study included 329 patients, of whom 242 were women and 87 were men. The mean age of these individuals was 79.7, with a standard deviation of 10.5 years. The investigators spoke with surviving patients regarding their ability to function after surgical intervention. These patients were at 12 months out from their fracture. The study looked at the number of patients who underwent a bone density scan, as well as the number of patients in whom a vitamin D level was checked. They also noted the number of people actually treated for osteoporosis following hip fracture. In this patient population, 12-month mortality was 26%, with a higher mortality in men than in women regardless of age or fracture type. Twelve to 24 months following fracture, 27% of patients still had pain and 60% had worsened mobility secondary to the fracture. Only 15%, or 32 people, were tested for vitamin D deficiency, of which 69%, or 22 people, were indeed found to be deficient. The study concluded that there is significant morbidity and mortality secondary to hip fracture (particularly in men) and that vitamin D deficiency often goes unrecognized.

12. **Olsson C, Petersson C, Nordquist A.** Increased mortality after fracture of the surgical neck of the humerus: A case-control study of 253 patients with a 12-year follow-up. Acta Orthop Scand 2003;74:714–717.

This study is a long-term follow-up case-control mortality study of 253 patients with a fracture of the surgical neck of the humerus during the year 1987 (study conducted in 1999). The mean patient age was 72 years. The study found a median survival time of 8.9 years in those with fracture compared with 12 years in controls with a p value of 0.005. This corresponds to a cumulative survival difference of 16%. Survival difference was more remarkable in men, with a median survival time of 6.5 years in male patients who sustained fracture compared with 12 years in their male controls, with a p value of 0.02. Mortality following fracture was higher in women as well, but only slightly (p value = 0.06). The most common cause of death in both populations (those who had sustained a fracture of the humerus and their controls) was cardiovascular disease and malignancy.

13. **Varney LF, Parker RA, Vincelette A,** et al. Classification of osteoporosis and osteopenia in postmenopausal women is dependent on site-specific analysis. J Clin Densitom 1999;2:275–283.

This study included 115 ambulatory, community-dwelling white, postmenopausal women in whom bone density was measured at the hip, posteroanterior spine, forearm, and finger by dual-energy x-ray absorptiometry, and at the calcaneus using ultrasound. The study assessed the ability of a bone density measurement at a single site to accurately predict a diagnosis of osteoporosis. When only the trochanteric region was evaluated, 4% of the study population were found to have osteoporosis, compared with 34% when Ward triangle measurements were utilized. In addition, looking at calcaneus measurements alone leads to a diagnosis of osteoporosis in 17%, and using the finger leads to a diagnosis in 13%. If, however, multiple standard central sites were taken into account, then 28% of women had osteoporosis (based on one osteoporotic value among the three sites). Within this subpopulation, the use of the Sahara Clinical Bone Sonometer did not make the diagnosis in 16% of patients with osteoporosis. Thirty-four percent of these patients were misdiagnosed as being "normal" using the accuDEXA Bone Mineral Density (BMD) Assessment System.

14. **Pacheco EM, Harrison EJ, Ward KA,** et al. Detection of osteoporosis by dual-energy X-ray absorptiometry (DXA) of the calcaneus: Is the WHO criterion applicable? Calcif Tissue Int 2002;70:475–482.

This study included 202 women with a mean age of 55.2 (SD = 13.7) in whom bone density was measured using a new peripheral dual-energy x-ray absorptiometry (DXA) scanner applied to the calcaneus. Measurements taken by this new scanner were found to be precise (0.48% *in vitro*, 1.40% *in vivo*), with little variation despite differences in operator, foot size, or body mass index. The calcaneus bone mineral density (BMD) measurements correlated with axial BMD measurements, with $r = 0.494$ to 0.690, $p < 0.001$. The specificity of the calcaneus measurements in predicting osteoporosis at axial sites was high (96.5%–97.1%). However, the test lacked sensitivity (20.3%–58.8%). The authors therefore propose the utilization of a different T-score threshold (–1.4) based on results of calcaneus measurements, when determining who should be referred for axial DXA.

15. **Siris ES, Miller PD, Barrett-Connor E,** et al. Identification and fracture outcomes of undiagnosed low bone mineral density in postmenopausal women: results from the National Osteoporosis Risk Assessment. JAMA 2001;286:2815–2822.

This is a longitudinal observational study undertaken from September 1997 to March 1999, with 12 months of follow-up. The study population was drawn from 4,236 primary care practices in 34 states and included 200,160 ambulatory postmenopausal women 50 years or older who carried no previous diagnosis of osteoporosis. Peripheral bone densitometry at the heel, finger, or forearm was used to establish a baseline bone mineral density (BMD) T-score for each patient. In addition, each participant filled out a questionnaire regarding risk factors for osteoporosis. Clinical fracture rates were derived at 12-month follow-up. A total of 39.6% of participants were found to have osteopenia by World Health Organization criteria, and 7.2% were found to have osteoporosis. Risk factors identified for the disease included age, history of fracture, Asian or Hispanic heritage, smoking, and cortisone. There was a lower incidence of osteoporosis in those of African American heritage, those using estrogen or diuretics, and in those who exercised or consumed alcohol. The rate of fracture in those with osteoporosis was 4 times higher than in those with a normal BMD (rate ratio, 4.03; 95% CI, 3.59–4.53). The rate of fracture in those with osteopenia was 1.8-fold higher (95% CI, 1.49–2.18). The study stressed the importance of identifying osteoporosis in the primary care setting in order to provide appropriate therapy to decrease the risk of fracture.

2

Pathogenesis

Pauline M. Camacho

Bone Remodeling Cycle, 15
Postmenopausal Osteoporosis, 16
Male Osteoporosis, 18
Glucocorticoid-induced Osteoporosis, 18

BONE REMODELING CYCLE

Bone is in a constant state of turnover or activity throughout life. Remodeling is the process of renewing bone by breaking down old bone and forming new bone. At the very core of this process is a unit, or group of cells, called the bone-remodeling unit (BRU). There are four distinct stages of bone remodeling, specifically, activation, resorption, reversal, and formation (Fig. 2.1).

Activation is initiated by the recruitment of osteoclast precursors into the areas that need to be resorbed. It is not yet exactly clear how the body determines which areas need to be remodeled. The precursor (mononucleated) cells fuse to become preosteoclast (multinucleated) cells and mature further into osteoclasts. The factors that are thought to regulate the process of osteoclast maturity include local factors such as receptor activator of nuclear factor-κB ligand (RANKL), interleukin-1 and -6 (IL-1, IL-6), colony-stimulating factors (CSF-1), tumor necrosis factor (TNF), transforming growth factor β (TGF-β), and systemic factors such as parathyroid hormone (PTH), 1,25-hydroxyvitamin D (OHD), and calcitonin [1–5]. Once activated, the osteoclasts acidify and release resorptive enzymes, leading to the formation of resorption cavities. After their job is finished, the osteoclasts undergo apoptosis.

This process is followed by the reversal stage, during which coupling signals are sent to attract osteoblasts into the resorptive sites. Resorption is then turned off, and the formation stage follows. The osteoblasts synthesize bone matrix and facilitate its mineralization. Calcium and phosphate ions are deposited into the matrix, leading to hardening of the bone. Osteoblasts undergo apoptosis, become encased within the mineralized matrix to become osteocytes, or evolve into bone-lining cells. The osteocytes maintain communication with each other, and they likely play a role in sensing the areas that need to be remodeled, transmitting information to other cells, and initiating the bone-remodeling process. The end product is the formation of new bone; this is where a negative balance may occur, leading to osteoporosis.

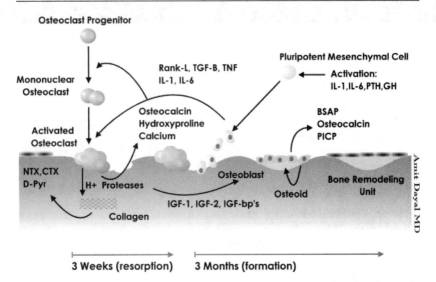

Figure 2.1.   The bone remodeling cycle. Rank-L, receptor activator of nuclear factor-κB ligand; TGF, transforming growth factor; TNF, tumor necrosis factor; IL, interleukin; PTH, parathyroid hormone; GH, growth hormone; BSAP, bone-specific alkaline phosphatase; PICP, procollagen I carboxyterminal propeptide; IGF, insulin-like growth factor; D-Pyr, urinary deoxypyridinoline; NTX, N-telopeptide; CTX, C-telopeptide.

POSTMENOPAUSAL OSTEOPOROSIS

The basic pathology in osteoporosis is an imbalance between bone resorption and bone formation. The most common cause of this imbalance is menopause. The bone mass of an elderly woman is the product of her peak bone mass and bone loss that she has incurred for various reasons (Table 2.1).

Peak Bone Mass

Puberty is characterized by rapid gain in bone brought on by surges in sex hormone levels. This gain continues until the peak is reached, at age 20 to 30 years (Fig. 2.2). Approximately 50% to 80% of a woman's peak bone mass is determined by her genetic predisposition [6], but other factors such as calcium, vitamin D intake, activity level, low body weight, illnesses, or delayed puberty also contribute to the overall product.

TABLE 2.1.   Factors that play a role in osteoporotic bone loss

- Age
- Genetics
- Estrogen
- Androgens
- Calcium, vitamin D, parathyroid hormone
- Thyroid hormones
- Glucocorticoids
- Local cytokines and growth factors
- Growth hormone

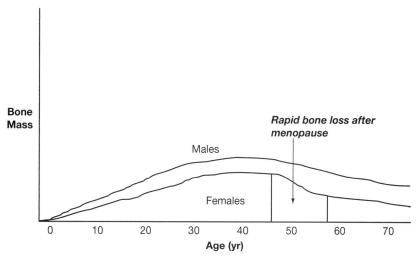

Figure 2.2.   Normal bone mass among males and females.

Period of Bone Loss

After peak bone mass is reached, the bone remodeling process is in a state of equilibrium until menopause. Cessation of estrogen production leads to rapid bone loss of approximately 2% to 3% per year in the spine for up to 6 to 8 years, which accounts for 50% of the total spinal bone loss among normal women [7]. This is then followed by a slower rate of bone loss (0.5%/year), which is attributed to aging (Fig. 2.2) [7].

Why does estrogen deficiency lead to acceleration of bone loss? Estrogen deficiency causes an increase in activation frequency, perhaps due to local growth factors and cytokines, which affect osteoblastic and osteoclastic action, with the net effect being a negative bone balance at the end of each remodeling cycle. This is further supported by the fact that after menopause, markers of both bone resorption and formation increase, and a greater increase is seen in bone resorption markers.

Even among men, it is now known that estrogen deficiency plays a big role in bone loss, perhaps an even bigger role than played by testosterone [8]. Studies among osteoporotic males have shown a closer correlation between estradiol levels and bone mineral density (BMD) than testosterone and BMD. A finding that men with osteoporosis may have low estradiol yet normal testosterone levels further supported this correlation [9].

Age-related bone loss is attributable to various factors (Fig. 2.3). Decline in kidney function leads to decreased 1α hydroxylation of vitamin D, decrease in gut calcium absorption, secondary hyperparathyroidism, and subsequent increase in bone resorption. Estrogen deficiency also contributes to diminished calcium absorption from the gastrointestinal tract and secondary hyperparathyroidism. Other factors that occur with aging include decrease in physical activity and in growth hormone secretion, ultimately leading to diminished osteoblastic function [7].

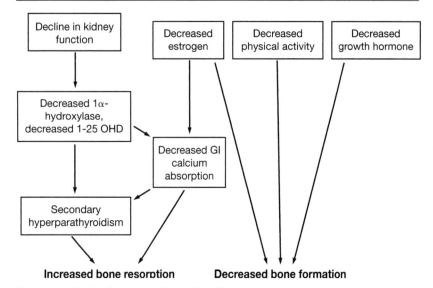

Figure 2.3. Pathophysiology of age-related bone loss among women.
GI, gastrointestinal.

MALE OSTEOPOROSIS

Most men develop osteoporosis because of secondary causes of bone loss (which will be discussed in more detail in Chapter 6). Like bone gain in women, bone gain in men accelerates during adolescence, but the peak bone mass is reached a little later in life. Contrary to the situation in women, however, there is no period of dramatic and accelerated bone loss; rather, there is a steady decline, similar to what occurs after the menopausal years. In general, clear differences in the bone structure of men and women protect men from osteoporosis. Specifically, their bones are larger and the cortices thicker.

The age-related changes in women described previously also occur in men. Bone loss is similarly more pronounced in trabecular bone. Slight cortical thinning in the long bones does occur but does not appear to contribute much to an increased risk of fracture, as there is an increase in periosteal bone expansion that preserves bone strength [10].

Hypogonadism, whether idiopathic or induced by medications, is an increasing cause of osteoporosis among men. The use of androgen deprivation therapy has been clearly associated with bone loss among men with prostate cancer [11–16]. Bone loss occurs at a rate of 3% to 4% per year and can continue for up to 10 years of therapy [13].

GLUCOCORTICOID-INDUCED OSTEOPOROSIS

The most common cause of secondary osteoporosis is the use of glucocorticoids. These agents have adverse effects both on bone formation and on bone resorption (Table 2.2). Glucocorticoids appear to have a direct inhibitory effect on the growth and differentiation of osteoblasts [17]. This has

TABLE 2.2.   Glucocorticoid effects on bone

- Decreased osteoblast growth, differentiation, and function, and increased apoptosis
- Increased osteoclast life through increase in receptor activator of nuclear factor $\kappa\beta$ ligand (RANKL) and decrease in osteoprotegerin (OPG)
- Decreased gonadal steroids
- Increased calcium excretion and secondary hyperparathyroidism

also been observed in histomorphometric studies [18]. They negatively affect the synthesis of local regulators such as insulin-like growth factor I (IGF-I), they decrease IGF-II receptor expression in osteoblasts [17,19], and they decrease levels of osteocalcin. Not only do glucocorticoids affect the differentiation of osteoblasts, but they also cause premature osteoblast and osteocyte apoptosis [19].

The effect of glucocorticoids on bone resorption is probably of equal magnitude to their detrimental effect on bone formation. Glucocorticoids increase RANKL and decrease osteoprotegerin (OPG), which leads to decreased osteoclastic apoptosis [20]. These agents also decrease intestinal calcium absorption [21,22] and increase urinary calcium and phosphate loss [23,24], thus causing secondary hyperparathyroidism. The results of studies on the effects of glucocorticoids on vitamin D metabolism are not consistent; thus, it is likely the effects on calcium metabolism that trigger the release of PTH.

Other effects of glucocorticoids include decreased secretion of gonadal steroids [25], decreased muscle mass and muscle strength, and a resultant decrease in physical activity.

REFERENCES
Annotations by Leslie Dalaza

1. **Blair HC, Athanasou NA.** Recent advances in osteoclast biology and pathological bone resorption. Histol Histopathol 2004;19:189–199.

   Osteoclasts are polykaryons that degrade bone. Studies of the processes that resorb bone have been done, and it was found that osteoclasts are derived from precursor monocytes or from macrophages. It is found that the contact between high concentrations of mononuclear phagocyte colony-stimulating factor (M-CSF) and mesenchymal cells with the tumor necrosis factor (TNF) family ligand of receptor activator of nuclear factor-κB ligand (RANKL) drives the formation of osteoclasts. Osteoclast precursors that express receptor activator of NF-κB (RANK) also interact with RANKL to increase osteoclast activity, resulting in bone resorption diseases, inflammation, arthritis, and malignant bone absorption. The expression of RANK and RANKL can be altered by parathyroid hormone (PTH), glucocorticoids, and humoral factors. TNFα, interleukin (IL)-6, and IL-11 contribute to osteoclast formation. Osteoclasts express proteins such as vacuolar type H+–adenosine triphosphatase (ATPase), which drives HCl secretion for bone resorption. The 116VO subunit of v-ATPase has many isoforms, but TCLRG1 is specifically upregulated in osteoclasts. Thus, the causes of osteoporosis are the following: chloride channel homologue defects, defects in phagocytosis, and defects in key ion transporters/enzymes that play a role in bone degradation.

2. **Boyle WJ, Simonet WS, Lacey DL.** Osteoclast differentiation and activation. Nature 2003;423:337–342.

   Osteoclasts are derived from the monocyte/macrophage hematopoietic lineage in the bone matrix, which secretes acid that degrades bone. Osteoclasts contain RANKL-signaling pathways that are active in bone resorption. Further studies of this RANKL pathway are under way, to better treat osteoporosis.

3. **Roodman GD.** Cell biology of the osteoclast. Exp Hematol 1999;27:1229–1241.

   Osteoclasts are derived from the granulocyte/macrophage colony-forming units (CFU-GM) and monocyte-macrophage lineage. The marrow environment is important for the production of RANKL, the differentiation factor for osteoclasts. Osteoprotegerin is known to be an inhibitor of osteoclast formation. The oncogenes c-fos and pp60 c-src offer insights into the regulation of the osteoclast pathways, specifically differentiation and bone resorption. Studies are now in progress to see how hormones or cytokines affect the osteoclast-signaling pathway.

4. **Roodman GD.** Mechanisms of bone metastasis. N Engl J Med 2004;350:1655–1664.

5. **Troen BR.** Molecular mechanisms underlying osteoclast formation and activation. Exp Gerontol 2003;38:605–614.

   Osteoporosis is a disease characterized by bone loss and the decrease in bone density. RANKL regulates osteoclast differentiation and activation, whereas tumor receptor–associated factors (TRAFS) regulate osteoclastogenesis. Cathepsin K and the sex steroids also affect osteoclastogenesis. This review discusses the various cytokines, growth factors, and hormones that regulate bone homeostasis, or the equilibrium between osteoblasts and osteoclasts.

6. **Jin H, Ralston SH.** Genetics of osteoporosis. Curr Rheumatol Rep 2005;7:66–70.

7. **Riggs BL, Khosla S, Melton LJ III.** Sex steroids and the construction and conservation of the adult skeleton. Endocr Rev 2002;23:279–302.

   This review article discusses the role of estrogen in regulating bone loss. Here, it is found that estrogen deficiency causes bone loss in both sexes, whereas in conjunction with growth hormone and insulin-like growth factor I (IGF-I), a 3- to 4-year growth spurt occurs in puberty—thus doubling the skeletal mass. Testosterone, however, accounts for the thicker cortices in the male skeleton. In women, there are two phases of bone loss—one that begins in menopause, as the loss of cancellous bone, and a faster phase, which increases cortical bone and results in secondary hyperparathyroidism. Overall, it is believed that the amount of biological estrogen is the major predictor of bone loss.

8. **Khosla S, Melton LJ III, Riggs BL.** Clinical review 144: Estrogen and the male skeleton. J Clin Endocrinol Metab 2002;87:1443–1450.

   It has been thought that estrogen in women, and testosterone in men, is responsible for bone turnover. However, it was found that in estrogen receptor (ER)–deficient and aromatase-deficient men, high bone turnover and osteopenia resulted. Thus, knock-out mice were developed that obliterated the ER-α and -aromatase genes. From this, it was found that estrogen is involved in the growth and maturation of the male skeleton. However, the distinction between the role of estrogen and testosterone was not defined. It is thought that estrogen is dominant in regulating bone metabolism in men. Thus, treatments that involve estrogen modulators or testosterone replacement, that mediate via the aromatization to estrogen, may treat men who are losing bone.

9. **Carlsen CG, Soerensen TH, Eriksen EF.** Prevalence of low serum estradiol levels in male osteoporosis. Osteoporos Int 2000;11:697–701.

   Of 63 men who participated in this study, 36 had low-energy spine fractures with bone mineral density (BMD) less than 2.5, 47 had lumbar BMD less than 2.5, and a hip BMD T-score less than 2.5. Of the 63 men, 42 were found to have primary osteoporosis; of those 42 men, 33% were found to have serum estradiol levels below normal ($p < 0.001$), whereas 3% had male hypogonadism in which their serum testosterone levels were below normal. Of the 63 men, 27 had their estrogen status available; of the 37, 26 had primary osteoporosis, none showed signs of hypogonadism, and 38% had undetectable levels of serum estradiol (<48 pM). Thus, estrogen deficiency can result in male osteoporosis. In further screenings for osteoporosis, men should have their serum estradiol levels screened.

10. **Seeman E.** Pathogenesis of bone fragility in women and men. Lancet 2002;359:1841–1850.

    It is thought that genetics and environmental factors play roles in bone fragility. As individuals get older, more bone is resorbed than formed—thus resulting in bone loss. In women, estrogen deficiency in menopause results in bone loss. Twenty percent to 30% of men with hypogonadism experience bone loss. In both men and women, hyperparathy-roidism increases bone remodeling, thus increasing the incidence of hip fractures. How-ever, in men, bone cortical formation compensates for bone loss. Women, however, are more architecturally sensitive to bone fractures.

11. **Daniell HW.** Osteoporosis due to androgen deprivation therapy in men with prostate cancer. Urology 2001;58(Suppl 1):101–107.

It is found that androgen deprivation therapy (ADT), usually in the treatment of prostate cancer, increases instances of osteoporosis in men. The relationship between bone mineral density (BMD) and development of osteoporotic fractures is discussed. Regular exercise and the administration of calcium, vitamin D, bisphosphonates, and calcitonin, as well as the cessation of smoking, are thought to be good therapies in preventing bone loss. How-ever, further studies are necessary in order to find the best therapeutic techniques in pre-venting osteoporosis in men with prostate cancer.

12. **Daniell HW, Dunn SR, Ferguson DW,** et al. Progressive osteoporosis during andro-gen deprivation therapy for prostate cancer. J Urol 2000;163:181–186.

A risk factor for osteoporosis in older men is hypogonadism. Femoral neck bone mineral density (BMD) was measured in 26 men before chemical castration and at 6-month inter-vals for 6 to 42 months. The BMDs of 16 men were measured at 12- to 24-month intervals beginning 3 to 8 years after castration, and bone loss was compared with the measurement in 12 control subjects. It was found that men who had been untreated by androgen depri-vation therapy (ADT) had higher BMD, which remained unchanged for 2 years. After cas-tration, BMD decreased by 2.4% to 7.4% in years 1 and 2 and by 2.5% to 17% in year 2. The average BMD loss during years 3 through 8 was found to be 1.4% to 2.6%. It was found that bone loss increased in obese men who did not exercise. Thus, men who were younger than 75 and chemically castrated could expect bone loss to follow. Therefore, age, obesity, and exercise influences bone loss in men undergoing ADT for prostate cancer.

13. **Kiratli BJ, Srinivas S, Perkash I,** et al. Progressive decrease in bone density over 10 years of androgen deprivation therapy in patients with prostate cancer. Urology 2001;57:127–132.

The longitudinal effects of androgen deprivation therapy (ADT) were studied in men with prostate cancer. In this study, hip and spine bone mineral density (BMD) was measured in 36 male prostate cancer patients at the following times: year 0 ($n = 0$), year 2 ($n = 6$), year 4 ($n = 7$), year 6 ($n = 5$), year 8 ($n = 5$), and year 10 ($n = 5$) of ADT therapy. It was found that as the years of ADT increased, BMD decreased ($r = 0.46$, $p = 0.00008$), and hip BMD de-creased among age-related subjects [$r = 0.55$, $p = 0.5 \times 10$ (–16)]. Thus, the hip BMD de-creased (mean BMD 0.0802 g/cm^2 on ADT compared with men's hip BMD without ADT (mean 0.935 g/cm^2]. It was also found that the decrease of BMD was more drastic for cas-tration than medical ADT ($p = 0.08$). Thus, continuous ADT and castration as therapeutic agents for men with prostate cancer prove deleterious, for these therapies decrease their bone density.

14. **Ross RW, Small EJ.** Osteoporosis in men treated with androgen deprivation ther-apy for prostate cancer. J Urol 2002;167:1952–1956.

The literature was searched on androgen deprivation therapy's (ADT's) effect on the onset of secondary osteoporosis. It is thought that male osteoporosis, fracture incidence, and de-creased bone mineral density (BMD) are possible side effects of ADT. It is widely accepted that hypogonadism results in osteoporosis—possibly through antitestosterone effects. It is noted that there is a 3% to 5% loss of bone yearly and an increased incidence of fractures of ADT. Bisphosphatates may have positive effects on preventing bone loss. However, more data are needed on the correlation between ADT and male osteoporosis. Until then, it is best that men on ADT receive calcium and vitamin D, and partake in moderate exercise.

15. **Stoch SA, Parker RA, Chen L,** et al. Bone loss in men with prostate cancer treated with gonadotropin-releasing hormone agonists. J Clin Endocrinol Metab 2001; 86:2787–2791.

The tumors of prostate cancer are thought to be testosterone dependent; thus, go-nadotropin-releasing hormone (GnRH) agonists (GnRH-a), which cause hypogonadism, are often used as therapy. It is hypothesized that GnRH-a has a negative effect on bone density. This study involved 60 men with prostate cancer, 19 of them receiving GnRH-a therapy and 41 of them eugonadal. The factors measured were the following: bone mineral density (BMD), markers for bone turnover (urinary N-telopeptides), and body composition (total body fat and lean body mass). They were compared with 197 controls of similar age. The BMD in men receiving GnRH-a decreased [lateral spine (0.69 ± 0.17 vs. 0.83 ± 0.20 g/cm^2; $p < 0.01$), total hip (0.94 ± 0.14 vs. 1.05 ± 0.16 g/cm^2; $p < 0.05$), and forearm (0.67 ± 0.11 vs. 0.78 ± 0.07 g/cm^2; $p < 0.01$)] compared with eugonadonal men with prostate cancer, whose BMD values were similar to that of the control. The bone turnover markers were found in increased levels in men receiving GnRH-a therapy, compared with the eugonadal men. Also, it was found that men receiving GnRH-a therapy experienced an increase in body fat and body weight (29 ± 5% vs. 25 ± 5%; $p < 0.01$) and lower percent lean body weight (71 ± 5% vs. 75 ± 5%; $p < 0.01$) compared with eugonadal men. Thus, men receiving GnRH-a therapy had a decrease in bone mass and an increase in bone turnover, which increased the risk of fractures.

16. **Wei JT, Gross M, Jaffe CA,** et al. Androgen deprivation therapy for prostate cancer results in significant loss of bone density. Urology 1999;54:607–611.

The long-term effects of androgen deprivation therapy (ADT) on bone mineral density (BMD) was studied in 32 men with prostate cancer. It was hypothesized that with ADT therapy, there would be a measurable loss in BMD. The 32 men consisted of those about to begin ADT therapy and those who had been receiving ADT therapy for more than a year. BMD was measured in the lumbar spine and hip. It was found that 63% of the men who had not received ADT and 88% of those who had received ADT for more than 1 year had osteopenia or osteoporosis at more than one site. Also, ADT therapy decreased lumbar spine BMD more so for men treated with ADT than for men without ADT ($p < 0.05$). Thus, ADT therapy and its duration are associated with decreased BMD in men with prostate cancer.

17. **Canalis E, Bilezikian JP, Angeli A,** et al. Perspectives on glucocorticoid-induced osteoporosis. Bone 2004;34:593–598.

18. **Dalle Carbonare L, Arlot ME, Chavassieux PM,** et al . Comparison of trabecular bone microarchitecture and remodeling in glucocorticoid-induced and postmenopausal osteoporosis. J Bone Miner Res 2001;16:97–103.

In this study, the effect of long-term use of glucocorticoids on cancellous bone remodeling was studied. It was hypothesized that glucocorticoid treatments increase bone loss and the incidence of fractures. To test this hypothesis, 22 transiliac biopsy specimens were taken from postmenopausal women (65 ± 6 years) receiving glucocorticoids (≥7.5 mg/day, for at least 6 months); also 22 age-matched specimens were taken from untreated postmenopausal women with osteoporosis (T-score < –2.5). It was found that glucocorticoid-induced osteoporosis decreased bone volume, trabecular thickness, wall thickness, osteoid thickness, and bone formation rate, whereas it increased resorption. The women with glucocorticoid-induced osteoporosis were divided into two groups: one group receiving a high cumulative dose of glucocorticoids (23.7 ± 9.7 g) and the other group receiving a low cumulative dose of glucocorticoids (2.7 ± 1.2 g). It was found that in comparison, those receiving the high cumulative dose of glucocorticoids had lower wall thickness ($p < 0.05$), lower bone volume ($p < 0.001$), lower trabecular number ($p < 0.05$), lower formation period ($p < 0.05$), increased Euler number and tissue volume ($p < 0.05$), increased interconnectivity index, and increased trabecular bone pattern. And women with glucocorticoid-induced osteoporosis had similar results, compared with women with postmenopausal osteoporosis, except that marrow volume was higher ($p < 0.005$). Thus, in postmenopausal osteoporosis, there is decreased formation and increased resorption of bone.

19. **Weinstein RS, Jilka RL, Parfitt AM,** et al. Inhibition of osteoblastogenesis and promotion of apoptosis of osteoblasts and osteocytes by glucocorticoids. Potential mechanisms of their deleterious effects on bone. J Clin Invest 1998;102:274–282.

Glucocorticoid-induced bone disease is the third most common cause of osteoporosis, thus leading to decreased bone formation and osteonecrosis. A study was performed in which 7-month-old mice were given prednisolone for 27 days. It was found that bone density, osteocalcin, and cancellous bone decreased and trabecular bone narrowed. Also, impaired osteoblastogenesis and osteoclastogenesis were seen in bone marrow cultures. There was a threefold increase in obsteoblast and osteocyte apoptosis. The accumulation of apoptotic osteocytes may explain osteonecrosis. Thus, glucocorticoid-induced bone disease results from changes in the number of bone cells.

20. **Hofbauer LC, Gori F, Riggs BL,** et al. Stimulation of osteoprotegerin ligand and inhibition of osteoprotegerin production by glucocorticoids in human osteoblastic lineage cells: Potential paracrine mechanisms of glucocorticoid-induced osteoporosis. Endocrinology 1999;140:4382–4389.

It is thought that osteoporosis, or the increased resorption of bone, can be a complication of systemic glucocorticoid use. Osteoprotegerin ligand (OPG-L) is known to be the final effector of osteoclastogenesis, whereas the soluble receptor for osteoprotegerin (OPG) opposes this. Through Northern analysis, reverse transcription polymerase chain reaction (RT-PCR), and enzyme-linked immunosorbent assay (ELISA), the regulatory effect of OPG and OPG-L was studied. Dexamethasone was found to inhibit the production of constitutive messenger ribonucleic acid (mRNA) OPG 70% to 90% of the time in stromal cells, primary trabecular osteoblasts, fetal osteoblasts, and osteosarcoma cells; these cells are not affected by cycloheximide. In fetal osteoblasts, it was found that 90% of constitutive mRNA for OPG was inhibited. Also dexamethasone (10^{-10} M–10^{-7} M) inhibited the concentration of OPG protein in cells from 2.5 ± 0.02 ng/mL to 0.30 ± 0.01 ng/mL (88% inhibition, $p < 0.001$). It was found that dexamethasone also stimulated the OPG-L mRNA steady-state levels in primary and fetal osteoblast cells by two- to fourfold. When murine marrow culture was treated with the medium from dexamethasone-treated osteosarcoma cells, it was found that the activity of tartrate-resistant acid phosphatase (TRAP) increased by 54% ($p < 0.005$) compared with control. In addition, dexamethasone (10^{-8} M) promoted osteoclast formation by 2.5-fold in TRAP cell lysates. In conclusion, glucocorticoids do increase osteoclastogenesis, which is inhibited by OPG and stimulated by OPG-L. Thus, bone resorption is enhanced by glucocorticoids.

21. **Klein RG, Arnaud SB, Gallagher JC,** et al. Intestinal calcium absorption in exogenous hypercortisonism. Role of 25-hydroxyvitamin D and corticosteroid dose. J Clin Invest 1977;60:253–259.

22. **Morris HA, Need AG, O'Loughlin PD,** et al. Malabsorption of calcium in corticosteroid-induced osteoporosis. Calcif Tissue Int 1990;46:305–308.

Calcium malabsorption in 60 postmenopausal women on corticosteroid therapy was studied. Specifically, radiocalcium in conjunction with serum 1,25-dihydroxyvitamin D [1,25$(OH)_2D_3$] was studied, where calcium is a function of 1,25$(OH)_2D_3$. These 60 postmenopausal women were compared with 31 normal, age-matched postmenopausal women and normal, corticosteroid-treated women. It was found that reduced serum levels of 1,25$(OH)_2D_3$ did not explain decreased calcium levels. The Z-score was reduced in the osteoporotic group. Vertebral mineral density (VMD) of the women was measured, and the results produced the same conclusion.

23. **Cosman F, Nieves J, Herbert J,** et al. High-dose glucocorticoids in multiple sclerosis patients exert direct effects on the kidney and skeleton. J Bone Miner Res 1994;9: 1097–1105.

24. **Reid IR, Ibbertson HK.** Evidence for decreased tubular reabsorption of calcium in glucocorticoid-treated asthmatics. Horm Res 1987;27:200–204.

Calcium levels were measured in 15 fasting asthma patients who were on glucocorticoid therapy; they were compared with age- and sex-matched controls not receiving treatment. It was found that the mean calcium/creatinine ratio and calcium excretion per liter of glomerular filtrate (CaE) was twice that of the control ($p < 0.005$). CaE was plotted against serum calcium, and it was found that the mean values exceeded that of control ($p < 0.05$). This finding suggests that there is a decrease in tubular calcium absorption. Thus, glucocorticoids inhibit tubular reabsorption, increasing the possibility of the development of osteoporosis.

25. **Kuhn JM, Gay D, Lemercier JP,** et al. Testicular function during prolonged corticotherapy. Presse Med 1986;15:559–562.

Because corticosteroid therapy may result in protein catabolism, short-term treatment of adrenocorticotropic hormone (ACTH) and/or glucocorticoids may decrease testosterone levels—resulting in hypogonadism. Eighteen men on prolonged glucocorticoid treatment were followed up, and it was found that in fewer than 3 months, the mean testosterone levels were not too different from those of controls (5.9 ± 0.8 ng/mL and 7.5 ± 0.5 ng/mL, respectively, where $p < 0.05$). Also, luteinizing hormone (LH) was found to be higher in these men after 3 months than the control (8.2 ± 1.9 mIU/mL and 3.6 ± 1 mIU/mL, respectively, with $p < 0.001$). After 2 years, it was found that the testosterone levels were below that of the control (3.8 ± 0.6 ng/mL, where $p < 0.001$). Also, the LH levels were noted to be normal. It was found that there was a negative correlation between plasma testosterone levels and glucocorticoids ($r = -0.01$, $p < 0.0001$). This finding suggests that glucocorticoids influence gonadotrophic function as well as testicular function and may lead to hypoandrogenism.

3

Assessment of Fracture Risk

Paul D. Miller

Use of Bone Mineral Density for Fracture Risk Assessment, 25
History of Fragility Fractures, 25
Effect of Age on Fracture Risk, 28
Combined Effect of Risk Factors, 28
The World Health Organization Absolute Risk Project, 29
Risk Determined by Vertebral Fracture Assessment, 30
Conclusions, 32

USE OF BONE MINERAL DENSITY FOR FRACTURE RISK ASSESSMENT

As pointed out in Chapter 1, the T-score has (and will remain) an important "number" for the diagnosis of osteoporosis in nonfractured patients. The impact on the T-score value for fracture risk prediction depends heavily on how the T-score is interpreted [1,2]. A low T-score [or bone mineral density (BMD)] has very different risk prediction implications at age 50 years than it does at age 80 years [3]. Hence, in isolation, a T-score is not a T-score is not a T-score (Fig. 3.1). A low BMD predicts an increased risk for fracture, but increased age is even a greater predictor of risk at equivalent levels of BMD. Why increased age conveys a greater fracture risk at the same BMD value is unclear, except that perhaps older people may fall more often than younger people, and, that there are changes in bone quality (cortical shell and porosity, crystal size, collagen maturation, microarchitecture) that render the older bone more fragile than the younger bone at the same T-score [3–5]. The combination of a T-score and additional risk factors for fracture provides a more refined quantitative assessment of fracture risk than can be obtained by a low BMD alone. It is important to stress, however, that the diagnosis of osteoporosis can also be made based on the presence of a fragility (low-trauma) fracture, regardless of the level of the T-score, which is the manner in which osteoporosis was diagnosed before the World Health Organization (WHO) criteria were developed.

HISTORY OF FRAGILITY FRACTURES

A prior fragility fracture is predictive of a high risk for future fracture. In the field of osteoporosis, a fragility fracture is defined as a fracture that occurs spontaneously or from a fall equal to or less than one's standing height.

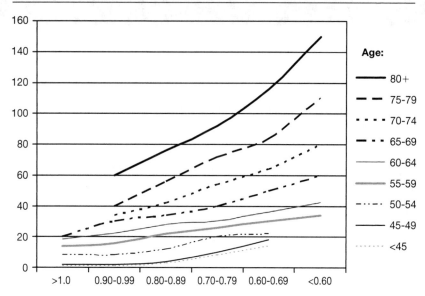

Figure 3.1. The effect of age on fracture risk at equivalent levels of bone mineral density. In this example, forearm SPA predicts nonspinal fractures in 521 white women followed up for 6.5 years. (Adapted from Hui SL, Slemenda CW, Johnston CC Jr. Age and bone mass as predictors of fracture in a prospective study. J Clin Invest 1988;81:1804–1809, with permission.)

Fractures that are predictive of a higher risk for future fracture in population studies as well as placebo arms of pharmacological clinical trials are vertebral compression fractures (VCF), hip fractures, wrist and forearm fractures, humeral and shoulder fractures, and rib fractures (Table 3.1) [6–15]. Fragility fractures at these sites are predictive of future fracture

Table 3.1.   Metaanalysis of the effect of prior fracture on subsequent relative risk for future fracture risk

Fracture History	Increase in Future Fracture Risk		
	Wrist	Spine	Hip
Wrist	3–4	2–7	1–2
Spine	1–2	4–19	2–3
Hip	NA	2–3	1–2

From **Klotzbuecher CM, Ross PD, Landsman PB,** et al. Patients with prior fractures have an increased risk of future fractures: a summary of the literature and statistical synthesis. J Bone Miner Res 2000;15:721–739. Based on data from **Hasserius R, Karlsson MK, Nilsson BE,** et al. Prevalent vertebral deformities predict increased mortality and increased fracture rate in both men and women: A 10-year population-based study of 598 individuals from the Swedish cohort in the European Vertebral Osteoporosis Study. Osteoporosis Int 2003;14:61–68; **Naves M, Dias-Lopez JB, Gomez C,** et al. The effect of vertebral fractures as a risk factor for osteoporotic fracture and mortality in a Spanish population. Osteoporosis Int 2003;14:520–524; and **Lindsay R, Silverman SL, Cooper C,** et al. Risk of new vertebral fracture in the year following a fracture. JAMA 2001;285:320–323.

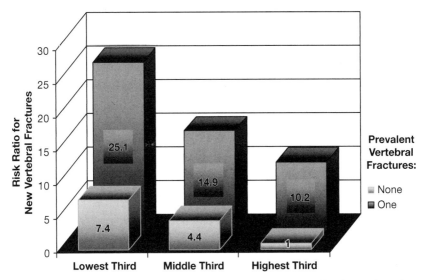

Figure 3.2. Effect of prevalent morphometric vertebral fracture or low bone mineral density on future fracture risk. (After Ross PD, Davis JW, Epstein RS, Wasnich RD. Preexisting fractures and bone mass predict vertebral fracture incidence in women. Ann Intern Med 1991;114:919–923, with permission.)

risk independent of the BMD. Forearm fractures, previously shown to be predictive of a high risk for other nonforearm fractures, have recently been shown to also predict a high risk for other fractures in the large, longitudinal National Osteoporosis Risk Assessment (NORA) database. In NORA, all (global) fragility fractures were captured after the age of 45 years, before as well as after the first 1 to 5 years after entry into NORA. There were 8,554 prior wrist fractures for end of year 1 captured in NORA [16]. In these postmenopausal women, a prior wrist fracture was associated with a large increase in the incidence of another fracture, even at distant skeletal sites (e.g., hip), within a brief period of time. Just why a prior fragility fracture conveys a high risk for fracture at other skeletal sites is not clear, except to suggest that a fragility fracture is symbolic of systemic skeletal fragility.

It was recognized in 1991 that the presence of a morphometric VCF increased the risk of future fractures of the vertebrae independent of the baseline BMD, and the presence of an existing VCF in combination with low BMD increased the future fracture risk far more that the risk predicted by either a VCF or low BMD alone [15] (Fig. 3.2).

Low BMD as measured by central or peripheral dual-energy x-ray absorptiometry (DXA), peripheral ultrasound, or spine quantitative computed tomography (QCT) is predictive of an increased risk for fractures at any other skeletal site [17–27].

In addition, from individual longitudinal studies, including population studies, and from metaanalysis, all these BMD measuring devices predict an increased risk of fracture in postmenopausal women or elderly men with an overlapping relative risk (RR) predictability: Risk increases approximately 2 times for each 1.0 SD reduction in BMD calculated from T-scores, or the variance from the mean of an aged-matched population [17].

Fracture risk prediction can also be enhanced by incorporating additional risk factors into the assessment of fracture risk. As risk factors for fracture increase, the risk for fracture also increases above and beyond the risk predicted by low BMD and increased age alone. The validation of how additional risk factors should be added to BMD to enhance risk prediction is important, since the current DXA reports may be misleading in their subjective pronouncements of fracture risk.

EFFECT OF AGE ON FRACTURE RISK

It has been recognized since the forearm DXA studies of Hui et al [3] that fracture risk is dependent on the age of the patient (Fig. 3.1). Any given patient's risk for fracture increases as age increases, even at the same BMD or T-score level [28]. Thus, DXA measurements capture an important, albeit small, part of the fracture risk. Understanding this fundamental point is pivotal to the proper interpretation of BMD values. The reason why risk is greater as age increases is not completely understood, but the higher risk for falls in the elderly may account for a portion of this age-related greater risk for fracture [29,30]. Older bone has less strength to resist fracture than younger bone at the same BMD or T-score, and investigators dedicated to measuring bone quality are refining our understanding of these issues [31]. It is important to point out, however, that even though the absolute risk for fragility fracture increases at the same level of BMD or T-score as age increases [32], fractures at both hip and nonhip skeletal sites are not infrequent in the younger (50–64 years), postmenopausal population. In the NORA study nearly 37% of all fractures occurred in this younger, untreated, postmenopausal group and was lower the lower the T-score value [33].

COMBINED EFFECT OF RISK FACTORS

As previously mentioned, prior fracture in the postmenopausal population is an independent predictor of future fracture risk. Furthermore, combining a prevalent fracture (even an asymptomatic VCF) and low BMD translates into a much greater risk for future fracture than what would be predicted by low BMD or prior fracture alone [15]. Adding risk factors enhances risk prediction.

In 1993, data showed the interaction of risk factors captured in the Study of Osteoporotic Fractures (SOF) with low BMD to enhance fracture risk prediction for hip fractures [34]. More recently, data from multiple population studies have documented the strong association between the presence of nonvertebral or nonhip fractures and fragility fractures of other skeletal sites, including shoulder, wrist, and rib [13,14,35,36]. Therefore, in the elderly population, any fragility fracture is symbolic of systemic skeletal fragility.

Clinicians should, therefore, incorporate BMD, age, and prior fracture in their assessment of fracture risk and patient management. Recent software upgrades in central DXA machines may use these three risk factors to calculate fracture risk. Broad implementation of standardized DXA reports can only be realized when the independent risk factors for fragility fractures in the postmenopausal population are validated and endorsed at an international level.

THE WORLD HEALTH ORGANIZATION ABSOLUTE RISK PROJECT

The World Health Organization's (WHO's) absolute risk project is the large project assessing the long-term (10-year) risk for all fragility fractures as a function of validated risk factors from large international studies [28]. This work, spearheaded by Professor John Kanis, is still in progress and will require review and comment by the WHO per se before final publication and ultimate implementation [37]. Based on data that have already been presented at many scientific meetings, there are eight independent validated risk factors for fracture risk. Those that may be included in the implementation of standardized DXA reports are BMD, prior fragility fracture, age, and family history, since beyond 4 or 5 risk factors, the absolute risk level increases only slightly. The combined risk factor analysis refines risk stratification. When implemented, it is hoped that absolute risk prediction calculation will facilitate intervention decisions for the postmenopausal population based on risk beyond a T-score value alone. Risk stratification has been shown in previous analysis; however, they are either based on restricted population studies or use peripheral BMD technologies for risk assessment [38,39]. The WHO absolute risk study will link absolute risk for all fractures, calculated from validated population studies representing more than 90,000 postmenopausal women, to treatment intervention based on disutility costs of hip fracture using the current costs of drugs registered for the treatment of postmenopausal osteoporosis (PMO).

It is obvious that the government reimbursement plan will differ from nation to nation by the gross domestic product (GDP) of a given nation. The WHO project does not include other risk factors that clinicians might reasonably use in counseling patients: nonclinical (morphometric) vertebral fractures, bone turnover markers, hip axis length, hip structural analysis, and other risk factors that might become identified in smaller, less well-validated multination population studies [6,40–48]. Morphometric vertebral fractures, however, will be acknowledged by the National Osteoporosis Foundation (NOF) clinical implementation of the WHO absolute risk analysis as being a strong risk factor for future fracture. In addition, the WHO absolute risk model will provide broad generalizations that will focus on intervention strategies, but it will not eliminate individual clinician decisions. Nevertheless, the WHO risk project will take the field of osteoporosis to a level comparable to the cardiovascular field regarding intervention

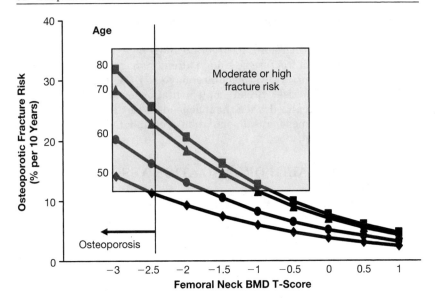

Figure 3.3. World Health Organization's 10 year validated absolute risk for all fractures in untreated postmenopausal women as a function of age and bone mineral density. (Data obtained from Kanis J. World Health Organization 10 year validated absolute fracture risk probabilities. International Osteoporosis Foundation. Toronto, 2006; Osteoporosis Int 2006; abstract.)

decisions. In addition, the WHO absolute risk assessment may advocate treatment of women whose lower T-scores or younger age might otherwise have discouraged their healthcare providers from prescribing treatment for them [27] (Fig. 3.3).

The WHO selected absolute risk rather than relative risk, even though both calculations of risk have value. The power of any given BMD measurement device to predict risk is based on its ability to predict RR. Yet, RR does not incorporate other risk factors; it is the ratio of the absolute risk for the disease event in a target population to the absolute risk in a population not at risk for the disease event (BMD, smoking, etc.). Absolute risk incorporates the discovered cumulative risk factors into the prediction of the risk for fractures over a given period of time [49] (Table 3.2). As shown in Table 3.2, the relative risk for fracture per SD reduction in BMD is constant over age, which is incorrect. As other risk factors are included in this calculation, the absolute risk will increase with age.

RISK DETERMINED BY VERTEBRAL FRACTURE ASSESSMENT

DXA is now a recognized technology for the identification of vertebral fractures. The presence of vertebral fractures, even if they are asymptomatic, is predictive of the risk for future (incident) vertebral fractures and nonvertebral fractures, independent of baseline BMD or T-score. In

Table 3.2. Limitations of relative risk

Age (y)	T-score	Relative Risk	Absolute Risk (%)
50	0	1	0.2
	−1	2	0.4
	−2	4	1.1
60	0	1	0.4
	−1	2	1.0
	−2	4	2.7
70	0	1	0.7
	−1	2	1.9
	−2	4	5.3

From **Blake GM, Knapp KM, Fogelman I.** Absolute fracture risk varies with bone densitometry technique used. J Clin Densit 2002;5:109–116, with permission.

addition, many patients without WHO-defined osteoporosis have prevalent VCFs [50]. The majority of prevalent VCFs are not recognized in postmenopausal women and elderly men. Population studies from the United States, Europe, Mexico, and Asia all suggest that VCF prevalence is similar across these ethnic groups and may be as high as 60% to 65% by the age of 65 years [51–55]. This suggests that osteoporosis is markedly underdiagnosed and that future fracture risk is markedly underestimated. Professor Harry Genant [56] has provided clinicians with a semiquantitative method for the identification of prevalent, as well as incident, vertebral clinical fracture (VCF) utilizing either plain radiography or DXA-based vertebral fracture assessment (VFA). The VFA technology for prevalent VCF detection by DXA has progressed to the point that it is becoming a standard of care in the risk assessment of the postmenopausal population. The International Society for Clinical Densitometry (ISCD) has provided guidelines for VFA determinations [57]. The ISCD indications for VFA by DXA are as follows [57]:

- Consider VFA when the results may influence clinical management.
- When BMD measurement is indicated, performance of VFA should be considered in clinical situations that may be associated with vertebral fractures. Examples include:
  - Documented height loss of more than 2 cm (0.75 in.) or historical height loss of more than 4 cm (1.5 in.) since young adulthood
  - History of fracture after age 50 years
  - Commitment to long-term oral or parenteral glucocorticoid therapy
  - History of findings suggestive of vertebral fracture not documented by prior radiologic study

If clinicians simply measure the height of their postmenopausal patients and perform a VFA in those who have lost more than 4 cm (1.5 in.) from their historical height, there is evidence that a large proportion of vertebral fractures will be detected [58].

Data suggest that all "grades" of prevalent vertebral fractures are predictive of future fracture and that this risk is increased within 12 months of the detection—even though the physician may not know when the prevalent vertebral fracture occurred [6,42,59,60]. The higher the grade (severity) of the existing vertebral fracture, or the more vertebral fractures present (one, two, or three), the greater the risk for future fractures. Furthermore, since these vertebral fractures, even those that are asymptomatic, are associated with a high risk of fractures even at nonvertebral sites, and are also associated with a higher morbidity and mortality as compared with age-matched patients without vertebral fractures, the detection of VCF will not only establish a diagnosis of osteoporosis regardless of the prevailing T-score [48] but will also identify a high risk for fracture group that merits treatment.

Thus, the advancements in DXA technology [61,62] that allow physicians to identify a prevalent VCF at the point of care when the BMD is done by DXA for diagnosis, risk assessment, or monitoring has improved the management and assessment of the osteoporotic patient.

CONCLUSIONS

A BMD measurement by DXA is the most important clinical tool to allow the field of osteoporosis to move from theory to practical application. Proper interpretation of BMD results, including the proper use of T-scores, fracture risk assessment, and monitoring BMD over time, provides the clinician with the best clinical information to use in the management of the osteoporotic patient. Central DXA utilization requires strict quality control of the measurements performed by DXA technologists and well-educated physicians who interpret the results [63–66]. The trust a clinician and patient place on DXA measurements lies in the appropriate interpretation of the result. The implementation of the validated WHO absolute fracture risk project should facilitate decision making for management of the patient with postmenopausal osteoporosis.

REFERENCES

Annotations by Elizabeth Dillard

1. **Miller PD, Bonnick SL, Rosen CJ.** Consensus of an international panel on the clinical utility of bone mass measurements in the detection of low bone mass in the adult population. Calcif Tissue Int 1996;58:207–214.

   This review article discusses whether, in the setting of the asymptomatic patient, low bone mass can predict fracture risk. Decreases in bone mass can be used for diagnosis when compared with normal controls, with prevention of the first fracture as a clinical goal. In patients with estrogen deficiency, vertebral abnormalities, radiographic osteopenia, asymptomatic primary hyperparathyroidism, or those patients with a history of long-term corticosteroid therapy, bone mass can be assessed for efficacy of therapy with serial measurements. A patient's risk factors can be used to identify the appropriate technique and skeletal site for bone mass measurements.

2. **Miller PD, Bonnick SL.** Clinical application of bone densitometry. In: Primer on the metabolic bone diseases and disorders of mineral metabolism, 4th ed. Philadelphia: Lippincott Williams & Wilkins; 1999:152–159.

   This handbook discusses disorders of mineral metabolism, metabolic bone diseases, and disorders of stone formation. The pathophysiology, diagnosis, and treatment of all bone and mineral disorders are discussed. In addition, the new WHO definition of osteoporosis is utilized as a new approach for therapy and treatment.

3. **Hui SL, Slemenda CW, Johnston CC Jr.** Age and bone mass as predictors of fracture in a prospective study. J Clin Invest 1988;81:1804–1809.

In this prospective analysis on the effect of bone mass on the risk of fracture, 521 women were monitored with serial bone mass measurements over an average of 6.5 years; 138 nonspinal fractures were observed during follow-up. Increasing age and decreasing radius were both predictive of increased fracture risk. Hip fractures correlated more to age-related changes, whereas distal forearm fractures correlated more with midshaft radius bone mass. Bone mass can be a clinical predictor of fractures; however, other age-related factors must be taken into consideration when monitoring the efficacy of treatment.

4. **Diab T, Condon KW, Burr DB, Vashishth D.** Age-related change in the damage morphology of human cortical bone and its role in bone fragility. Bone 2006;38: 427–431.

In this study, age-related changes in bone morphology and microdamage were examined with bending fatigue testing. Histologic evaluation of the resultant tensile (diffuse damage) and compressive (linear microcracks) damage was monitored to identify the damage morphologies. Young donors (38 ± 9 years) had a longer fatigue life ($p < 0.05$) and produced more diffuse damage than the older donors (82 ± 5 years) ($p < 0.05$). However, old donors had a shorter fatigue life and produced more linear microcracks than the younger donors ($p < 0.05$). Linear microcracks were associated with weak lamellar interfaces. Younger donors had more areas of diffuse damage than in older donors ($p < 0.05$), and had no relationship to the lamellar arrangement of bone. The propensity of bone to form different damage morphology due to age and that young donors have diffuse damage over inter-lamellae linear microcracks may help to enlighten researchers on the way that fractures occur and the relationship with these changes in morphology and fracture production in adults.

5. **Russo CR, Lauretani F, Seeman E,** et al. Structural adaptations to bone loss in aging men and women. Bone 2006;38:112–118.

This prospective case-control study analyzed the sex-related differences in bone strength by identifying changes in cortical thickness and porosity. In this study, 688 women and 561 men (20–102 years old) were monitored for changes in cross-sectional area (tCSA), cortical thickness (Ct.Th), and distance to the cortex. Young adult men had greater total and medullary areas than young adult women. In men with advancing age, tCSA increased by 0.79 SD and medullary area increased by 0.54 SD; cortical area and cortical thickness were similar at all ages. In women, tCSA increased by 0.2 SD, whereas medullary area increased by 2.6 SD; this caused cortical area and thickness, and the moments of inertia diminished. The volumetric bone mineral density (vBMD) of women decreased more (by 3.1 SD) than that of men (which decreased by 0.5 SD). In both sexes, the lower the cortical apparent vBMD, the higher the tCSA (women $R^2 = 0.13$, men $R^2 = 0.16$, both $p < 0.0001$), whereas the lower the Ct.Th, the lower the tCSA (women $R^2 = 0.30$, men $R^2 = 0.32$, both $p < 0.0001$). Cortical thickness is reduced with bone loss; intracortical porosity similarly is increased by bone loss. Men appear to compensate for these changes more greatly than women, which could be a mechanism for the sex-related differences in bone strength.

6. **Lindsay R, Silverman SL, Cooper C,** et al. Risk of new vertebral fracture in the year following a fracture. JAMA 2001;285:320–323.

This metaanalysis discusses trials studying the risk of further vertebral fractures during the first year following a vertebral fracture. Postmenopausal women were enrolled if vertebral fracture status was known at entry ($n = 2,725$). Vertebral fractures that were identified by radiograph during the year following an incident vertebral fracture were analyzed, and it was found that 6.6% of women had new vertebral fractures within the first year. If the patient had one or more vertebral fractures at baseline, there was a fivefold increased risk of sustaining another vertebral fracture [relative risk (RR), 5.1; 95% confidence interval (CI), 3.1–8.4; $p < 0.001$]. With the 381 participants who had an incident vertebral fracture, the incidence of a new vertebral fracture within the next year was 19.2% (95% CI, 13.6%–24.8%). This risk was also increased in the presence of prevalent vertebral fractures (RR, 9.3; 95% CI, 1.2–71.6; $p = 0.03$). This suggests that women who sustain one vertebral fracture have a significantly increased risk of another vertebral fracture within the first year.

7. **Ross PD, Genant HK, Davis JW,** et al. Predicting vertebral fracture incidence from prevalent fractures and bone density among nonblack, osteoporotic women. Osteoporos Int 1993;3:120–126.

   In this randomized, placebo-controlled, clinical trial of bisphosphonate (etidronate), the ability of bone density and vertebral fractures to predict further vertebral fracture risk was analyzed. Three-hundred-eighty postmenopausal women (mean age 65 years) treated with bisphosphonate (etidronate) or placebo were monitored, and baseline measurements of bone mineral density were obtained. Serial spine radiographs monitored vertebral fractures. One or two fractures at baseline increased the rate of new vertebral fractures 7.4-fold (95% CI = 1.0 to 55.9). A decrease of 2 SD in spinal bone density by absorptiometry was associated with a 5.8-fold increase in fracture rate (95% CI = 2.9 to 11.6). The lowest and highest quintiles of bone density had absolute fracture rates of 120 and 6 cases per 1,000 patient-years, respectively. The use of two predictors (bone density and prevalent fractures or two bone density measurements) together can help with fracture prediction, when compared with the use of a single predictor. Both bone density and prevalent vertebral fractures are strong, complementary predictors of vertebral fracture risk.

8. **Kotowicz MA, Melton LJ III, Cooper C,** et al. Risk of hip fracture in women with vertebral fracture. J Bone Miner Res 1994;9:599–605.

   This population-based cohort study followed up Rochester women aged 35 to 69 years with one or more vertebral fractures for subsequent hip fractures. In the 336 women with no history of hip fracture at the time of their vertebral fracture, 52 proximal femur fractures in 4,788 person-years of follow-up were noted. Intertrochanteric femoral fractures had a higher standardized morbidity ratio (SMR) of expected hip fractures than cervical femoral fractures (SMR, 2.3 vs. 1.3; $p = 0.07$). Hip fracture risk among women with symptomatic vertebral fractures was slightly less than in those with asymptomatic vertebral fractures (SMR, 1.8 vs. 2.3; not significant). Younger women had no higher risk of a subsequent hip fracture than women who were 60 or more years of age at the time of their vertebral fracture (SMR, 1.4 vs. 1.8; not significant). Heterogeneity of osteoporotic fractures can help explain the results of this study.

9. **Schousboe JT, Fink HA, Taylor BC,** et al. Association between self-reported prior wrist fractures and risk of subsequent hip and radiographic vertebral fractures in older women: A prospective study. J Bone Miner Res 2005;20:100–106.

   This prospective cohort study of elderly women discussed prior wrist fracture and incident hip and radiographic vertebral fractures relationships when adjusted for bone mineral density (BMD); 9,704 elderly women, with known wrist fracture history since age 50, were measured with calcaneal and hip BMD and followed up for 10.1 years. A 72% increased odds ratio of incident radiographic vertebral fractures was associated with prior fractures [odds ratio (OR), 1.72; 95% CI, 1.31–2.25]. Even after specific calcaneal BMD was taken into consideration, the association of prior wrist fracture with incident radiographic vertebral fracture was attenuated (OR, 1.39; 95% CI, 1.05–1.83). A similar association of prior wrist fractures and a 43% excess rate of incident hip fracture was obtained [hazards ratio (HR), 1.43; 95% CI, 1.17–1.74]. However, after adjustment for hip BMD, prior wrist fracture was not a statistically significant predictor of incident hip (HR, 1.12; 95% CI, 0.92–1.38). Prior wrist fracture, according to this study, can be a risk factor for vertebral fractures alone, whereas with hip fractures, the hip BMD must be taken into consideration.

10. **Papaioannou A, Joseph L, Ioannidis G,** et al. Risk factors associated with incident clinical vertebral and nonvertebral fractures in postmenopausal women: The Canadian Multicentre Osteoporosis Study (CaMos). Osteoporos Int 2005;16:568–578.

    This analysis used data from the Canadian Multicentre Osteoporosis Study (CaMos) to examine potential risk factors and the occurrence of incident vertebral and nonvertebral fractures; 5,143 postmenopausal women were followed up for 3 years. The subjects were stratified into four groups according to fracture status during the years of follow-up. These groups included those without a new fracture; those with a new clinically recognized vertebral fracture; those with an incident nonvertebral fracture at the wrist, hip, humerus, pelvis, or ribs (main nonvertebral fracture group); and those with any new nonvertebral fracture (any-nonvertebral-fracture group). Thirty-four, 163, and 280 women developed a vertebral, a main nonvertebral, or any nonvertebral fracture, respectively, throughout the 3 years of follow-up. Predictive models associated a five-point lower quality of life (as measured by the SF-36 physical component summary score) when associated with relative risks of 1.21 (95% CI, 1.02–1.44), 1.17 (95% CI, 1.07–1.28), and 1.19 (95% CI, 1.11–1.27) for incident vertebral, main nonvertebral, and all nonvertebral fractures, respectively. With lower femoral neck bone mineral density (BMD), even by one standard deviation (SD = 0.12), the relative risks for incident vertebral, main nonvertebral, and any nonvertebral fractures increased by 2.73 (95% CI, 1.74–4.28), 1.39 (95% CI, 1.06–1.82), and 1.34 (95% CI, 1.09–1.65), respectively. This paper identified several risk factors that should be monitored in postmenopausal women with regard to osteoporosis risk.

11. **Klotzbuecher CM, Ross PD, Landsman PB,** et al. Patients with prior fractures have an increased risk of future fractures: A summary of the literature and statistical synthesis. J Bone Miner Res 2000;15:721–739.

In this review, a statistical analysis of the risk of future fracture in women with prior fracture was performed. Prior and subsequent vertebral fractures had the highest risk relationship; women with preexisting vertebral fractures (identified at baseline by vertebral morphometry) had a 4 times greater risk of subsequent vertebral fractures than those without prior fractures. The number of prior fractures is proportional to that increase in risk. In general, combinations of prior and future fracture sites (hip, spine, wrist, or any site) increased relative risk of fracture by about 2. In comparison to women who did not have a prior fracture, both peri- and postmenopausal women with prior fractures had 2.0 (95% CI = 1.8, 2.1) times the risk of subsequent fractures. This study recommends that patients with prior fracture history should have increased awareness of future fracture risk.

12. **Siris ES, Brenneman S, Barrett-Conner E,** et al. The effect of age and bone mineral density on the absolute, excess and relative risk of fracture in postmenopausal women age 50–99: Results from the National Osteoporosis Risk Assessment. Osteoporos Int 2005;17:565–574.

In the National Osteoporosis Risk Assessment (NORA) cohort study, 170,083 women, aged 50 to 99 years, were monitored for risk of incident fractures for 3 years. Bone mineral density (BMD) T-scores at the heel, forearm, or finger were obtained at baseline; new fractures at the hip, spine, rib, wrist, and forearm were obtained from questionnaires at 1- and 3-year follow-ups; 5,312 women reported 5,676 fractures (868 hip, 2,420 wrist/forearm, 1,531 rib, and 857 spine). Age-related risk of fracture increased at all fracture sites but was most evident at the hip; low BMD increased the risk of hip fracture 2× for each increase in decade of life. However, relative risk for any fracture per 1 SD decrease in BMD was similar across age groups ($p > 0.07$), and those subjects with low BMD (T-score < -1.0) had a similar relative risk for fracture regardless of age. BMD decreases were associated with both the absolute fracture risk and the excess fracture risk with advancing age, even though the relative risk of fracture for low bone mass was consistent across all age groups.

13. **Johnell O, Kanis JA.** Epidemiology of osteoporotic fractures. Osteoporos Int 2005;16(Suppl 2):S3–S7.

This review article discussed the incidence and prevalence of osteoporotic fractures with regard to recently updated definitions of osteoporosis and age-related changes. Forty percent to 50% of women and 13% to 22% of men over their lifetime have risk of osteoporotic fractures. Multiplying the morbidity of hip fractures according to age group should be used to calculate true burden of osteoporotic fractures. In women aged 50 to 54 years, the disability caused by osteoporotic fractures is 6.07 times that accounted for by hip fracture alone, whereas for women aged 80 to 84 years, the incidence of hip fractures should be multiplied by 1.55. In men aged 50 to 54 years, the incidence of hip fractures should be multiplied by 4.48, and for those aged 80 to 84 years by 1.50 to determine true osteoporotic fracture burden.

14. **Kanis JA, Johnell O, De Laet C,** et al. A metaanalysis of previous fracture and subsequent fracture risk. Bone 2004;35:375–382.

In a metaanalysis of 11 cohort studies, previous fracture was analyzed as a risk factor for future fracture in regard to age, sex, and bone mineral density (BMD). Weighted beta-coefficients were used to merge results of the different studies. In comparison to subjects without prior fracture, those with previous fracture history had a significantly increased risk of any fracture (RR = 1.86; 95% CI = 1.75–1.98). The risk ratio was similar for the outcome of osteoporotic fracture or for hip fracture. No significant changes were noted between men and women with regard to risk. When adjusted for BMD, the risk ratio (RR) had a downward adjustment. Low BMD explained a minority of the risk for any fracture (8%); 22% of hip fractures were attributed to low BMD. Only hip fracture outcome was associated with age-related changes in risk ratio. Previous history of fracture increases the risk of fracture that cannot be completely explained by changes in BMD.

15. **Ross PD, Davis JW, Epstein RS, Wasnich RD.** Pre-existing fractures and bone mass predict vertebral fracture incidence in women. Ann Intern Med 1991;114: 919–923.

    This cohort study of postmenopausal Japanese-American women analyzed bone mass changes and existing fractures as risk factors for new fractures over a mean follow-up period of 4.7 years. Changes of 2 SD in bone mass were associated with fourfold to sixfold increase in the risk for new vertebral fractures. Baseline fractures increased the risk for new vertebral fractures; there was a fivefold increased risk with one fracture at baseline, and a 12-fold risk increase with two or more fractures. When combining the risk factors, low bone mass (below the 33rd percentile) and two or more prevalent fractures at baseline increased the risk 75-fold, when compared with women with higher bone mass (above the 67th percentile) and who had no prevalent fractures. Fracture incidence did not change with differences in stature, body mass index, arm span, and spinal conditions (such as scoliosis, osteoarthritis, and sacroiliitis; $p > 0.05$). Weight was predictive ($p = 0.04$) of fracture incidence, but after bone mass was added into the analysis, the effect was not predictive ($p \geq 0.05$). Using both bone mass and prevalent fracture as clinical indicators can increase the value for predicting new fractures than either variable alone.

16. **Barrett-Conner E, Siris E, Miller PD,** et al. Association of wrist fracture with subsequent hip, spine, rib, and wrist or forearm fractures in postmenopausal women: Results from National Osteoporosis Risk Assessment (NORA). Menopause 2005;13:Abstract 350048.

17. **Marshall D, Johnell O, Wedel H**. Meta-analysis of how well measurements of bone mineral density predict the occurrence of osteoporotic fractures. BMJ 1996;312: 1254–1259.

    In this metaanalysis of prospective cohort studies, the researchers discussed bone density measurements and their ability to predict subsequent fractures. Case control studies of hip fractures were also analyzed for comparison. All measuring sites had similar predictive abilities [relative risk 1.5 (95% CI, 1.4–1.6)] for decrease in bone mineral density; however, spinal measurements for predicting vertebral fractures [RR, 2.3 (1.9–2.8)] and measurement at hip for hip fractures [2.6 (2.0–3.5)] were somewhat different. The case-control studies had similar results. Measurements of bone mineral density can only predict fracture risk but will not identify individuals who will have a fracture, and therefore should not be used as a screening tool for osteoporosis.

18. **Blake GM, Fogelman I.** Peripheral or central densitometry: Does it matter which technique we use? J Clin Densit 2001;4:83–96.

    This review article analyzes the use of new equipment for monitoring bone density in peripheral sites in comparison to dual x-ray absorptiometry (DXA). To compare the value of different techniques, the relative risk (RR) of fracture analyzed from prospective studies should be used. Hip bone mineral density can be used in comparison with peripheral measurements for predicting hip fracture risk. Using receiver operating characteristic curves, guidelines adopted for scan interpretation are necessary to monitor efficacy of readings. Setting thresholds for peripheral devices that target either the same percentage of the population or the same percentage of future fracture cases as femur DXA can have the greatest correlation. Different methods select different groups of individuals from the total pool of patients who will later sustain a fracture, with the most successful technique being the one with the largest RR value. The emphasis placed by many studies on validating new techniques by studying their correlation with DXA may lead to the clinical value of peripheral devices being underestimated when the key datum is the RR value inferred from prospective fracture studies.

19. **Miller PD, Njeh C, Jankowski LG, Lenchik L.** What are the standards by which bone mass measurement at peripheral skeletal sites should be used in the diagnosis of osteoporosis? J Clin Densitomet 2002;5(S1):S39–S45.

    This article discusses the International Society for Clinical Densitometry (ISCD) Position Development Conference conclusions about peripheral BMD testing as a way to monitor osteoporosis. The ISCD recommends that the WHO T-score criteria should not be used with peripheral devices, and that for peripheral BMD measurements above which osteoporosis is unlikely, device-specific cut points for peripheral BMD should be identified that have 90% sensitivity for identifying patients who have osteoporosis (T-score of -2.5 or below) based on measurements of the spine and hip. Patients who have peripheral BMD below the 90% sensitivity level should have a central BMD measurement, if available. Postmenopausal women are the best subject population for the use of peripheral BMD testing.

20. **Greenspan SL, Cheng S, Miller PD, Orwoll ES, for the QUS-2 PMA Trials Group.** Clinical performance of a highly portable, scanning calcaneal ultrasonometer. Osteoporos Int 2001;12:391–398.

This study attempted to identify clinical usage efficacy for scanning calcaneal ultrasonometer (QUS-2) to monitor for fracture and low bone mass; 1,401 women, including 794 healthy women 25 to 84 years of age evenly distributed per 10-year period to establish a normative database, were monitored. Mean calcaneal broadband ultrasound attenuation (BUA) was constant in healthy women from 25 to 54 years of age and decreased with increasing age. Short-term precision, with and without repositioning of the heel, and long-term precision yielded comparable results [BUA SDs of 2.1–2.4 dB/MHz, coefficients of variations (CVs) of 2.5%–2.9%]. In 698 women, calcaneal BUA was significantly correlated with BMD of the total hip (TH), femoral neck (FN), and lumbar spine (LS) in 698 women ($r = 0.6$–0.7, all $p < 0.0001$). A similar relationship was observed for LS BMD compared with either TH or FN BMD ($r = 0.7$, $p < 0.0001$). Using the WHO criteria, the prevalence of osteoporosis was 20%, 17%, 21%, and 24% for BUA, BMD of the TH, FN, and LS, respectively. Age-adjusted values for a 1 SD reduction in calcaneal BUA and TH and FN BMD predicted prevalent fractures of the spine, forearm, and hip with significant ($p < 0.05$) odds ratios of 2.3, 2.0, and 2.1, respectively. Age-adjusted bone mass values predicting prevalent fracture were 0.62 for BUA, 0.59 for TH BMD, 0.60 for FN BMD, and 0.57 for LS BMD—all statistically equivalent. This analysis states that the QUS-2 calcaneal ultrasonometer has similar reproducibility to the use of BMD of the spine and hip to identify those women with increased fracture risk.

21. **Kanis JA, Gluer C-C, for the Committee of Scientific Advisors, International Osteoporosis Foundation.** An update on the diagnosis and assessment of osteoporosis with densitometry. Osteoporos Int 2000;11:92–202.

This review article uses literature to analyze the 1994 WHO guidelines for the diagnosis of osteoporosis. The problems of uncertainties in the optimal site for examination, inaccuracies in the different measurements from site to site, as well as threshold readings for men, are discussed and recommendations are made.

22. **Gluer C-C for the International Quantitative Ultrasound Consensus Group.** Quantitative ultrasound techniques for the assessment of osteoporosis: Expert agreement on current status. J Bone Miner Res 1997;12:1280–1288.

This discussion details the use of ultrasound techniques for the assessment of osteoporosis. There are a variety of bone densitometry measurement techniques, which can be interpreted in different ways. This paper suggests that the results should be used along with clinical examination results. All measurements should be analyzed with careful quality assurance recommendations.

23. **Baran DT, Faulkner KG, Genant HK,** et al. Diagnosis and management of osteoporosis: Guidelines for the utilization of bone densitometry. Calcif Tissue Int 1997;61:433–440.

This review article discusses practical guidelines for the use of bone densitometry methods in the analysis of osteoporosis and fracture risk in patients. The current capabilities of densitometry methods, as well as the risk reduction of single or multiple site analysis, are delineated. The use of each bone densitometry technique depends on the nature of the issue and the age of the patient, as well as cost, availability, and patient population. The paper recommends the use of dual x-ray absorptiometry (DXA), as well as spinal and peripheral quantitative computer tomography (QCT/pQCT), together to evaluate fracture risk prediction.

24. **Miller P, Siris E, Barrett-Connor E,** et al. Prediction of fracture risk in postmenopausal white women with peripheral bone densitometry: Evidence from the National Osteoporosis Risk Assessment (NORA) program. J Bone Miner Res 2002;17:2222–2230.

This cohort study analyzed the association between bone mineral density (BMD) measurements at peripheral sites and subsequent fracture risk at the hip, wrist or forearm, spine, and rib in 149,524 postmenopausal white women who did not carry the diagnosis of osteoporosis. New fractures of the hip, wrist or forearm, spine, or rib within the first 12 months after testing was the primary outcome measurement. After 1 year, 2,259 women reported 2,340 new fractures. T-scores less than or equal to -2.5 SD were 2.15 (finger) to 3.94 [heel ultrasound (US)] times more predictive of fracture than normal BMD. All measurement sites and devices predicted fracture equally, and risk prediction was similar whether calculated from the manufacturers' young normal values (T-scores) or using SDs from the mean age of the National Osteoporosis Risk Assessment (NORA) population. Low BMD found by peripheral technologies, regardless of the site measured, is associated with at least a twofold increased risk of fracture within 1 year, regardless of where the fracture occurs.

25. **Hans D, Dargent Molina P, Schott AM,** et al. Ultrasonographic heel measurements predict hip fracture in elderly women: the EPIDOS prospective study. Lancet 1996;348:511–514.

    This prospective study analysis assesses the value of measurements with ultrasound in predicting the risk of hip fracture. Researchers analyzed the bone quality of 5,662 elderly women (mean age 80.4 years) with baseline calcaneal ultrasonography measurements and femoral radiography (dual-photon x-ray absorptiometry, DPXA). They recorded 115 incident hip fractures during a mean follow-up duration of 2 years. Low calcaneal ultrasonographic variables were associated with increased risk of hip fracture; in comparison with the accuracy of bone mineral density (BMD) obtained by DPXA, the results were similar. The relative risk of hip fracture for 1 SD reduction was 2.0 (95% CI, 1.6–2.4) for ultrasound attenuation and 1.7 (1.4–2.1) for speed of sound, compared with 1.9 (1.6–2.4) for BMD. Even with controlling for femoral neck BMD, ultrasonographic variables continued to predict hip fracture. The incidence of hip fracture among women with values greater than the median for both calcaneal ultrasound attenuation and femoral neck BMD was 2.7 per 1,000 woman-years, compared with 19.6 per 1,000 woman-years for those with values lower than the median for both measures. The os calcis ultrasound measurements were able to predict the risk of hip fracture in elderly women, as well as DPXA of the hip; combination of both methods can identify women at both high- and low-risk categories.

26. **Hans D, Hartl F, Krieg MA.** Device-specific weighted T-score for two quantitative ultrasounds: operational propositions for the management of osteoporosis for 65 years and older women in Switzerland. Osteoporos Int 2003;14:251–258.

    This review of the use of quantitative ultrasound (QUS) along with dual x-ray absorptiometry (DXA) to predict fracture risk discusses the clinical recommendations of the Swiss Quality Assurance Project. Using two different ultrasound devices, device-specific weighted "T-scores" based on the risk of osteoporotic hip fractures, as well as on the prediction of DXA osteoporosis at the hip, according to the WHO definition of osteoporosis, were calculated for the Achilles (Lunar, General Electric, Madison, WI) and Sahara (Hologic, Waltham, MA) ultrasound devices. Several studies were used to calculate age-adjusted odd ratios (OR) and area under the receiver operating curve (AUC) for the prediction of osteoporotic fracture. The ORs were 2.4 (1.9–3.2) and AUC 0.72 (0.66–0.77), respectively, for the Achilles, and 2.3 (1.7–3.1) and 0.75 (0.68–0.82), respectively, for the Sahara device. Ninety percent sensitivity was used to define low fracture and low osteoporosis risk, and a specificity of 80% was used to define subjects as being at high risk of fracture or having osteoporosis at the hip. From the combination of the fracture model with the hip DXA osteoporotic model, a T-score threshold of -1.2 and -2.5 for the stiffness (Achilles) determined, respectively, the low- and high-risk subjects. Similarly, T-scores at -1.0 and -2.2 for the QUI index (Sahara) were identified in the same fashion. QUS, DXA, and clinical factors can be used together to identify women who would need treatment for osteoporotic risk.

27. **Blake GM, Knapp KM, Spector TD, Fogelman I.** Predicting the risk of fracture at any site in the skeleton: Are all bone mineral density measurement sites equally effective? Calcif Tissue Int 2006;78:9–17.

    This review article discusses the association between bone densitometry (BMD) and relative risk (RR) of fracture incidence. The larger the value of RR, the more effective measurements are at identifying patients at risk of fracture, and RR values for predicting the risk of any fracture are approximately the same for all BMD measurement sites. This study attempts to hypothesize whether a lower limit on RR at distant BMD sites is necessary.

28. **Kanis JA, Johnell O, Oden A,** et al. Ten year probabilities of osteoporotic fractures according to BMD and diagnostic thresholds. J Bone Miner Res 2001;16:S194.

    This prospective cohort study used the NHANES III population to establish a 10-year probability of osteoporotic fractures in men and women with regard to bone mineral density (BMD) and age. The 10-year probability of any fracture was determined from the proportion of individuals fracture-free from the age of 45 years. With the exception of forearm fractures in men, 10-year probabilities for fracture increased with age and changes in T-score. Fracture probabilities between men and women were similar for any age if the subject had low BMD. Age as an independent risk, regardless of BMD, calls into consideration that other variables should be monitored as well with fracture prediction.

29. **Dargent-Molina P, Favier F, Grandjean H,** et al. Fall-related factors and risk of hip fracture: the EPIDOS prospective study. Lancet 1996;348:145–149.

    This prospective cohort study compared the factor of bone mineral density (BMD) and the roll of fall-related factors to predict hip fracture risk. Researchers followed up 7,575 women, aged 75 years or older, with no history of hip fracture, an average of 1.9 years. During that time, 154 women suffered a first hip fracture. Four independent fall-related predictors of hip fracture: slower gait speed [relative risk = 1.4 for 1 SD decrease (95% CI, 1.1–1.6)]; difficulty in doing a tandem (heel-to-toe) walk [1.2 for 1 point on the difficulty score (1.0–1.5)]; reduced visual acuity [2.0 for acuity $\leq$2/10 (1.1–3.7)]; and small calf circumference [1.5 (1.0–2.2)] were identified. When adjusted for femoral-neck BMD, neuromuscular impairment—gait speed, tandem walk—and poor vision remained significantly associated with an increased risk of subsequent hip fracture. Hip fracture among women classified as high risk (based on fall risk and low BMD) was 29 per 1,000 woman-years, compared with 11 per 1,000 for women classified as high risk by either a high fall-risk status or low BMD alone; for women classified as low-risk-based on both criteria the rate was 5 per 1,000.

30. **Riggs BL, Melton JL III, Robb RA,** et al. Population-based analysis of the relationship of whole bone strength indices and fall-related loads to age- and sex-specific patterns of hip and wrist fractures. J Bone Miner Res 2006;21:315–323.

    This cohort study estimated fall-related loads and bone strength in ultradistal radius (UDR) and femoral neck (FN) to identify sex- and age-related changes. Using quantitative computer tomography (QCT), volumetric bone mineral density (vBMD), cross-sectional geometry, and axial (EA) and flexural (EI) rigidities (indices of bone's resistance to compressive and bending loads, respectively) were assessed at the ultradistal radius (UDR) and femoral neck (FN), and estimates of the loads applied to the wrist and hip during a fall were made. Fall load (FL)/bone strength ratios estimated fracture risk. vBMD in young adults was similar between sexes; decreases in vBMD over life were also similar (30% and 28%) at UDR but were somewhat greater (46% and 34%) at FN in women versus men, respectively. FL/strength ratios at UDR were 32% to 51% lower (better) in young adult men than in young adult women and increased (worsened) over life less in men (+4%–+22%) than in women (+20%–+33%). In young adults, FL/strength ratios at FN were only marginally better in men than in women but worsened less over life in men (+22%–+36%) than in women (+40%–+62%). The increased number of wrist fractures in women versus men can be explained by the more favorable FL/strength ratio at UDR in young adult men (because of larger bone size and more favorable geometry) versus women and to maintaining this advantage over life. The twofold lower incidence of hip fractures in men versus women is largely explained by age-related increases (worsening) of FL/bone strength ratios that are only one-half the increases in women.

31. **Bouxsein ML.** Bone quality: Where do we go from here? Osteoporos Int 2003;14 (Suppl 5):118–127.

    In this review summary, literature is discussed to identify and describe new insights to bone fragility and structural features. The author attempts to highlight areas of consensus and those of continued controversy, and to identify areas in need of future research.

32. **Siris ES, Brenneman S, Barrett-Conner E,** et al. The effect of age and bone mineral density on the absolute, excess, and relative risk of fracture in postmenopausal women age 50–99: Results from the National Osteoporosis Risk Assessment. Osteoporos Int 2006;7:565–574.

    In this further analysis of the National Osteoporosis Risk Assessment (NORA) cohort study, 170,083 women, aged 50 to 99 years, were monitored for risk of incident fractures for 3 years. Bone mineral density (BMD) T-scores at the heel, forearm, or finger were obtained at baseline; new fractures at the hip, spine, rib, wrist, and forearm were obtained from questionnaires at 1- and 3-year follow-ups. In these questionnaires, 5,312 women reported 5,676 fractures (868 hip; 2,420 wrist or forearm; 1,531 rib; and 857 spine). Age-related risk of fracture increased at all fracture sites but was most evident at the hip; low BMD increased the risk of hip fracture 2 times for each increase in decade of life. However, relative risk for any fracture per 1 SD decrease in BMD was similar across age groups (p > 0.07), and those subjects with low BMD (T-score < -1.0) had a similar relative risk for fracture regardless of age. BMD decreases were associated with both the absolute fracture risk and the excess fracture risk with advancing age, even though the relative risk of fracture for low bone mass was consistent across all age groups.

33. **Siris ES, Brenneman SK, Miller PD,** et al. Predictive value of low BMD for 1-year fracture outcomes is similar for postmenopausal women ages 50–64 and 65 and older: Results from the National Osteoporosis Risk Assessment (NORA). J Bone Miner Res 2004; 19:1215–1220.

    In another analysis of the National Osteoporosis Risk Assessment (NORA) trial, the frequency of low bone mass and the subsequent association with fracture in women 50 to 64 years of age were observed in comparison with women 65 years of age or older. The NORA trial enrolled women without prior diagnosis of osteoporosis; baseline bone mineral density (BMD) was measured at the heel, forearm, or finger. A survey requesting incident fractures since baseline after 1 year was completed by 163,935 women, 87,594 (53%) of whom were 50 to 64 years of age. Thirty-one percent of women 50 to 64 years of age had low bone mass (T-scores ≤1.0) compared with 62% of women 65 years of age or older. In the study, 2,440 women reported fractures of wrist or forearm, rib, spine, or hip, including 440 hip fractures in the first year of follow-up. Nine hundred four women 50 to 64 years of age reported fractures, including 86 hip fractures, accounting for 37% of fractures and 20% of hip fractures reported in the entire NORA cohort. Osteoporotic fracture risk was increased 1.5 for each SD decrease in BMD for both the younger and older groups of women.

34. **Cummings SR, Nevitt MC, Browner WS,** et al. Risk factors for hip fracture in white women. Study of Osteoporotic Fractures Research Group. N Engl J Med 1995;332:767–773.

    In this prospective study, 9,516 white women with no history of previous fracture 65 years of age or older were enrolled; 4.1 years of follow-up were monitored to determine frequency of incidence hip fracture. During that time, 192 women had first hip fractures not due to motor vehicle accidents. In multivariable, age-adjusted analyses, history of maternal hip fracture doubled the risk of hip fracture (relative risk, 2.0; 95% CI, 1.4–2.9), even after adjustment for bone density. Women who had gained weight since the age of 25 had a lower risk. The risk was higher among women who had previous fractures of any type after the age of 50, were tall at the age of 25, rated their own health as fair or poor, had previous hyperthyroidism, had been treated with long-acting benzodiazepines or anticonvulsant drugs, ingested greater amounts of caffeine, or spent 4 hours a day or less on their feet. An increased risk was associated with the inability to rise from a chair without using one's arms, poor depth perception, poor contrast sensitivity, and tachycardia at rest. Low calcaneal bone density was also an independent risk factor. The incidence of hip fracture ranged from 1.1 (95% CI, 0.5–1.6) per 1,000 woman-years among women with no more than two risk factors and normal calcaneal bone density for their age to 27 (95% CI, 20–34) per 1,000 woman-years among those with five or more risk factors and bone density in the lowest third for their age.

35. **Haentjens P, Autier P, Collins J,** et al. Colles fracture, spine fracture, and subsequent risk of hip fracture in men and women: a metaanalysis. J Bone Joint Surg 2003;85A:1936–1943.

    This metaanalysis of cohort studies discussed the history of any fracture as an independent risk factor for future fracture. Among postmenopausal women, the relative risks for a future fracture of the hip after a fracture of the wrist or spine were 1.53 (95% CI, 1.34–1.74; p < 0.001) and 2.20 (95% CI, 1.92–2.51; p < 0.001), respectively. In older men, the relative risks after wrist or spine fracture were 3.26 (95% CI, 2.08–5.11; p < 0.001) and 3.54 (95% CI, 2.01–6.23; p < 0.001), respectively. Men had a more significant increase in risk of fracture after the distal part of the radius was fractured than women (p = 0.002). However, the impact of a spine fracture did not differ between genders (p = 0.11). Previous spine fracture had an equally important impact on the risk of a subsequent hip fracture in both genders. Men who had a Colles fracture and then a subsequent hip fracture had more of an association than women.

36. **Looker AC, Wahner HW, Dunn WL,** et al. Updated data on proximal femur bone mineral levels of US adults. Osteoporos Int 1998;8:468–489.

This paper analyzed bone mineral levels in the proximal femur of US adults based on the third National Health and Nutrition Examination Survey (NHANES III, 1988–1994). The data were collected from 14,646 men and women aged 20 years and older using dual-energy x-ray absorptiometry and included bone mineral density (BMD) and bone mineral content (BMC). Area of bone was scanned in four selected regions of interest (ROI) in the proximal femur: femur neck, trochanter, intertrochanter, and total. The variables are provided separately by age and sex for non-Hispanic whites (NHW), non-Hispanic blacks (NHB), and Mexican Americans (MA). NHW in the southern United States had slightly lower BMD levels than NHW in other U.S. regions; however, differences were not large enough to stop pooling of these subjects for data analysis. This updated data provide reference data on femur bone mineral levels of non-institutionalized adults.

37. **Kanis J, Borgstrom F, Delaet C, et al.** Assessment of fracture risk. Osteoporos Int 2005;16:581–589.

38. **Black DM, Steinbuch M, Palmero L,** et al. An assessment tool for predicting fracture risk in postmenopausal women. Osteoporos Int 2001;12:519–528.

This investigation attempted to determine a clinical assessment tool based on risk factors identified in the Study of Osteoporotic Fractures (SOF): 7,782 women age 65 years and older were monitored for bone mineral density (BMD) measurements and baseline risk factors. Two models, one using BMD T-scores and one without T-scores, identified variables that could be assessed either by physicians or by self-administration. This FRACTURE Index uses seven variables that include age, BMD T-score, fracture after age 50 years, maternal hip fracture after age 50, weight less than or equal to 125 lb (57 kg), smoking status, and use of arms to stand up from a chair. The Index is predictive of hip fracture, vertebral, and nonvertebral fractures. The EPIDOS fracture study validates these findings.

39. **Miller PD, Barlas S, Brenneman SK,** et al. An approach to identifying osteopenic women at increased short-term risk of fracture. Arch Intern Med 2004;164:1113–1120.

This prospective cohort study identifies a classification algorithm for women who are osteopenic and the subsequent risk of fracture. 57,421 postmenopausal white women with baseline peripheral T-scores of −2.5 to −1.0 were monitored for new fractures within 1 year. Risk factors were then analyzed to predict future fracture events. Previous fracture, T-score at a peripheral site of −1.8 or less, self-rated poor health status, and poor mobility were the most important determinants of short-term fracture. Of the women analyzed in the study, 55% were identified with increased fracture risk, even at osteopenic T-scores. Women with previous fracture, regardless of T-score, had a risk of 4.1%, followed by 2.2% in women with T-scores of −1.8 or less or with poor health status, and 1.9% for women with poor mobility; 74% of the women who had a fracture within the first year were identified by the algorithm produced by this study.

40. **Nevitt MC, Cummings SR, Stone KL,** et al. Risk factors for a first-incident radiographic vertebral fracture in women ≥65 years of age: The study of osteoporotic fractures. J Bone Miner Res 200520:131–140.

In this prospective cohort study, risk factors for an incident occurrence of vertebral fracture were identified in 5,822 women at or more than 65 years of age who had no fracture at baseline. Fractures were assessed by spine radiographs obtained at baseline and follow-up an average of 3.7 years later. Older age, previous nonspine fracture, low bone mineral density (BMD) at all sites, a low body-mass index (BMI), current smoking, low milk consumption during pregnancy, low levels of daily physical activity, having a fall, and regular use of aluminum-containing antacids all independently increased risk of vertebral facture as shown by multivariate analysis. Physical activity and estrogen use decreased risk. When adjusted for BMD, low BMI, smoking, use of estrogen and antacids, and previous fracture were partially diminished. Women in the lower third of wrist BMD with five or more risk factors had a 12-fold greater risk than women in the highest third of BMD who had zero to three risk factors. Sixty percent of the incident fractures were involved with 27% of women in the highest risk category. Older women have increased risk of developing a first vertebral fracture when identified with several modifiable risk factors and low BMD.

41. **Papaioannou A, Joseph L, Ioannidis G,** et al. Risk factors associated with incident clinical vertebral and nonvertebral fractures in postmenopausal women: The Canadian Multicentre Osteoporosis Study (CaMos). Osteoporos Int 2005;16:568–578.

This analysis used data from the Canadian Multicentre Osteoporosis Study (CaMos) to examine potential risk factors and the occurrence of incident vertebral and nonvertebral fractures; 5,143 postmenopausal women were followed up for 3 years. The subjects were stratified into four groups according to fracture status during the years of follow-up. These groups included those without a new fracture; those with a new clinically recognized vertebral fracture; those with an incident nonvertebral fracture at the wrist, hip, humerus, pelvis, or ribs (main nonvertebral fracture group); and those with any new nonvertebral fracture (any nonvertebral-fracture group). Thirty-four, 163, and 280 women developed a vertebral, a main nonvertebral, or any nonvertebral fracture, respectively, throughout the 3 years of follow-up. Predictive models associated a five-point lower quality of life (as measured by the SF-36 physical component summary score) when associated with relative risks of 1.21 (95% CI, 1.02–1.44), 1.17 (95% CI, 1.07–1.28), and 1.19 (95% CI, 1.11–1.27) for incident vertebral, main nonvertebral, and all nonvertebral fractures, respectively. With lower femoral neck bone mineral density (BMD), even by 1 SD (SD = 0.12), the relative risks for incident vertebral, main nonvertebral, and any nonvertebral fractures increased by 2.73 (95% CI, 1.74–4.28), 1.39 (95% CI, 1.06–1.82), and 1.34 (95% CI, 1.09–1.65), respectively. This paper identified several risk factors that should be monitored with postmenopausal women with regard to osteoporosis risk.

42. **Gallagher JC, Genant HK, Crans GG,** et al. Teriparatide reduces the fracture risk associated with increasing number and severity of osteoporotic fractures. J Clin Endocrinol Metab 2005;90:1583–1587.

The Fracture Prevention Trial, a randomized, double-blind control study, evaluated 931 postmenopausal women with prevalent vertebral fractures randomized to daily placebo or teriparatide (20 μg) for new fracture incidence. After a mean follow-up time of 21 months, placebo patients with one, two, or three or more prevalent vertebral fractures, 7%, 16%, and 23%, respectively, developed vertebral fractures ($p < 0.001$), and 3%, 9%, and 17% developed moderate or severe vertebral fractures ($p < 0.001$). Among placebo patients with mild, moderate, or severe prevalent vertebral fractures, 10%, 13%, and 28%, respectively, developed vertebral fractures ($p < 0.001$), and 4%, 8%, and 23% developed moderate or severe vertebral fractures ($p < 0.001$). Placebo patients with zero, one, or two or more prior nonvertebral fragility fractures, 4%, 8%, and 18%, respectively, developed nonvertebral fragility fractures ($p < 0.001$). However, in the teriparatide-treated group, there was no significant increase in vertebral or nonvertebral fracture risk in these subgroups. New vertebral fracture risk was predicted by the number and severity of previous fractures independent of other risk factors; similar results were not found in the teriparatide group.

43. **Garnero P, Delmas P.** Contribution of bone mineral density and bone turnover markers to the estimation of risk of osteoporotic fracture in postmenopausal women. J Musculoskelet Neuronal Interact 2004;4:50–63.

This review article addresses the need for consistent and accurate identification of patients with osteoporosis at risk for fracture. Although bone mineral density (BMD) measured by various techniques has been shown to be a predictor of fracture risk in postmenopausal women, many patients with incident fractures have BMD values above threshold for diagnostic criteria. Several prospective studies associate increased bone resorption, as determined by specific biochemical markers, with increased risk of the hip, spine, and nonvertebral fractures, regardless of BMD. The Os des Femmes de Lyon (OFELY) study included 668 postmenopausal women followed up over 9 years and identified that within the 115 incident fractures, 54 (47%) actually occurred in nonosteoporotic women. Bone markers and previous fracture history were highly predictive of fracture risk. The increasing knowledge of bone matrix biochemistry, most notably of post-translational modifications in type I collagen, can identify biochemical markers that reflect changes in the material property of bone. The extent of post-translational modifications of collagen could identify cortical bone competency, regardless of BMD.

44. **Faulkner KG, Wacker WK, Barden HS,** et al. Femur strength index predicts hip fracture independent of bone density and hip axis length. Osteoporos Int 2006;17:593–599.

This cohort study analyzed femoral bone density, structure, and strength assessments obtained from dual-energy x-ray absorptiometry (DXA) measurements in women with and without hip fracture to determine hip fracture risk. DXA measurements of the proximal femur were obtained from 2,506 women 50 years of age or older, 365 with prior hip fracture, and 2,141 controls. Structural variables were determined using the Hip Strength Analysis program, including hip axis length (HAL), cross-sectional moment of inertia (CSMI), and the femur strength index (FSI) (a ratio of estimated compressive yield strength of the femoral neck to the expected compressive stress of a fall on the greater trochanter). Those women with previous fractures had a significantly lower femoral neck BMD and significantly higher HAL. In comparison with CSMI, there were no significant difference between the two groups after controlling for BMD and HAL. FSI was significantly lower in the fracture group, even after controlling for T-score and HAL. Therefore, BMD, HAL, and FSI can be used as independent risk factors of hip fracture.

45. **Mayhew PM, Thomas CD, Clement JG,** et al. Relation between age, femoral neck cortical stability, and hip fracture risk. Lancet 2005;366:129–135.

This cohort study measured the computed tomography distribution of bone in the mid-femoral neck of 77 deceased patients, and calculated cortical stress to determine elasticity and stability. In normal aging bone, the thin cortical zone in the upper femoral neck became significantly thinner. Relative to mean values at age 60 years, female cortical thickness declined by 6.4% (SD 1.1) per decade ($p < 0.0001$), and critical stress by 13.2% (4.3) per decade ($p = 0.004$) in the superoposterior octant compressed most in a sideways fall. Similar, but not as great, changes were found in men ($p = 0.004$). The capacity of the femur to absorb energy was independently decreased because of these changes. As women age, hip fragility increases because underloading of the superolateral cortex leads to atrophic thinning. These fragile zones may need strength training, rather than just walking, to decrease fracture risk.

46. **Uusi-Rasi K, Semanick LM, Zanchetta JR,** et al. Effects of teriparatide [rhPTH (1–34)] treatment on structural geometry of the proximal femur in elderly osteoporotic women. Bone 2005;36:948–958.

This randomized double-blind placebo-controlled study evaluated effects of teriparatide injection on hip structure in 558 patients enrolled in the Fracture Prevention Trial. Both treatment groups of 20 µg and 40 µg of teriparatide had increased bone mass and improved bone strength compared with placebo. Compared with placebo, the mean difference (95% CI) in bone cross-sectional area (CSA) in the TPTD20 was 3.5% (1.8%–5.3%), and 6.3% (4.5%–8.2%) in TPTD40 at study termination. Teriparatide treatment increased bending strength, with the mean difference in section modulus being 3.6% (1.4%–5.8%) and 6.8% (4.6%–9.1%) greater in the TPTD20 and TPTD40 groups, respectively. Local cortical instability characterized by the buckling ratio decreased by 5.5% (3.5% to 7.5%) and 8.6% (6.6% to 10.5%) in the TPTD20 and TPTD40 groups, respectively. Teriparatide increased cortical thickness and stability at the femoral neck and intertrochanteric region, while improving axial and bending strength.

47. **Khoo BC, Beck TJ, Qiao QH,** et al. In vivo short-term precision of hip structure analysis variables in comparison with bone mineral density using paired dual-energy X-ray absorptiometry scans from multi-center clinical trials. Bone 2005;37:112–121.

This article discusses hip structural analysis (HSA) in use with dual-energy x-ray absorptiometry (DXA) to extract strength-related structural dimensions of bone cross-sections from two-dimensional hip scan images. The first precision analysis of HSA variables is discussed here, in comparison with that of conventional bone mineral density (BMD). One HSA variable, section modulus (Z), which is indicative of bone strength during bending, had a short-term precision percentage coefficient of variation (CV%) in the femoral neck of 3.4% to 10.1%; differences were due to the different manufacturer and model of DXA equipment. Cross-sectional area (CSA), a determinant of bone strength during axial loading and closely aligned with conventional DXA bone mineral content, had a range of CV% from 2.8% to 7.9%. Poorer precision was associated with inadequate inclusion of the femoral shaft or femoral head in the DXA-scanned hip region. Precision of HSA-derived BMD varied between 2.4% and 6.4%. Precision of DXA manufacturer-derived BMD varied between 1.9% and 3.4%, arising from the larger analysis region of interest (ROI). The magnitude, subject height, weight, or conventional femoral neck densitometric variables were not necessary to determine precision. The poorer precision of key HSA variables than conventional DXA-derived BMD stresses the need for adequate and appropriately positioned ROI.

48. **Greenspan SL, von Stetten E, Emond SK,** et al. Instant vertebral assessment: A noninvasive dual X-ray absorptiometry technique to avoid misclassification and clinical mismanagement of osteoporosis. J Clin Densitom 2001;4:373–380.

This cohort study of 482 participants with no previous history of fracture analyzed the Instant Vertebral Assessment (IVA) technology, which uses dual x-ray absorptiometry (DXA) to assess fracture. Bone mineral density (BMD) at the spine, total hip, femoral neck, or combination of these sites was used to classify patients. Subjects were classified as osteoporotic if they had vertebral fractures independent of low bone density. The vertebral fractures that were identified by IVA were found in 18.3% of asymptomatic postmenopausal women. BMD alone using either a vertebral fracture or low BMD to identify osteoporotic individuals ranged from 40% to 74%. Using IVA, from 26% to 60% of osteoporotic individuals, may have been overlooked. However, 11.0% to 18.7% of clinically osteoporotic individuals would have been classified as normal by BMD criteria alone. IVA may be a useful tool in conjunction with BMD to determine osteoporotic individuals.

49. **Blake GM, Knapp KM, Fogelman I.** Absolute fracture risk varies with bone densitometry technique used. J Clin Densitom 2002;5:109–116.

In this cohort study, peripheral bone mineral density (BMD) measurements are discussed and how these measurements should be interpreted is analyzed. Thresholds (equivalent T-scores) defined to have the same absolute fracture risk as a femoral neck T-score of −2.5 could be used clinically; however, the fracture risk for a population has to be determined, regardless of which technique was used for measurement. Sixty-three postmenopausal women with Colles fracture and 191 control subjects were monitored for *in vivo* measurements of fracture risk prediction. A theoretical analysis identified that if the normal population has a Gaussian BMD distribution, fracture risk varies exponentially with Z-score as $\exp(-\text{beta } Z)$, then patients who experience a low-trauma fracture have a fracture risk that is larger by a factor $\exp(\text{beta}(2))$ compared with the fracture risk of the whole population. When individual subjects were analyzed for fracture risk, the Colles group varied between 1.03 times larger risk (for tibial SOS) and 2.77 times larger risk (for total hip BMD) than the average fracture risk for the whole population. As predicted by the theoretical study, fracture risk varied depending on the odds ratio determined by logistic regression analysis. Estimates of fracture risk in the same group of patients changed as much as three times, depending on the type of measurement. Equating different scan absolute fracture risk estimates cannot be the basis of deriving equivalent T-scores.

50. **Papaioannou A, Joseph L, Ioannidis G,** et al. Risk factors associated with incident clinical vertebral and nonvertebral fractures in postmenopausal women: The Canadian Multicentre Osteoporosis Study (CaMos). Osteoporos Int 2005;16:568–578.

This analysis used data from the Canadian Multicentre Osteoporosis Study (CaMos) to examine potential risk factors and the occurrence of incident vertebral and nonvertebral fractures; 5,143 postmenopausal women were followed up for 3 years. The subjects were stratified into four groups, according to fracture status during the years of follow-up. These groups included those without a new fracture; those with a new clinically recognized vertebral fracture; those with an incident nonvertebral fracture at the wrist, hip, humerus, pelvis, or ribs (main nonvertebral fracture group); and those with any new nonvertebral fracture (any nonvertebral-fracture group). Thirty-four, 163, and 280 women developed a vertebral, a main nonvertebral, or any nonvertebral fracture, respectively, throughout the 3 years of follow-up. Predictive models associated a five-point lower quality of life (as measured by the SF-36 physical component summary score) when associated with relative risks of 1.21 (95% CI, 1.02–1.44), 1.17 (95% CI, 1.07–1.28), and 1.19 (95% CI, 1.11–1.27) for incident vertebral, main nonvertebral, and all nonvertebral fractures, respectively. With lower femoral neck BMD, even by 1 SD (SD = 0.12), the relative risks for incident vertebral, main nonvertebral, and any nonvertebral fractures increased by 2.73 (95% CI, 1.74–4.28), 1.39 (95% CI, 1.06–1.82), and 1.34 (95% CI, 1.09–1.65), respectively. This paper identified several risk factors that should be monitored with postmenopausal women in regard to osteoporosis risk.

51. **Melton LJ III, Lane AW, Cooper C,** et al. Prevalence and incidence of vertebral deformities. Osteoporos Int 1993;3:113–119.

This continued cohort analysis of 762 Rochester, Minnesota, women was extended to identify vertebral deformities. Changes in the method of measuring vertebral heights, changes in the source of normal values for vertebral measurements, and changes in the criteria for assessing vertebral deformity had little impact on estimated prevalence and incidence in this population. Any vertebral deformity was prevalent in 25.3 per 100 Rochester women aged 50 years and older (95% CI, 22.3–28.2); the incidence of a new deformity in this group was estimated at 17.8 per 1,000 person-years (95% CI, 16.0–19.7). This suggests that, when the analysis is projected nationally, more than 500,000 white women develop vertebral deformities for the first time each year; more than 7 million white women aged 50 years and older might be affected at any given time. Because of the lack of gold standard analysis of morphometric data to determine false-positive and -negative rates, these estimates are limited.

52. **O'Neill TW, Felsenberg D, Varlow J,** et al. The prevalence of vertebral deformity in European men and women: The European Vertebral Osteoporosis Study. J Bone Miner Res 1996;11:1010–1018.

In this study, a cross-sectional population-based survey was utilized to monitor the prevalence of radiographically identified vertebral deformities: 15,570 males and females aged 50 to 79 years were monitored with lateral spinal radiographs. The published methodology of McCloskey and Eastell defined vertebral deformities. Based on this method, the mean center prevalence was 12% in females (range 6%–21%) and 12% in males (range 8%–20%) for all deformities. Both sexes had an increase in vertebral deformities due to age; however, this change was greater in females. There were also changes in prevalence due to geographical region, with the highest prevalence in Scandinavian countries.

53. **Spector TD, McCloskey EV, Doyle DV, Kanis JA.** Prevalence of vertebral fracture in women and the relationship with bone density and symptoms: The Chingford Study. J Bone Miner Res 1993;8:817–822.

In this study, a population survey was utilized to estimate prevalence of vertebral fractures. The relationship to symptoms and bone density was analyzed to identify risk factors. 1,035 women aged 45 to 69 (mean 55.4 years, response rate 77%) were used for the study; thoracic and lumbar spine x-rays, as well as bone mineral density (BMD) of lumbar spine L1-4 and neck of femur, were quantitated. One hundred forty-seven, 14.2% (95% CI, 12.0%–16.2%) of the 1,035 women, had minor fractures (at least two vertebral ratios 22.99 SD below the mean) and 20, 1.9% (95% CI, 1.2%–3.0%) of the total, had severe fractures (at least two ratios more than 3 SD below the mean). The bone density of the spine was not significantly lower in those women who had minor fractures than in the other 868 women; back pain or loss of height was not more prevalent. Multiple minor fractures correlated with lower bone density, by 0.4 SD. In the 20 women with severe fracture, bone density was significantly lower, by 0.6 SD. Loss of height was more common in severe fractures; however, back pain was not. Minor fractures were not associated with back pain or loss of height.

54. **Ross PD, Fujiwara S, Huang C,** et al. Vertebral fracture prevalence in women in Hiroshima compared with Caucasians or Japanese in the US. Int J Epidemiol 1995;24:1171–1177.

This prospective cohort study compared prevalence of vertebral fractures in U.S. Caucasians with native Japanese and Japanese immigrants in Hawaii. In comparison with Japanese-Americans, odds ratios (OR) and 95% confidence intervals (CI) for prevalent vertebral fractures were 1.8 (95% CI, 1.3–2.5) for native Japanese women and 1.5 (95% CI: 1.1–2.1) for Minnesota Caucasians. OR analysis appeared to be higher in women with two or more fractures: OR = 3.2 (95% CI, 2.0–5.3) for native Japanese and OR = 1.9 (95% CI, 1.2–3.2) for Minnesota Caucasians. Similar results were observed for native Japanese using a fracture definition of greater than or equal to 4 SD below the mean, but the OR for Caucasians was reduced to 1.2 (95% CI, 0.6–2.3). Spine fracture prevalence appears to be greatest among native Japanese; this implies that risk factors may be different for different populations of patients.

55. **Cooper C, O'Neill T, Silman A.** The epidemiology of vertebral fractures. European Vertebral Osteoporosis Study Group. Bone 1993;14(Suppl 1):S89–S97.

This review article compares the vertebral fracture data and analysis of the European Vertebral Osteoporosis Study Group to that of a series of studies using patients from Rochester, Minnesota. The results of the Rochester study suggest a prevalence rate of vertebral deformity of 25.3 per 100 Rochester women aged 50 years and older (95% CI, 22.3–28.2), with an estimated incidence of 17.8 per 1,000 person-years. However, the incidence of diagnosed vertebral fractures among women in the same population was 5.3 per 1,000 person-years; this implies that only 30% of such deformities in women receive clinical attention. Morphometric measurement on the radiographs of women with clinically diagnosed fractures revealed that 80% had grade 2 (>4 SD) deformities. The European Vertebral Osteoporosis Study (EVOS) is a multicenter epidemiologic study designed to monitor 300 men and 300 women over the age of 50 for prevalence of vertebral deformities.

56. **Genant HK, Li J, Wu CY, Shepherd JA.** Vertebral fractures in osteoporosis: A new method for clinical assessment. J Clin Densitom 2000;3:281–290.

    This review article discusses the necessity for vertebral fractures to be assessed as part of a clinical work-up for osteoporosis. The standard of care for assessment of fractures is radiographic analysis; however, this is not utilized for osteoporosis assessment. Most patients are asymptomatic, which leads to difficult clinical diagnosis. High-resolution lateral spine images, obtained on advanced fan-beam dual x-ray absorptiometry (DXA) systems, provide a practical, low-radiation dose, point-of-care methodology for assessment of vertebral fractures. Clinical data are reviewed that support the visual evaluation of lateral spine images obtained from a fan-beam DXA system as another measurement of osteoporotic risk.

57. **Vokes T, Bachman D, Baim S,** et al. Vertebral fracture assessment: The 2005 ISCD official positions. J Clin Densitom 2006;9:37–46.

    Vertebral Fracture Assessment (VFA) is utilized to image the thoracolumbar spine using bone densitometers. This review of the International Society for Clinical Densitometry (ISCD) positions concerning VFA, indications for using VFA, methodology for diagnosing vertebral fractures using VFA, and indications for additional imaging after VFA use gives evidence for these positional statements.

58. **Siminoski K, Warshawski RS, Jen H, Lee K.** The accuracy of historical height loss for the detection of vertebral fractures in postmenopausal women. Osteoporos Int 2006;17:290–296.

    This cohort study of postmenopausal women aged 50 or older who have been assessed by a specialist for osteoporotic risk determined the accuracy of historical height loss (HHL) to detect vertebral fracture development ($n = 323$; average age 66.0 ± 9.2 years; range 50–92 years). With HHL from 6.1 to 8.0 cm, the positive Likelihood Ratio (LR+) was 2.8 [95% confidence interval (95% CI), 1.3, 6.0]. When HHL was greater than 8.0 cm, the LR+ was 9.8 (95% CI, 3.0, 31.8). At a HHL of greater than 6.0 cm, sensitivity was 30% (95% CI, 22, 37%) and specificity was 94% (95% CI, 90, 97%). In the range of theoretical prevalence, the positive predictive value was low; however, the negative predictive value was high with prevalence data at the rates of most clinical practices. This study shows that a HHL of less than 6.0 cm rules out prevalent vertebral fracture with a high degree of accuracy; patients with a HHL greater than 6.0 cm should have spine radiographs to assess for the presence of vertebral fractures.

59. **Seeman E, Crans GG, Diez-Perez A,** et al. Anti-vertebral fracture efficacy of raloxifene: A meta-analysis. Osteoporos Int 2006;17:313–316.

    This metaanalysis of all randomized, double-blind, placebo-controlled studies analyzes whether the reduction in the risk for vertebral fracture is consistent among studies. A systematic review of the literature (MedLine, EMBASE) confirmed that all studies using raloxifene were included in this analysis. Raloxifene use of 60 mg/day (RLX60) and 120 mg/day pooled with 150 mg/day (RLX120/150) were analyzed by intention to treat. No heterogeneity among the studies included in the metaanalysis was identified. Odds ratio estimates (95% CI) were 0.60 (0.49, 0.74) for RLX60 and 0.51 (0.41, 0.64) for RLX120/150. In postmenopausal women, Raloxifene appears to consistently reduce vertebral fracture risk.

60. **Delmas P, Genant HK, Crans GG,** et al. Severity of prevalent vertebral fractures and the risk of subsequent vertebral and nonvertebral fractures: Results from the MORE trial. Bone 2003;33:522–532.

    This randomized, double-blind 3-year Multiple Outcomes of Raloxifene Evaluation (MORE) trial monitored 7,705 postmenopausal women with osteoporosis (low BMD or prevalent vertebral fractures) that were treated with placebo, raloxifene 60 mg/day, or raloxifene 120 mg/day for new vertebral and nonvertebral fractures. Women who had mild, moderate, and severe prevalent vertebral fractures—10.5%, 23.6%, and 38.1%, respectively—had new vertebral fractures, whereas 7.2%, 7.7%, and 13.8% respectively, experienced new nonvertebral fractures. Number of prevalent vertebral fractures and baseline BMD also predicted vertebral fracture risk; however, the severity of prevalent vertebral fractures only predicted nonvertebral fracture risk, even with adjustment for outlying variables. In those subjects with severe baseline vertebral fractures, raloxifene 60 mg/day decreased the risks of new vertebral [RR, 0.74 (95% CI, 0.54, 0.99); p = 0.048] and nonvertebral (clavicle, humerus, wrist, pelvis, hip, and leg) fractures [RH, 0.53 (95% CI, 0.29, 0.99); p = 0.046] at 3 years. Number needed to treat (NNT) analysis to prevent 1 new fracture at 3 years in women who had severe baseline vertebral fractures and who were treated with raloxifene 60 mg/day was 10 for vertebral and 18 for nonvertebral fractures. Similar results were observed in women receiving raloxifene 120 mg/day. The best independent predictor for new vertebral and nonvertebral fracture risk was baseline vertebral fracture severity. Raloxifene decreased new vertebral and nonvertebral fracture risk in the subgroup of women with severe vertebral fractures at baseline.

61. **Lenchik L, Rogers LF, Delmas P, Genant HK.** Diagnosis of osteoporotic vertebral fractures: Importance of recognition and description by radiologists. AJR Am J Roentgenol 2004;183:949–958.

62. **Duboeuf F, Bauer DC, Chapurlat RD,** et al. Assessment of vertebral fracture using densitometric morphometry. J Clin Densitom 2005;8:362–368.

This review article discusses the use of dual-energy x-ray absorptiometry (DXA) to diagnose vertebral fractures, and the accuracy and precision of other diagnostic techniques. Different techniques are using DXA as a basis for new morphometry analysis. DXA provides moderate sensitivity and excellent specificity in identifying vertebral deformities. However, image quality is lacking in DXA analysis. Therefore, improvements must be made to help with image quality.

63. **Kahn AA, Bachrach L, Brown JP,** et al. Standards and guidelines for performing central dual-energy x-ray absorptiometry in premenopausal women, men, and children. J Clin Densitom 2004;7:51–64.

This review article discusses the Canadian Panel of the International Society for Clinical Densitometry and their guidelines for dual-energy x-ray absorptiometry (DXA). The use of this densitometry in men, premenopausal women, and children is also discussed.

64. **Miller PD.** Pitfalls in bone mineral density measurements. Curr Osteoporos Rep 2004;2:59–64.

In this review article, bone mineral density (BMD) measurements are discussed in regard to their clinical use, efficacy, and problems in using BMD measurements for risk assessment and diagnosis. Proper clinical interpretation of BMD as well as quality control measures must be used to help ensure correct use of BMD data.

65. **Miller PD.** Review: Bone mineral density—clinical use and application. Endocrinol Metab Clin North Am 2003;32:159–179.

This review article discusses the use of bone densitometry to predict fracture risk for men, postmenopausal women, and those patients using glucocorticoids. It appears that bone densitometry can be used as a marker to assess efficacy of therapies.

66. **Miller PD, Zapalowski C, Kulak CAM, Bilezikian JP.** Bone densitometry: The best way to detect osteoporosis and to monitor therapy. J Clin Endocrinol Metab 1999;84:1867–1871.

This review advocates for the use of bone mass measurements to assess for the risk of osteoporosis in the general population. This measurement can be used to help identify those patients with osteoporosis, as well as the efficacy of treatment protocols.

4

Bone Densitometry: Using Dual-energy X-ray Absorptiometry for Monitoring

Paul D. Miller

Determining the Least Significant Change, 51
Effect of Anabolic Therapy on Areal Versus Volumetric Bone Mineral Density Measurement, 51

Central dual-energy x-ray absorptiometry (DXA) has been the foundation for monitoring patients with osteoporosis. Monitoring is useful for following the effects of diseases that may negatively affect bone, such as primary hyperparathyroidism; of drugs that may negatively affect bone, such as glucocorticoids; and of pharmacological agents for the treatment of postmenopausal osteoporosis (PMO).

Although there has been widespread acceptance of the use of bone mineral density (BMD) for monitoring disease states or in patients who are taking drugs that may cause bone loss (such as glucocorticoids) [1–4], there has been much debate regarding the utility of BMD to monitor the pharmacological response to osteoporosis therapies [5–15]. The debate has focused on the contribution that pharmacologically mediated changes in BMD make to a reduction in fracture risk. The use of the change in BMD as a surrogate marker for a change in bone strength is clouded by the fact that the increase in BMD mediated by current osteoporosis treatments as it relates to reduction in fracture risk is neither linear nor proportional and by the statistical methods applied to examine the relationship between BMD change and fracture risk reduction. Summary statistics (metaanalysis) [10] (Fig. 4.1) have suggested that this relationship is closer to being linear than the nonlinear relationship defined by individual clinical trial analysis defined by Freedman et al. [14,15] (Table 4.1). In addition, the U.S. Surgeon General's report on America's bone health has stated that surrogate markers can be used within the context of clinical trials to reflect drug-induced improvements in bone strength. Finally, the Food and Drug Administration (FDA) approval of intermittent bisphosphonate dosing intervals (weekly, monthly, quarterly) has been allowed, based on the trust that changes in BMD reflect equal fracture risk reduction as compared with the daily dosing regimens, which were required to prove fracture reduction ("bridging concept") [16–19]. Nevertheless, other factors lead to fracture risk reduction mediated by osteoporosis-specific pharmacological agents independent of change in BMD [20–23]. In

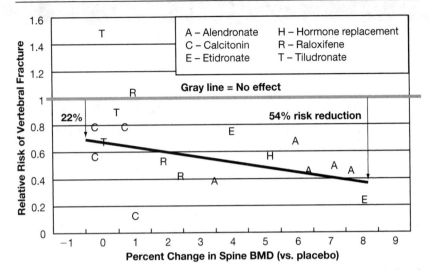

Figure 4.1. A metaanalysis examining the relationship between antiresorptive-induced changes in spine bone mineral density and risk reduction. (After Wasnich RD, Miller PD. Antifracture efficacy of antiresortive agents are related to changes in bone density. J Clin Endocrinol Metab 2000;85:1–6, with permission.)

addition, head-to-head randomized studies, either comparing BMD changes of alendronate to that of risedronate or alendronate to that of teriparatide, have no prospective fracture data to know if differences in BMD increase render a bone stronger [24,25].

Therefore, the debate continues regarding the value of measuring change in DXA-derived BMD as a surrogate marker for fracture risk. This debate, mostly driven by marketing, has clouded the value of BMD monitoring in patients being treated for osteoporosis. Without measuring BMD over time, patients would never receive any feedback to determine if their long-term therapy of an often asymptomatic condition is worth their commitment and

Table 4.1.   Relationship between pharmacologically induced increases in bone mineral density and fracture risk reduction as assessed by Freedman's analysis from individual clinical trials

Drug	Proportion of Fracture Risk Change Explained by Changes in Bone Mineral Density (%)	Study
Alendronate	16	Cummings et al. (11)
Risedronate	28	Eastell et al. (7)
Raloxifene	4	Sarkar et al. (5)
Risedronate	28	Watts et al. (13)
Teriparitide	40	P. Chen et al. (39)

From **Miller PD.** Bone density and markers of bone turnover in predicting fracture risk and how changes in these measures predict fracture risk reduction. Curr Osteoporos Rep 2005;3:103–110, with permission.

expense. In addition, the discovery of a loss in BMD beyond the *in vivo* least significant change [26,27] should never become an acceptable standard of care in the management of the osteoporosis patient on treatment. A loss in BMD cannot be assumed to reflect a residual improvement in bone strength [28,29]. A loss of BMD may be due to poor patient compliance or adherence to treatment, or to previously unrecognized and possibly reversible secondary conditions that may be responsible for a loss of BMD (e.g., celiac disease). A loss in BMD may be reversed by providing an alternative route of administration (e.g., an intravenous or transdermal or subcutaneous route of administration) or a change in pharmacological agents [30–32].

DETERMINING THE LEAST SIGNIFICANT CHANGE

The application of the least significant change (LSC) to the practice of DXA use is so important that the International Society for Clinical Densitometry (ISCD) has not only stressed this important *in vivo* quality performance in their Position Development Conference (PDC) statements but has initiated a nationwide site accreditation process to give recognition to those DXA sites that have performed *in vivo* precision error studies [33,34]. Phantoms do not move in serial BMD measurements—patients do. Therefore, the manufacturer-supplied *in vitro* (phantom) precision error data are not applicable to *in vivo* quality control studies. To perform an *in vivo* precision study in order for a DXA site to know its LSC (the minimum change in BMD in absolute or relative terms) and know if a BMD change is significant or a measurement error, a site need only to measure 30 patients in duplicate. This is not research and should not require an IRB (Institutional Review Board) approval, since performing duplicate measurements is often the standard of care in may communities for DXA performance. Once the 30 patients are done in duplicate, the mathematical calculations to find one's LSC can easily be entered on the ISCD Web site (http://www.iscd.org), which takes just a few minutes to include the patient BMD data to derive a facility's LSC. Without knowing one's LSC, one can never know if a change in BMD is real or a measurement error—a fundamental requirement for competent DXA interpretation.

EFFECT OF ANABOLIC THERAPY ON AREAL VERSUS VOLUMETRIC BONE MINERAL DENSITY MEASUREMENT

A word should be said about monitoring the effect of teriparatide (recombinant human 1–34 parathyroid hormone). Teriparatide increases bone strength and reduces fracture risk in part by increasing periosteal bone formation [35,36]. Thus, teriparatide increases bone area. BMD as measured by DXA is a derived equation: BMD = bone mineral content (g)/bone area (cm^2) to give a two-dimensional areal measurement (g/cm^2). It is possible that patients treated with teriparatide may have a drop in areal BMD yet have an increase in bone strength [37,38]. In cynomogolus monkeys treated with teriparatide, forearm BMD measured by DXA declined, yet volumetric BMD measured by peripheral quantitative computed tomography increased and forearm bone strength increased as well [36]. The practical issue for patient management is that if the clinician is convinced that the patient being treated with teriparatide is compliant and that secondary factors that might mitigate a pharmacological response have been excluded, the patient on teriparatide needs reassurance and commitment to continuation of therapy.

REFERENCES
Annotations by Elizabeth Dillard

1. **Khosla S.** Surrogates for fracture end-points in clinical trials. J Bone Miner Res 2003;18:1146–1149.

   In this review article, the author discusses the use of bone mineral density (BMD) and bone turnover markers as ways to assess the efficacy of risk reduction in vertebral fracture trials. Traditionally, vertebral fractures were used as endpoints in clinical trials; however, the use of BMD as a surrogate marker could reduce the number of subjects necessary to achieve clinical significance. Models that incorporate changes in both BMD and bone turnover markers could prove to be more accurate predictors of fracture risk reduction.

2. **Miller PD.** Bone density and markers of bone turnover in predicting fracture risk and how changes in these measures predict fracture risk reduction. Curr Osteoporos Rep 2005;3:103–110.

   This review article discusses the assessment of markers such as bone mineral density (BMD) and bone turnover markers (BTM) used to determine the clinical response to pharmacological therapy of osteoporosis. Changes in either measurement can be indicative of reductions in nonvertebral and vertebral fracture risk. An assessment of BTM change earlier in therapy can provide a clinician with information on compliance and the physiologic effects of drug therapy. Increases in BMD after 12 to 24 months also correlates with increase in bone strength, and no change in BMD can be associated with risk reduction in certain clinical trials. Fluctuations in BMD and BTM can be used together to determine efficacy of pharmacological management.

3. **Miller PD, Bilezikian JP.** Bone densitometry in asymptomatic hyperparathyroidism. J Bone Miner Res 2002;17(Suppl 2):N98–N102.

4. **Miller PD, Hochberg MC, Wehren LE,** et al. How useful are measures of BMD and bone turnover? Curr Med Res Opin 2005;4:545–554.

   In this review, the recent questioning of bone mineral density (BMD) and biochemical markers of bone turnover as useful in the diagnosis and treament of osteoporosis is analyzed. BMD is the current gold standard for the diagnosis of osteoporosis and prediction of fracture risk. Bone turnover has been shown to be of limited usefulness in predicting fracture risk, due to the inability to measure markers routinely. However, in research applications, both BMD and markers of bone turnover are used to identify optimal candidates for clinical trials. Head-to-head comparisons of treatments that use these measurements can be used instead of fracture endpoint trials, which would statistically need to be large and complex. Those studies that suggest change in BMD or bone turnover not correlated with fraction risk reduction appear to be flawed. BMD and bone turnover markers are the best studies to follow for response to treatment at this time.

5. **Sarkar S, Reginster JY, Crans GG,** et al. Relationship between changes in biochemical markers of bone turnover and BMD to predict vertebral fracture risk. J Bone Miner Res 2004;19:394–401.

   The Multiple Outcomes of Raloxifene Evaluation (MORE) trial was a randomized, placebo-controlled trial of 7,705 women with osteoporosis treated with raloxifene 60 or 120 mg/day for 3 years. This retrospective analysis of the MORE trial analyzed markers of bone turnover measured in one-third of the study population ($n = 2,503$). Logistic regression models constructed used 1-year percent changes in bone mineral density (BMD) and bone turnover and relevant baseline demographics to predict the risk of vertebral fracture with pooled raloxifene therapy at 3 years. All variables were standardized before analysis. Independent predictors of fracture risk in raloxifene-treated patients included prevalent vertebral fracture status ($p < 0.0001$), baseline lumbar spine BMD ($p < 0.0001$), and number of years postmenopausal ($p = 0.0005$). Therapy-by-change in femoral neck BMD ($p = 0.02$) and therapy-by-change in osteocalcin (OC; $p = 0.01$) were also significant for all treatment groups. Another model included significant baseline variables and significant change in OC ($p = 0.01$); change in femoral neck BMD in the same model was not significant. Changes in BMD and OC have different effects on fracture risk for the placebo versus pooled raloxifene groups. After adjustment of each significant baseline variable in patients treated with raloxifene, the percent change in OC predicted reduction in vertebral fracture risk more accurately than the percent change in femoral neck BMD.

6. **Delmas PD, Seeman E.** Changes in bone mineral density explain little of the reduction in vertebral or nonvertebral fracture risk with anti-resorptive therapy. Bone 2004;34:599–604.

In this review article, the basis for the decrease in vertebral and nonvertebral fracture risk in patients using antiresorptive therapy is discussed. Several metaanalyses failed to detect a significant association between vertebral fracture risk reduction and increases in bone mineral density (BMD) or reported that only a small proportion of the vertebral fracture risk reduction was explained by changes in BMD. This questions the previous ideology that BMD correlated with vertebral fracture risk. One report of the risk of nonvertebral fractures decreasing with antiresorptive treatment correlated with an increase in BMD [J Clin Endrocrinol Metab 2002;87:1586]. However, after correcting for issues in reported BMD and person-year data, a new analysis suggested that the reductions in nonvertebral fracture risk did not correlate in magnitude with increases in BMD at the end of the first year or at completion of the studies. This analysis concludes that only a fraction of the reduction in fracture risk can be explained by changes in BMD. Further studies are needed to define the structural basis of the fracture risk reduction.

7. **Eastell R, Delmas PD.** How to interpret surrogate markers of efficacy in osteoporosis. J Bone Miner Res 2005;20:1261–1262.

In this letter to the editor, the authors examine the use of bone mineral density (BMD) and bone turnover markers to determine clinical efficacy of treatments for osteoporosis. Their comments conclude that there are several issues that need to be resolved before making these surrogates alternatives to fractures the primary endpoint in clinical trials.

8. **Garnero P, Delmas PD.** Contribution of bone mineral density and bone turnover markers to the estimation of risk of osteoporotic fracture in postmenopausal women. J Musculoskelet Neuronal Interact 2004;4:50–63.

This metaanalysis discussed several studies that show that an increased bone resorption monitored with biochemical markers was associated with increased risk of the hip, spine, and nonvertebral fractures, regardless of the bone mineral density (BMD) of the patient. In the Os des Femmes de Lyons (OFELY) study, including 668 postmenopausal women followed prospectively over 9 years, in the 115 incident fractures found, 54 (47%) occurred in nonosteoporotic women. Within this group, bone markers and history of previous fracture were predictive of fracture risk. Thus, bone markers could be clinically relevant in assessing fracture risk in selected cases in which BMD does not change. Different post-translational modifications of type I collagen could reflect variations in bone strength, as determined by the material property of bone. Preliminary *in vitro* studies indicate that the extent of these modifications of collagen plays a role independent of BMD in determining the mechanical competence of cortical bone.

9. **Hochberg M, Greenspan S, Wasnich R,** et al. Changes in bone density and turnover explain the reductions in incidence of nonvertebral fractures that occur during treatment with antiresorptive agents. J Clin Endocrinol Metab 2002;87:1586–1592.

Within this metaanalysis of all randomized, placebo-controlled trials of antiresorptive agents conducted in postmenopausal women with osteoporosis (i.e., prior vertebral fracture or low BMD) with relevant data, the changes in bone mineral density (BMD) and biochemical markers (BCM) of bone turnover during antiresorptive therapy were analyzed in respect to reduction in nonvertebral fractures. In 18 trials, a total of 2,415 women with incident nonvertebral fractures over 69,369 woman-years of follow-up were found. Poisson regression was used to estimate the association between changes in BMD or BCM during the first year and overall reductions in risk of nonvertebral fractures (vs. the placebo group) across all trials. Greater reductions in nonvertebral fracture risk were found with larger increases in BMD and larger reductions in BCM. Each 1% increase in spine BMD at 1 year was associated with an 8% reduction in nonvertebral fracture risk ($p = 0.02$). Agents that increase spine BMD by 6% at 1 year reduced nonvertebral fracture risk by about 39%, and an agent that increases hip BMD by 3% at 1 year reduces nonvertebral fracture risk by about 46%. A 70% reduction in resorption BCM would reduce risk of fracture by 40%, and a 50% reduction in formation BCM would reduce risk by 44%. These data demonstrate that larger increases in BMD at both the spine and hip and larger reductions in both formation and resorption BCM are associated with greater reductions in the risk of nonvertebral fractures.

10. **Wasnich RD, Miller PD.** Antifracture efficacy of antiresorptive agents are related to changes in bone density. J Clin Endocrinol Metab 2000;85:1–6.

This metaanalysis of clinical trials of antiresorptive agents assessed the relative risk of vertebral fractures against the average change in bone mineral density (BMD) for each trial. The data were analyzed to determine the correlation between (BMD) and antifracture efficacy for antiresorptive therapy. There was marked variability in antifracture efficacy at any given level of change in BMD; similarly, wide ranges of confidence intervals were discovered. However, trials that reported larger increases in BMD tended to observe greater reductions in vertebral fracture risk. Poisson regression was used to quantify this relationship. The model predicts that treatments that increase spine BMD by 8% would reduce risk by 54%; most of the total effect of treatment was explained by the 8% increase in BMD (41% risk reduction). These findings are consistent with the short-term predictions of the conceptual model and with reports from randomized trials. The small but significant reductions in risk that were not explained by measurable changes in BMD might be related to publication bias, measurement errors, or limitations of current BMD technology.

11. **Cummings SR, Karpf DB, Harris F,** et al. Improvement in spine bone density and reduction in risk of vertebral fractures during treatment with anti-resorptive drugs. Am J Med 2002;112:281–289.

In a metaanalysis of 12 clinical trials, the researchers attempted to determine the relationship between improvement in bone and reduction in risk of vertebral fracture in postmenopausal women. The Fracture Intervention Trial was analyzed with logistic models to quantify changes in risk of vertebral fracture with alendronate in relation to improved bone mineral density (BMD). A decrease in the relative risk (RR) of vertebral fracture by 0.03 correlated with a 1% improvement in spine BMD [95% confidence interval (CI): 0.02 to 0.05]. The improvement in BMD caused a greater relative risk of fraction reduction than the logistic model anticipated. The model predicted that treatments would reduce fracture risk by 20% (RR = 0.80), however. The increase in bone mineral density reduced the risk of fracture by about 45% (RR = 0.55). In patients treated with alendronate, the Fracture Intervention Trial showed that improved spine bone mineral density accounted for 16% (95% CI: 11%–27%) of the reduction in the risk of vertebral fracture. Increases in BMD after treatment with antiresorptive drugs is only one portion of the reduction of risk of vertebral fracture.

12. **Delmas PD, Li Z, Cooper C.** Relationship between changes in bone mineral density and fracture risk reduction with antiresorptive drugs: some issues with metaanalyses. J Bone Miner Res 2004;19:330–337.

This study examined the effects of study selection or the use of summary statistics or individual patient data (IPD) as the basis for inconsistant analysis of metaanalyses of clinical trials investigating the relationship between bone mineral density (BMD) and fracture risk reduction with antiresorptive therapy. Poisson regression analyses were used to evaluate effects of study selection. IPD were created to match summary statistics for published trials to evaluate the effects of using individual patient data instead of summary statistics. These results were compared with those based on metaregression using summary statistics. The effect of varying the BMD increase with treatment (3%–8%) used in predicting the fracture risk reductions in these simulations was also analyzed. Though the Poisson regression originally found in a metaanalysis of 18 trials a statistically significant relationship between nonvertebral fracture risk and spinal BMD ($p = 0.02$), this relationship was not significant when analyses were based on 7 studies that were at least 3 years in duration and placebo controlled. Simulated IPD metaanalysis of 12 trials of six antiresorptive agents produced accurate results indeterminant of the proportion of vertebral risk reduction related to BMD change; however, metaregression using summary statistics consistently produced an estimate around 50%, regardless of the statistics. When this technique was applied to actual data from two risedronate studies, the metaregression of summary statistics demonstrated an increase in the correlation between BMD change and fracture risk reduction over the IPD analysis. The prediction of fracture risk reduction due to BMD gain was proportional to the percentage of gain; the average BMD gain (3%) observed produced an overall fracture risk reduction similar to the clinical presentation. However, the use of larger BMD gains (8%) produced substantially higher estimated fracture risk reduction and skewed a higher proportion of fracture risk reduction attributed to BMD gains. Caution should be used in interpreting the results of such analyses when exploring the relationship between BMD changes and fracture risk reduction with antiresorptive therapy of osteoporosis.

13. **Watts NB, Cooper C, Linday R,** et al. Relationship between changes in bone mineral density and vertebral fracture risk associated with risedronate: greater increases in bone mineral density do not relate to greater decreases in fracture risk. J Clin Densitom 2004;7:255–261.

This metaanalysis compared three risedronate trials to determine the relationship between bone mineral density (BMD) change and fracture risk in postmenopausal osteoporotic women receiving antiresorptive treatment. For 3 years, women received risedronate ($n = 2,047$) or placebo ($n = 1,177$) daily. The BMD and vertebral radiographs were assessed periodically throughout that time period. Patients whose BMD increased and those whose BMD decreased were compared with each other in respect to fracture risk reduction. Risedronate-treated patients whose BMD decreased were at a significantly greater risk ($p = 0.003$) of sustaining a vertebral fracture than patients whose BMD increased. The degree of increase of BMD was not statistically significant; risedronate-treated patients whose increases in BMD were less than 5% (the median change from baseline) and those whose increases were greater than or equal to 5% had similar fracture risk reduction ($p = 0.453$). Only 18% of risedronate's vertebral fracture efficacy was determined by changes in lumbar spine BMD [95% confidence interval (CI), 10%, 26%; $p < 0.001$]. Greater increases in BMD did not necessarily predict greater decreases in fracture risk, even though increases in BMD did correlate with lower fracture risk.

14. **Freedman LS, Graubard BI, Schatzkin A.** Statistical validation of intermediate endpoints for chronic diseases. Stat Med 1992;11:167–178.

This paper discusses the criterion for statistical validation of intermediate endpoints for chronic disease. A cohort or intervention study would be adjusted for the intermediate endpoint, and reduced to zero. For example, to examine whether serum cholesterol level is an intermediate endpoint for coronary heart disease (CHD), investigations of the effect of the cholesterol-lowering drug cholestyramine on CHD incidence would be adjusted for serum cholesterol levels. When the unadjusted exposure or treatment effect is less than four times its standard error, the analysis usually leads to weak validation. This suggests that the data are not inconsistent with a validation criterion. The more significant exposure effect, the more powerful the validation criteria.

15. **Shih J, Bauer DC, Orloff J,** et al. Proportion of fracture risk reduction explained by BMD changes using Freeman's analysis depends on choice of predictors. Osteoporos Int 2002;13(Suppl 3):538–539.

16. **Schnitzer T, Bone H, Crepasldi G,** et al. Therapeutic equivalence of alendronate 70 mg once-weekly and alendronate 10 mg daily in the treatment of osteoporosis. Aging Clin Exp Res 2000;12:1–12.

This double-blind, multicenter study of postmenopausal women (ages 42 to 95) with osteoporosis, as defined by bone mineral density (BMD) of either lumbar spine or femoral neck at least 2.5 SDs below peak premenopausal mean, or prior vertebral or hip fracture, analyzed the efficacy and safety of treatment with oral once-weekly alendronate 70 mg ($n = 519$), twice-weekly alendronate 35 mg ($n = 369$), and daily alendronate 10 mg ($n = 370$). The primary endpoint compared increases in lumbar spine BMD, using predefined equivalence criteria. Secondary endpoints included changes in BMD at the hip and total body and rate of bone turnover, monitored with biochemical markers. Mean increases in lumbar spine BMD at 12 months were 5.1% (95% CI 4.8, 5.4) in the 70 mg once-weekly group, 5.2% (4.9, 5.6) in the 35 mg twice-weekly group, and 5.4% (5.0, 5.8) in the 10 mg daily treatment group. All three dosing regimens had statistically similar increases in BMD at the total hip, femoral neck, trochanter, and total body. Biochemical markers of bone resorption (urinary N-telopeptides of type I collagen) and bone formation (serum bone-specific alkaline phosphatase) were reduced by all three treatment groups in similar significance. Similar incidences of upper gastrointestinal (GI) adverse experiences were found in the three treatment groups; however, fewer serious upper GI adverse experiences were found in the once-weekly group compared to the once-daily group. These data are consistent with preclinical animal models, and suggest that once-weekly dosing has the potential for improved upper GI tolerability. The alendronate 70 mg once-weekly dosing regimen may enhance compliance and long-term persistence with therapy due to decrease in adverse GI effects.

17. **Brown JP, Kendler DL, McClung MR,** et al. The efficacy and tolerability of risedronate once a week for the treatment of postmenopausal osteoporosis. Calcif Tissue Int 2002;71:103–111.

In a randomized, double-blind, active-controlled study, risedronate once a week (35 mg and 50 mg) therapy and risedronate 5 mg once daily therapy were compared in women with osteoporosis with regard to efficacy and patient compliance. The study was conducted for 2 years; the primary efficacy of percent change in lumber spine bone mineral density (BMD) assessment was performed after 1 year. Women aged 50 years or older who had been postmenopausal for at least 5 years were enrolled in the study. Subjects had either a BMD T-score of –2.5 or lower (lumbar spine or proximal femur) or a T-score lower than −2 and at least one prevalent vertebral fracture. Risedronate therapy regimens of 5 mg once daily, 35 mg once a week, or 50 mg once a week were compared. Calcium and vitamin D supplementation was given to participants. A total of 1,456 women were randomized and received medication; 1,209 (83%) completed 1 year of the study. The mean percent change (SE) in lumbar spine BMD after 12 months was 4.0% (0.2%) in the 5-mg daily group, 3.9% (0.2%) in the 35-mg group, and 4.2% (0.2%) in the 50-mg group. Secondary outcomes of efficacy and side effects were also similar in all three groups after 12 months. Risedronate 35 mg and 50 mg once a week provides the same efficacy and safety as the daily 5-mg regimen. The lower dose regimen of 35 mg once a week is considered optimal for women with postmenopausal osteoporosis.

18. **Miller PD, McClung M, Macovei L,** et al. Monthly oral ibandronate therapy in postmenopausal osteoporosis: One year results from the MOBILE study. J Bone Miner Res 2005;20:1315–1322.

The MOBILE study is a 2-year, randomized, double-blind, phase III, noninferiority trial; 1,609 women with postmenopausal osteoporosis were administered one of the following oral ibandronate regimens: 2.5 mg daily, 50 mg/50 mg monthly (single doses, consecutive days), 100 mg monthly, or 150 mg monthly. Lumbar spine bone mineral density (BMD) increased by 3.9%, 4.3%, 4.1%, and 4.9% in the 2.5-, 50/50-, 100-, and 150-mg arms, respectively, after 1 year. The 150-mg regimen was superior, though all monthly regimens were not inferior, to daily regimen. All monthly regimens showed a larger increase in BMD than the daily regimen. All regimens similarly decreased serum levels of C-telopeptide, a biochemical marker of bone resorption. A significantly larger proportion of women receiving the 100-mg and 150-mg monthly regimens reached the predefined threshold levels for percent change from baseline in lumbar spine (6%) or total hip BMD (3%) than the daily regimen group. All regimens were similarly well tolerated. Therefore, monthly ibandronate is at least as effective and just as well tolerated as the current daily ibandronate regimen in postmenopausal osteoporosis.

19. **Miller PD.** Optimizing the management of postmenopausal osteoporosis with bisphosphonates: the emerging role of intermittent therapy. Clin Ther 2005;27:1–16.

This analysis reviewed the available data relative to the efficacy and tolerability of intermittent (less frequent than weekly) bisphosphonate dosing regimens for the treatment of postmenopausal osteoporosis. When administered intermittently, several bisphosphonates have shown efficacy with increases in bone mineral density (BMD) and decreases in markers of bone turnover. Evidence of fracture benefit from a less frequent bisphosphonate dosing regimen has been demonstrated. Ibandronate, a nitrogen-containing bisphosphonate, was shown to be associated with a significant decrease in vertebral fracture risk even if administered intermittently ($p < 0.001$ vs. placebo). Bisphosphonate therapy using intermittent schedules longer than 1 week can be capable of reducing the risk of fracture, improving BMD, and suppressing biochemical markers of bone turnover, as shown by the ibandronate study.

20. **Borah B, Dufresne TE, Chmielewski PA,** et al. Risedronate preserves trabecular architecture and increases bone strength in vertebra of ovariectomized minipigs as measured by three-dimensional microcomputed tomography. J Bone Miner Res 2002; 17:1139–1147.

This study of ovariectomized minipigs monitored the effects of risedronate on trabecular bone mass and architecture, and the contribution of mass and architecture to strengthen the minipigs. The minipigs were OVX at 18 months of age and were treated daily for 18 months with either vehicle or risedronate at doses of 0.5 mg/kg/day or 2.5 mg/kg/day. The three-dimensional (3D) microcomputed tomography (μCT) evaluated the 3D bone architecture of L4 vertebral cores of the minipigs. In comparison to the OVX control, both treated groups had higher vertebral bone volume [bone volume/tissue volume (BV/TV)] ($p < 0.05$). The 2.5 mg/kg dose had more significant architectural changes, and these changes were more prevalent at the cranial-caudal ends compared with the midsection. A significant preservation of trabeculae orthogonal to the cranial-caudal axis was confirmed by a decrease in the degree of anisotropy (DA) and an increase in the percent Cross-strut (% Cross-strut; $p < 0.05$) in the 2.5 mg/kg group. At the higher dose, the trabecular thickness (Tb.Th), trabecular number (Tb.N), and connectivity were higher, and marrow star volume (Ma.St.V) and trabecular separation (Tb.Sp) were lower ($p < 0.05$). An approximate structural variations measurement, the trabecular separation variation index (TSVI), was smaller in the 2.5 mg/kg treated group ($p < 0.05$). Normalized maximum load (strength) and stiffness of the vertebral cores were higher in the 2.5 mg/kg risedronate group compared with the OVX group ($p < 0.05$). The combination of bone volume and architectural variables explained more than 90% of the bone strength. BV per TV alone appeared to explain 76% of the variability of the strength. Trabecular architecture in the vertebra of OVX minipigs was preserved by risedronate therapy, and bone mass and architecture directly affect strength of bone.

21. **Roschger P, Rinnerthaler S, Yates J,** et al. Alendronate increases degree and uniformity of mineralization in cancellous bone and decreases the porosity in cortical bone of osteoporotic women. Bone 2001;29:185–191.
This analysis studied the Phase III Alendronate (Aln) 10 mg/day trials (6 subjects per group; placebo and Aln after 2 and 3 years of treatment). The mineral structures of 24 transiliac bone biopsies were investigated. Quantitative backscattered electron imaging (qBEI) and scanning small-angle x-ray scattering (scanning-SAXS) monitored the bone mineralization density distribution (BMDD), and the size and arrangement of the mineral particles in bone, respectively. The relative calcium content of osteoporotic bone was significantly lower than that of database controls. With Aln treatment, mineralization improved and was more uniform. The size and characteristics of the mineral particles did not differ in placebo versus Aln-treated groups; however, the porosity of cortical bone was reduced significantly by Aln treatment. Aln treatment appears to increase the degree and uniformity of bone matrix mineralization while preserving the size and habitus of the mineral crystals.

22. **Eastell R, Barton I, Hannon RA,** et al. Relationship of early changes in bone resorption to the reduction in fracture risk with risedronate. J Bone Miner Res 2003; 18:1051–1056.
Biochemical markers of bone resorption were analyzed in conjunction with risedronate treatment to determine whether changes in these markers correlated with the efficacy of risedronate therapy with regard to fractures. Two bone resorption markers, the C-telopeptide of type I collagen (CTX) and the N-telopeptide of type I collagen (NTX), in osteoporotic patients given risedronate were measured. Six hundred ninety-three women with at least one vertebral deformity (mean age, 69 ± 7 years) received calcium (and vitamin D if required) and placebo or risedronate 5 mg daily for 3 years. Urinary CTX (median, 60%) and NTX (51%) at 3 to 6 months with risedronate therapy was significantly associated ($p < 0.05$) with the reduction in vertebral fracture risk (75% over 1 year and 50% over 3 years). The changes in both CTX and NTX were associated with one-half (CTX, 55%; NTX, 49%) of risedronate's reduction of vertebral fractures in the first year and approximately two-thirds (CTX, 67%; NTX, 66%) over 3 years compared with placebo. In comparison, the changes in CTX and NTX accounted for 77% and 54%, respectively, of risedronate's effect in reducing the risk of nonvertebral fractures over 3 years compared with placebo. There was no linear relationship between vertebral fracture risk and changes from baseline in CTX and NTX ($p < 0.05$). Little improvement in fracture benefit occurred with decreases of 55% to 60% for CTX and 35% to 40% for NTX. Risedronate therapy's reduction in fracture risk correlates largely to the decrease in bone resorption; however, there may be a maximal level of benefit to decreasing bone resorption.

23. **Bauer DC, Black DM, Ganero P,** et al. Change in bone turnover and hip, nonspine and vertebral fractures in alendronate treated women: Fracture Intervention Trial. J Bone Miner Res 2004;19:1250–1258.
This analysis of the Fracture Intervention Trial assessed the change in bone turnover after 1 year of alendronate or placebo in relationship to hip, nonspine, and spine fracture risk

among 6,186 postmenopausal women by monitoring biochemical markers of bone turnover [bone-specific alkaline phosphatase (bone ALP), intact N-terminal propeptide of type I collagen, and C-terminal crosslinked telopeptide of type 1 collagen] and bone mineral density (BMD) of the spine and hip at baseline and after 1 year of alendronate or placebo. Seventy-two hip, 786 nonspine, and 336 vertebral fractures were documented within 3.6 years of follow-up. With each SD reduction in 1-year change in bone ALP, fewer spine (odds ratio = 0.74; CI: 0.63, 0.87), nonspine [relative hazard (RH) = 0.89; CI: 0.78, 1.00; $p < 0.050$], and hip fractures (RH = 0.61; CI: 0.46, 0.78) were documented. A 30% reduction in bone ALP in alendronate-treated women correlated with a lower risk of non-spine (RH = 0.72; CI: 0.55, 0.92) and hip fractures (RH = 0.26; CI: 0.08, 0.83) compared with those with reductions less than 30%. The greater reductions in bone turnover with alendronate therapy are associated with fewer hip, nonspine, and vertebral fractures.

24. **Rosen CJ, Hochberg M, Bonnick S,** et al. Treatment with once-weekly alendronate 70 mg compared with once-weekly risedronate 35 mg in women with postmenopausal osteoporosis: A randomized, double-blind study. J Bone Miner Res 2005; 20:141–151.

    A double-blind, randomized control trial analyzed a total of 1,053 postmenopausal women with low bone mineral density (BMD) from 78 U.S. sites. The subjects were randomized to OW alendronate 70 mg ($n = 520$) or risedronate 35 mg ($n = 533$). Significantly greater increases in hip trochanter BMD were seen with alendronate (3.4%) than risedronate (2.1%) at 12 months (difference, 1.4%; $p < 0.001$) as well as 6 months (difference, 1.3%; $p < 0.001$). Significantly greater gains in BMD were seen with alendronate at all BMD sites measured (1 year difference: total hip, 1.0%; femoral neck, 0.7%; LS, 1.2%). Changes in BMD were seen starting at 6 months of treatment. A greater percentage of patients had greater than or equal to 0% ($p < 0.001$) and greater than or equal to 3% ($p < 0.01$) gain in trochanter and spine BMD at 12 months with alendronate than risedronate. Significantly greater ($p < 0.001$) reductions in all biochemical markers of bone turnover occurred with alendronate, compared with risedronate by 3 months. There were no differences between treatment with side effects or number of subjects who discontinued therapy. In as early as 3 months of therapy, alendronate produced greater gains in BMD and greater reductions in markers of bone turnover than risedronate.

25. **McClung M, San Martin J, Miller PD,** et al. Teriparatide and alendronate increase bone mass by opposite effects on bone remodeling. Arch Intern Med 2005;165: 1762–1768.

    In this randomized double-blind study, women with osteoporosis were assessed to determine the effects of daily doses of 20 µg of teriparatide and 10 mg of alendronate sodium on bone mineral density (BMD) and markers of bone turnover; 203 subjects were monitored for 18 months. Teriparatide significantly increased markers of bone turnover (serum procollagen type I N-terminal propeptide, 218%, and urinary N-telopeptide corrected for creatinine, 58%; $p < 0.001$); this increase peaked at 6 months of treatment. However, alendronate significantly decreased the markers at 6 months (-67% and -72%, respectively; $p < 0.001$). At the endpoint of 18 months, areal and volumetric spine BMDs were significantly higher in the teriparatide group than with alendronate [10.3% vs. 5.5% ($p < 0.001$) and 19.0% vs. 3.8% ($p < 0.01$), respectively]. Femoral neck BMD was significantly higher than baseline in both groups (3.9% and 3.5%, respectively). No significant differences were found in trabecular femoral neck BMD between the teriparatide and alendronate groups (4.9% and 2.2%, respectively). Cortical volumetric femoral neck BMD was significantly different between the teriparatide and alendronate groups (-1.2% and 7.7%, respectively; $p = 0.05$). These different options for the management of osteoporosis increase BMD through opposite mechanisms of action on bone remodeling.

26. **Bonnick SL, Johnston CC Jr, Kleerekoper M,** et al. Importance of precision in bone density measurements. J Clin Densitom 2001;4:105–110.

    This review article examines the necessity of reproducible bone densitometry. The precision of each densitometry facility should be quantified with precision studies of the various skeletal sites. The precision, as the root-mean-square standard deviation or root-mean-square coefficient of variation, can determine the change in bone density that signifies the amount of significant change and the minimum interval between follow-up measurements. Without these precision studies, the least significant change cannot be determined for any level of statistical confidence, making the interpretation of serial studies impossible.

27. **Lenchick L, Leib ES, Hamdy RC,** et al. Executive summary International Society for Clinical Densitometry position development conference, Denver, Colorado, July 20 22, 2001. J Clin Densitom 2002;5(Suppl 1):S1–S3

In this summary of the International Society for Clinical Densitometry (ISCD), the controversy of interpretation of bone densitometry to assess skeletal strength is addressed, and the ISCD makes their recommendations on the management of these interpretations.

28. **Chapurlat RD, Palmero L, Ramsay P, Cummongs SR.** Risk of fracture among women who lose bone density during treatment with alendronate. The Fracture Intervention Trial. Osteoporos Int 2005;16:842–848.

In the Fracture Intervention Trial, a randomized double-blind control study, 6,459 women were assigned to treatment with alendronate or placebo and bone mineral density (BMD), and new spine fractures were analyzed as endpoints. In the group of women who took at least 70% of the study, drug, hip, and spine BMD were measured after 1 and 2 years of treatment and compared with reductions in risk of spine fractures at end of follow-up (3 or 4 years). Women in the alendronate group who "lost" BMD at the lumbar spine (0% to 4%) continued to have a reduction of 60% in vertebral fracture risk [OR = 0.40 (0.16, 0.99)] compared with placebo. However, those that lost more than 4% did not have a significant benefit [OR = 0.15 (0.02, 1.29)]. Those who "gained" BMD (0% to 4%) during treatment had a reduction in risk of 51% [OR = 0.49 (0.30, 0.78)]. Women on alendronate who "lost" total hip BMD (0% to 4%) had a 53% decreased risk of vertebral fracture compared with placebo [OR = 0.47 (0.27, 0.81)]; "gaining" BMD (0% to 4%) had a similar risk reduction [OR = 0.49 (0.34, 0.71)]. Again, women who lost more than 4% did not show benefit [OR = 0.61 (0.11, 3.45)]. When losing BMD at both the hip and spine, there was no protective benefit with alendronate. It appears, due to these conclusions, that the alendronate's reduction in bone turnover could be more important than BMD changes in predicting fracture risk reduction.

29. **Watts NB, Guesens P, Barton IP, Felsenberg D.** Relationship between changes in BMD and nonvertebral fracture incidence associated with risedronate: reduction in risk of nonvertebral fracture is not related to change in BMD. J Bone Miner Res 2005;20:2097–2104.

A post hoc analysis is utilized in this study, which combined data from three pivotal risedronate fracture endpoint trials. Risedronate 2.5 or 5 mg ($n = 2,561$) or placebo ($n = 1,418$) was given to women daily for up to 3 years. Bone mineral density (BMD) and nonvertebral fractures confirmed by radiograph (hip, wrist, pelvis, humerus, clavicle, and leg) were assessed independently. The incidence of nonvertebral fractures in risedronate-treated patients did not differ between patients whose spine BMD decreased (7.8%) and those whose spine BMD increased [6.4%; hazard ratio to subgroup of patients who lost BMD (HR), 0.79; 95% CI, 0.50, 1.25] or between those whose femoral neck BMD decreased (7.6%) and those whose femoral neck BMD increased (7.5%; HR, 0.93; 95% CI, 0.68, 1.28). Changes in lumbar spine and femoral neck BMD explained only 12% (95% CI, 2%, 21%; $p = 0.014$) and 7% (95% CI, 2%, 13%; $p = 0.005$), respectively, of risedronate's nonvertebral fracture efficacy. The degree of risk reduction of nonvertebral fractures when treated with risedronate did not correlate with changes in BMD.

30. **Lewiecki EM.** Nonresponders to osteoporosis therapy. J Clin Densitom 2003;6: 307–314.

This review article investigates the necessity for testing fracture reduction in patients with osteoporosis, due to the silent nature of the disease. When using bone mineral density (BMD) as a measure of unresponsiveness to therapy, one definition of nonresponse could be as follows: A decrease in BMD greater than the least significant change at the 95% level of confidence. This least significant change relates to the standard of care. Other components for measuring responsiveness to therapy, such as biochemical markers of bone metabolism, are not as standardized or validated as BMD. Poor adherence, calcium and vitamin D deficiency, malabsorption, comorbidity, metabolic factors, wrong dose, wrong dosing interval, and lack of efficacy can all contribute to a nonresponse. Fracture risk reduction is associated with BMD increase or stability, and decreases in BMD could be associated with treatment failure. Patients who may require additional medical intervention or changes in management can be identified with this unresponsiveness criteria.

31. **Hodgson SF, Watts NB, Bilezikian JP, et al., for the AACE Osteoporosis Task Force.** American Association of Clinical Endocrinologists medical guidelines for clinical practice for the prevention and treatment of postmenopausal osteoporosis: 2001 edition, with selected updates for 2003. Endocr Pract 2003;9:544–564.

These guidelines produced by the American Association of Clinical Endocrinologists (AACE) in 2001 discuss the prevention, diagnosis, and management of postmenopausal osteoporosis. The goals of these guidelines are to help patients and physicians use the most effective and efficient methods of treatment and prevention to ensure the skeletal health and quality of life of patients with osteoporosis.

32. **Tannenbaum C, Clark J, Schwartzman K,** et al. Yield of laboratory testing to identify secondary contributors to osteoporosis in otherwise healthy women. J Clin Endocrinol Metab 2002;87:4431–4437.

This cross-sectional study examined useful and cost-efficient screening techniques for underlying pathology of bone and mineral metabolism in osteoporotic women. Six hundred sixty-four postmenopausal women with osteoporosis were identified. Previously undiagnosed disorders of bone and mineral metabolism were identified in 55 of 173 (32%) women who met the inclusion criteria. Hyperparathyroidism and calcium metabolism disorders were the most frequent diagnoses. Measurement of 24-hour urine calcium, serum calcium, and serum parathyroid hormone (PTH) for all women and serum thyroid-stimulating hormone (TSH) among women on thyroid replacement therapy would have diagnosed disorders in 47 of these 55 women (85%); an estimated cost of $75 per patient was associated with these tests. In healthy women with low bone density, there can be underlying disorders affecting skeleton stability.

33. **Leib E, Lewiecki M, Binkley N, Hamdy RC.** Official Positions of the International Society for Clinical Densitometry. J Clin Densitom 2004;7:1–6.

The International Society for Clinical Densitometry (ISCD) is a professional society that works to enhance the knowledge and quality of bone densitometry among healthcare professionals. In this position statement, the ISCD attempts to educate clinicians and technologists about new advances in bone densitometry. During the Position Development Conferences, the ISCD makes recommendations based on literature reviews on the techniques and methodology of bone densitometry. This paper discusses those recommendations.

34. **Binkley N, Bilezikian JP, Kendler DL,** et al. Official Positions of the International Society for Clinical Densitometry and Executive Summary of the 2005 Position Development. J Clin Densitom 2006;9:4–14.

This report describes the methodology of the 2005 Position Development Conference (PDC) for the International Society for Clinical Densitometry (ISCD). The ISCD convenes every two years to make recommendations on topics regarding bone densitometry. The expert panel includes representatives of the American Society for Bone and Mineral Research (ASBMR) and the International Osteoporosis Foundation (IOF). Topics discussed in the 2005 meeting included technical standardization, vertebral fracture assessment, and application of the 1994 World Health Organization (WHO) criteria to various skeletal sites and to populations other than postmenopausal white women. PDC presents a summary of all ISCD Official Positions in this paper.

35. **Misof BM, Roschger P, Cosman F,** et al. Effects of intermittent parathyroid hormone administration on bone mineralization density in iliac crest biopsies from patients with osteoporosis: a paired study before and after treatment. J Clin Endocrinol Metab 2003;88:1150–1156.

This study used quantitative backscattered electron imaging in men and women with osteoporosis who were treated for 18 to 36 months with parathyroid hormone (PTH) therapy. Bone mineral density was analyzed by bone biopsies. Comparison before and after treatment revealed a reduction in the typical calcium concentration in men ($-3.32\%; p = 0.02$, by paired t-test), but no change in women. The mineralization heterogeneity increased in both males and females [$+18.80\%$ ($p = 0.09$) and $+18.14\%$ ($p = 0.005$), respectively]. In cancellous bone, there was no change in the typical calcium concentration, but there was a greater heterogeneity of mineralization in both men and women [$+19.65\%$ ($p = 0.02$) and $+21.59\%$ ($p = 0.056$), respectively]. Small-angle x-ray scattering performed revealed normal collagen and mineral structure. The accepted ideal that PTH stimulates skeletal remodeling is supported by these data.

36. **Zanchetta JR, Bogado CE, Ferretti JL,** et al. Effects of teriparatide [recombinant human parathyroid hormone (1–34)] on cortical bone in postmenopausal women with osteoporosis. J Bone Miner Res 2003;18:539–543.

The following cross-sectional study analyzed cortical bone quality by peripheral quantitative computed tomography (pQCT) in the nondominant distal radius of 101 postmenopausal women with osteoporosis. The subjects were placed randomly in once-daily, self-administered subcutaneous injections of placebo ($n = 35$) or teriparatide 20 µg ($n = 38$) or 40 µg ($n = 28$). Bone circumferences, bone mineral content, bone area, and inertia data were collected. Subjects who received both 20 and 40 µg had higher bone mineral content, total and cortical bone areas, periosteal circumferences, and axial cross-sectional analysis than placebo; 40-µg treatment groups also had higher endocortical circumferences and axial moments of inertia than placebo. Total bone mineral density (BMD), cortical thickness, cortical bone mineral density, or cortical bone mineral content remained constant in all groups. Teriparatide induced beneficial changes in the structural architecture of bone without adverse effects on total bone mineral density or cortical bone mineral content.

37. **Miller PD, Bilezikian JP, Deal C,** et al. Clinical use of teriparatide in the real world: initial insights. Endocr Pract 2004;10:139–145.

This review article attempts to find acceptable clinical answers to questions regarding teriparatide therapy for osteoporosis in men and postmenopausal women.

38. **Hodsman AB, Bauer DC, Dempster D,** et al. Parathyroid hormone and teriparatide for the treatment of osteoporosis: A review of the evidence and suggested guidelines for its use. Endocr Rev 2005;10:2004–2006.

In a review of teriparatide as a new therapy for osteoporosis, several studies are discussed. In phase III trials, significant reductions in fracture rates have been demonstrated in women with at least one prevalent vertebral fracture before the onset of therapy. There has not been a cost–comparison analysis of teriparatide and bisphosphonate therapy with regard to efficacy and tolerance. In the subset of individuals on glucocorticoid therapy, teriparatide can be considered as an alternative for treatment. For high-risk subjects, including subjects who are younger than age 65 and who have particularly low bone mineral density (BMD) measurements (T-scores ≤3.5), teriparatide can also be used as an alternative. However, based on osteosarcoma studies in rat models, teriparatide therapy is not recommended for more than 2 years. Monitoring of serum calcium can be limited to measurement at 1 month of treatment; reducing the dosing frequency of PTH or withdrawing dietary calcium supplements can eliminate mild elevations in hypercalcemia.

39. **Chen P, Miller PD, Delmas PD, et al.** Change in lumbar spine BMD and vertebral fracture risk reduction in teriparatide-treated postmenopausal women with osteoporosis. J Bone Miner Res 2006;21:1785–1790.

5

Biochemical Evaluation

Pauline M. Camacho

Biochemical Tests, 63
Biochemical Markers of Bone Turnover, 67

Successful management of osteoporosis requires a careful choice of biochemical tests to determine the presence of secondary causes of osteoporosis. In addition, biochemical markers of bone turnover are increasingly used in the initial and follow-up evaluations of these patients. The arguments for and against using bone turnover markers will be discussed in this chapter.

BIOCHEMICAL TESTS

Complete Blood Count

Complete blood count (CBC) tests can detect anemia, which can be seen in many secondary causes of osteoporosis; these include celiac sprue and other malabsorptive states, chronic liver disease, chronic kidney failure, metastatic bone disease, and multiple myeloma.

Estimation of Kidney Function Using Serum Creatinine, Estimated Glomerular Filtration Rate, or 24-Hour Urine Creatinine Clearance

To ensure that occult renal insufficiency is detected among elderly patients, calculation of glomerular filtration rate (GFR) must be done (www.nephron.com; Table 5.1). Renal insufficiency often leads to a deficiency in 1–25 OH vitamin D deficiency and secondary hyperparathyroidism, which must be addressed prior to initiation of osteoporosis therapy. Kidney Disease Outcomes Quality Initiative or KDOQI guidelines (Table 5.2) outline parathyroid hormone (PTH) goals for various levels of renal dysfunction. Furthermore, bisphosphonates are contraindicated when GFR falls below 30 mg/24 hours. However, Miller reported the risedronate could be safely used even among those with GFR below this cut-off. In a post hoc review of the Vertebral Efficacy with Risedronate Therapy (VERT) data, adverse events and renal function related side effects were not different between risedronate and placebo, regardless of renal function [1]. Bisphosphonates are not FDA approved for patients with advanced renal disease.

TABLE 5.1. Formulas used in biochemical evaluation

Corrected Calcium

Corrected calcium (mg/dL) = total calcium (mg/dL) + 0.8 (4 − albumin in g/dL)

GFR Estimate by MDRD Formula

eGFR (mL/min/1.73 m^2) = 186 × [serum creatinine (μmol/L) × 0.0113]$^{-1.154}$ × age (y)$^{-0.203}$ (× 0.742 if female)[a]

Calculated Creatinine Clearance (Cockcroft and Gault) with Lean Body Mass Estimated from Patient Height

Creatinine clearance (mL/s) = (140 − age [y]) × (weight [kg] × F[b])/(plasma creatinine [μmol/L] × 48.816)

Fractional Excretion of Calcium

FECa = (urinary calcium × serum creatinine) / (urinary creatinine × serum calcium)

GFR, glomerular filtration rate; MDRD, Modification of Diet in Renal Disease Study Group.
[a]Automatic calculator available in www.nephron.com.
[b]F = 1 (males) or 0.85 (females).

Liver Function Tests
An alanine aminotransferase (ALT) test is the most cost-effective way to screen for liver disease among osteoporotic patients. Elevated ALT levels suggest liver dysfunction, which, regardless of the cause, increases the risk of vitamin D deficiency.

Serum Total or Ionized Calcium
Patients with low albumin levels will have falsely low serum calcium concentrations. Correction of serum calcium level must be done when patients have low or high albumin concentrations (Table 5.1). This formula, however, sometimes leads to incorrect results, and it is more reliable to order an ionized calcium for confirmation. A small proportion of patients with mild primary hyperparathyroidism may have normal corrected calcium and mildly elevated ionized calcium.

TABLE 5.2. Parathyroid hormone goals based on stage of chronic kidney disease

CKD Stage	GFR Range (mL/min/1.73 m^2)	Target Intact PTH (pg/mL)
3	30–59	35–70 (3.85–7.7 pmol/L)
4	15–29	70–110 (7.7–12.1 pmol/L)
5	<15 or dialysis	150–300 (16.5–33.0 pmol/L)

PTH, parathyroid hormone; CKD, chronic kidney disease; GFR, glomerular filtration rate.

It must be noted, however, that vitamin D and calcium deficiency usually leads to hypocalcemia only when the deficiency is severe. Hypocalciuria (to be discussed in this chapter) occurs sooner and is by far more common among those with mild to moderate deficiencies.

Serum Phosphorus

Phosphorus is an essential component of bone formation, as calcium phosphate is the primary substance in bone. Serum phosphorus must be part of the initial evaluation of osteoporotic patients or patients with low bone mass. The more common causes of low phosphorus concentrations include vitamin D deficiency, primary hyperparathyroidism, hypophosphatemic rickets, and nutritional deficiency (rare). Hyperphosphatemia is seen in chronic renal failure and hypoparathyroidism, and is one of the biochemical findings in hypophosphatasia.

25-Hydroxy Vitamin D

Vitamin D deficiency is very common among patients with low bone mass and osteoporosis, with recent reports of 30% to 50% prevalence [2–4]. As the storage form of vitamin D in the body, 25-OHD provides the most accurate assessment of vitamin D reserve. Measurement of 1–25-OHD can be misleading, since the levels may be high or high-normal in early stages of vitamin D deficiency due to upregulation of 1α hydroxylation by PTH.

In the past years, assay variabilities have led to some confusion about the correct interpretation of 25-OHD, with some reference labs reporting normal levels as low as 10 ng/mL. Studies have shown that when 25-OHD levels fall below 30 ng/mL, PTH levels start to rise, suggesting that 30 ng/mL differentiates an insufficient from a vitamin D–replete state [5,6]. Those with levels below 15 ng/mL to 20 ng/mL are frankly deficient. Some patients with this level or lower may even have osteomalacia, and this needs to be established prior to initiation of osteoporosis therapy.

It is not uncommon to see 25-OHD levels between 20 ng/mL and 30 ng/mL without concomitant secondary hyperparathyroidism. It is recommended that these levels be addressed, regardless of the presence or absence of secondary hyperparathyroidism, and for optimum bone health, one must aim to keep these levels at or above 30 ng/mL.

It is important to note that in patients with primary hyperparathyroidism, PTH increases 1α hydroxylase activity, which could lead to low 25-OHD and high-normal 1–25-OHD levels. However, concurrent vitamin D deficiency may be found among patients with primary hyperparathyroidism [7], but there is no consensus as to whether low 25-OHD states should be treated prior to parathyroidectomy, as hypercalcemia may worsen. The author recommends repeating the 25-OHD 6 to 8 weeks after parathyroidectomy to establish the patient's new levels. If patients are not candidates for surgery, careful replacement can be undertaken, with frequent monitoring of serum and urinary calcium levels to ensure that hypercalcemia and hypercalciuria do not worsen.

Intact Parathyroid Hormone

Intact parathyroid hormone levels are essential in the initial work-up of patients with osteoporosis. An elevation could suggest primary hyperparathyroidism, secondary hyperparathyroidism from deficiencies in calcium or vitamin D or renal insufficiency, and very rarely pseudohypoparathyroidism. An increasing number of patients are also being found to have normocalcemic hyperparathyroidism, that is, elevated PTH with no apparent deficiencies in calcium or vitamin D. These patients likely have very early mild primary hyperparathyroidism.

Recently, a new bio-intact PTH assay has become available that measures the whole PTH molecule and is not affected by fragments that build up during renal failure or insufficiency. The exact utility of the assay is not yet clearly established for osteoporosis patients but can be helpful among renal patients.

24-Hour Urine Calcium and Creatinine

The value of the 24-hour urine calcium and creatinine test tends to be underestimated in the work-up of osteoporosis. First and foremost, in order to ensure complete collection, it is important that patients are given detailed instructions and be made aware of the importance of the test. When urine is properly collected, urinary calcium excretion provides valuable information that can increase one's success in treating osteoporosis. The normal range quoted in the literature varies. In general, 1.5 to 3 mg/kg/24 hours provides a good estimate of normal urinary calcium excretion [8]. Most calcium and vitamin D–replete adults would fall between the levels of 150 mg and 300 mg/24 hours. Those who have values between 100 mg and 150 mg usually have mild degrees of calcium and vitamin D deficiency, which may be corrected by increasing elemental calcium intake to 1,200 to 1,500 mg/day and 800 IU of vitamin D per day. A level below 100 mg/24 hours is considered low.

Differentials for hypocalciuria include malabsorptive states such as celiac sprue, nutritional vitamin D and calcium deficiency, renal insufficiency, use of thiazide diuretics, and benign familial hypocalciuric hypercalcemia. Some individuals who have celiac sprue may have hypocalciuria with normal 25-OHD levels. This is usually associated with secondary elevation in PTH. Individuals who are found to be hypocalciuric should have their celiac antibodies tested, and if negative, duodenal biopsy should be done, because there are seronegative celiac patients [9,10]. Other malabsorptive disorders, such as inflammatory bowel disease (IBD), and bacterial overgrowth should be considered when work-up for celiac disease is negative.

On the opposite end of the spectrum, hypercalciuria (>300 mg/24 hours) may be due to aggressive calcium supplementation, vitamin D toxicity, use of loop diuretics, primary hyperparathyroidism, or idiopathic hypercalciuria. The first two conditions can usually be differentiated from the last based on the PTH levels. PTH is usually low-normal or suppressed when there is excess of calcium and vitamin D supplementation, whereas PTH is usually normal among patients with idiopathic hypercalciuria.

Celiac Antibodies

When malabsorption is suspected, celiac antibodies should be obtained. A panel consisting of transglutaminase antibodies, anti-gliadin, or anti-endomysial antibodies may detect the presence of celiac disease. Given biochemical findings suggestive of malabsorption, positive antibody testing may not require a duodenal biopsy before the necessary intervention. These levels can be falsely low when patients are already on a gluten-free diet.

A significant proportion of patients with celiac disease are sero-negative, and relying on positive celiac antibodies may lead to underdiagnosis [9,10]. These individuals should be referred to a gastroenterologist for a duodenal biopsy and evaluation for other malabsorptive conditions. Sero-negative patients often have milder disease and partial rather than complete villous atrophy.

Thyroid-stimulating Hormone

Hyperthyroidism and subclinical hyperthyroidism have both been shown to cause accelerated bone resorption [11–16]. Since most osteoporotic patients are elderly, the incidence of asymptomatic or apathetic hyperthyroidism is much higher. Clinical signs and symptoms will not suffice in ruling out hyperthyroidism, and thus, it is important to obtain a thyroid-stimulating hormone (TSH) level.

Serum Protein Electrophoresis and Urine Protein Electrophoresis

These should be ordered when dealing with male osteoporosis, or when bone loss in a woman appears to be advanced or inappropriate for her age. Although multiple myeloma has other clinical features, its initial presentation can also be solely as low bone mass.

Free Testosterone Panel

Males with osteoporosis are more likely to have secondary causes of bone loss than women. One of the most common causes is hypogonadism, which may present asymptomatically. Free testosterone panel [includes total, sex hormone globulin (SHBG), free and weakly bound testosterone] at 8:00 a.m. provides an accurate screen for hypogonadism among males. If levels are low, luteinizing hormone (LH) and/or follicle-stimulating hormone (FSH) levels must be obtained to determine the etiology.

Screening for Cushing Syndrome or Disease

One must be vigilant for mild cases or subclinical Cushing disease, which could lead to bone loss and yet have very subtle clinical findings [17]. When clinically indicated, screening for Cushing disease should be done with a 24-hour urine free cortisol and creatinine

BIOCHEMICAL MARKERS OF BONE TURNOVER

Although there has been controversy regarding the use of bone markers in the routine management of osteoporosis, they are now gaining acceptance for reasons discussed as follows.

TABLE 5.3.   Currently available bone biochemical markers

Bone Formation Markers

Serum
  Bone-specific alkaline phosphatase (BSAP)
  Osteocalcin (OC)
  Carboxyterminal propeptide of type I collagen (PICP)
  Aminoterminal propeptide of type I collagen (PINP)

Bone Resorption Markers

Urine
  Free and total pyridinolines (Pyd)
  Free and total deoxypyridinolines (Dpd)
  N-telopeptide of collagen cross-links (NTX)
  C-telopeptide of collagen cross-links (CTx)

Serum
  Cross-linked C-telopeptide of type I collagen (ICTP)
  Tartrate-resistant acid phosphatase 5b (TRACP5b)

From **Camacho P, Kleerekoper M.** Biochemical markers of bone turnover. In Favus M, ed.
Primer on the metabolic bone diseases and disorders of mineral metabolism, 6th ed. Washington,
DC: American Society for Bone and Mineral Research, 2006, with permission.

Bone is in a constant state of turnover, with formation and resorption occurring simultaneously. There are two major kinds of bone turnover biochemical markers (BTMs): those that measure the rate of bone formation
and those that measure bone resorption (Table 5.3). These dynamic measurements complement the static measurement provided by BMD in assessing and predicting fracture risk.

Utility of Bone Turnover Biochemical Markers in the Management of Osteoporosis

Monitoring Effectiveness of Therapy

The increases in bone density that may be seen within a few years of osteoporosis therapy are very small. These range from 2% to 5% when bisphosphonates are given [18–20] and are a bit more robust (9%) when teriparatide is used [20]. Two metaanalyses highlighted the small contribution of
bone mineral density (BMD) to fracture risk reduction (Chapter 4) [22,23].
In fact, for monitoring treatment, bone densitometry is more commonly utilized to look for stability rather than for significant increases in BMD.

Therefore, with bone quality changes accounting for the rest of fracture
risk reduction, it is important that we are able to quantify this. Currently,
the only clinically available determination of bone quality is the measurement of bone turnover markers.

Medicare allows BMD testing only once every 2 years, and in select situations, once a year. This can be quite frustrating for both the patient and the

physician. Most patients rely on a demonstrable result after therapy. With the use of bone markers, it is possible to detect significant changes within weeks for bone resorption markers and months for bone resorption markers [24,25]. With antiresorptive agents, a decline of anywhere from 20% to 80% has been reported [18,20,25–28], whereas the anabolic agent teriparatide can increase the bone formation marker, osteocalcin, by about 30% to 50% within 3 to 6 months of therapy [21]. This immediate feedback is not only emotionally rewarding for the patients, but it gives clinicians a clue when patients are not taking their medications.

Predicting Fracture Risk Reduction
BMD is indeed strongly correlated with fracture risk and is a strong predictor of fracture risk. However, as stated earlier, after therapy is initiated, BMD changes that can be seen are minimal. In a metaanalysis, it was shown that greater declines in markers of bone resorption after initiation of antiresorptive therapy are associated with greater reductions in fracture risk in nonvertebral sites [23]. Thus, it is possible to predict a reduction in fracture risk in response to therapy within months of initiation of treatment.

Determining Baseline Fracture Risk
Assessment of fracture risk of individual patients has moved away from considering BMD alone. It has been increasingly recognized that the same BMD in two individuals can signify very different fracture risks. Several studies have shown that baseline BTMs are independent predictors of fracture risk [29,30]. In a French study, high markers of bone resorption were associated with higher hip fracture risk, even after they were adjusted for BMD. Clearly, a negative association exists between high BTMs, low BMD, and the presence of osteoporosis [29].

Prediction of Bone Loss After Menopause
Rates of bone loss after menopause can be extremely variable. Whereas some women lose an average of 2% to 4% per year in the first 5 to 6 years of menopause, there are those whose bone mass remains steady for a few years. Baseline BMD determination alone will not predict who will lose bone faster. At least two studies [31,32] have documented the predictive ability of BTMs for postmenopausal bone loss. Garnero's study [31] showed that higher baseline levels of bone formation (serum osteocalcin and serum type I collagen N-terminal propeptide) and bone resorption markers (urinary N-telopeptides, urinary and serum C-telopeptides) were significantly associated with faster rates of postmenopausal bone loss ($r = -0.19$ to 0.30, $p < 0.001$). This effect was independent of age. The group of women with normal BTMs lost less than 1% BMD, whereas the group that had elevated BTMs lost 3 to 5 times the amount of bone.

Limitation of Bone Turnover Biochemical Markers
It is important to know that measurement of BTMs has inherent limitations. BTMs have a circadian rhythm, with peaks between 4:00 and 8:00 a.m., and nadirs in the late afternoon. However, reference ranges provided by most labs are adjusted and standardized for this circadian variation.

Urinary collections can be done either as second-void urine in the a.m. or as a 24-hour urine collection. Some experts even suggest doing a 3-day collection of second-void urine to improve result reproducibility, but we routinely do urinary N-telopeptide of collagen cross-links (NTX) on the same collection as the 24-hour urine calcium and creatinine.

Perhaps the most important limitation is the large precision error, which determines the least significant change (LSC) of the test. Whereas BMD has an LSC of around 3% to 4%, depending on which site is measured, the LSC of BTMs for urine markers can be as high as 30% to 40% [33]. The LSC of serum BTMs is much less. Bisphosphonates can decrease markers of bone resorption by as much as 50% to 60%, and given this high an expected change, it would be acceptable to use a test that has such a high LSC.

Selection of Biochemical Tests

To do all of the biochemical tests described here would be extremely expensive for the healthcare system. Thus, it is important that the clinician is able to stratify who will get which tests and the extent of testing for secondary causes. In general, the prevalence of vitamin D deficiency is so high that every patient with low bone mass should be screened for this condition. 25-OHD is the ideal screen, and it is usually helpful to have an intact PTH when the results are abnormal. Clinical history and bone density results can be used to guide clinicians in assessing the "age-appropriateness" of bone loss and subsequent metabolic bone work-up. A younger premenopausal or recently menopausal woman who has already suffered from fractures deserves comprehensive evaluation. Certain clinical data, such as very low body weight, intolerance to gluten, history of kidney stones, finding limbic calcifications, suggest secondary causes and thus would deserve a very thorough work-up. In our practice, Z-scores have effectively guided us in determining the extent of osteoporosis work-up and in predicting which individuals will have secondary causes of bone loss. We have found that secondary causes of bone loss are highly likely when the Z-scores are less than -1 [34]. However, individuals with milder degrees of vitamin D deficiency (25-OHD levels of 25–30 ng/mL) or mild primary hyperparathyroidism will generally have Z-scores that are higher than -1.

REFERENCES
Annotations by Alexandra Reiher

1. **Miller PD, Roux C, Boonen S**, et al. Safety and efficacy of risedronate in patients with age-related reduced renal function as estimated by the Cockcroft and Gault method: A pooled analysis of nine clinical trials. J Bone Miner Res 2005;20:2105–2115. This retrospective analysis combined data from nine randomized, double-blind, placebo-controlled phase III trials and studied women with osteoporosis and how renal function influences the efficacy and safety of risedronate. The patients in the trials had no strikingly abnormal laboratory values that were considered clinically significant or evidence of significant disease. Forty-five hundred women received placebo and 4,496 women received 5 mg risedronate for up to 3 years (average length of exposure was 2 years), and the enrolled women had creatinine clearances (CrCl) of less than 80 mL/min. Renal impairment was categorized as mild (CrCl ≥50 to <80 mL/min), moderate (CrCl ≥30 to <50 mL/min), or severe (CrCl <30 mL/min). The Cockcroft-Gault method was used to measure creatinine clearance, which is based on age, weight, and serum creatinine. At baseline, 48% had mild

renal impairment (mean creatinine 0.9 mg/dL, range 0.4–1.6 mg/dL), 45% had moderate impairment (mean creatinine 1.1 mg/dL, range 0.6–0.9 mg/dL), and 7% had severe renal impairment (mean creatinine 1.3 mg/dL, range 0.7–2.7 mg/dL). The patients with the most severe renal impairment had more severe osteoporosis and were older in both the placebo and risedronate groups. The incidence of overall adverse events was similar in the placebo and treatment groups regardless of renal function. No differences in changes from baseline serum creatinine at any point in time were observed between the placebo and risedronate groups. In both the placebo and risedronate group, risedronate was found to effectively maintain bone mineral density (BMD) and decrease the incidence of vertebral fractures.

2. **Gloth FM III, Gundberg CM, Hollis BW,** et al. Vitamin D deficiency in home-bound elderly persons. JAMA 1995;274:1683–1686.

A cohort analytic study examined 244 subjects at least 65 years old, with 116 (85 women and 31 men) having been confined indoors for at least 6 months, either in a teaching nursing home or a private residence in the community, and 128 control subjects. The control subjects came from the Baltimore Longitudinal Study on Aging and were free of diseases or medications that could interfere with their vitamin D status. All subjects had serum levels of 1,25-dihydroxyvitamin D [1,25-(OH)2D] and 25-hydroxyvitamin D (25-OHD) measured, and serum levels of intact PTH, ionized calcium, osteocalcin, and vitamin D intake (through 3-day food diaries) were measured in a subgroup of 80 subjects. Also, a randomly selected cohort of sunlight-deprived subjects had serum levels of vitamin D–binding protein measured. In sunlight-deprived subjects overall, the mean 25-OHD level was 30 nmol/L (12 ng/mL) and the mean 1,25-(OH)D level was 52 pmol/L (20 pg/mL). In the sunlight-deprived individuals, serum levels of 25-OHD were below 25 nmol/L (10 ng/mL) in 38% of the nursing home residents and 54% of the community residents. When 25-OHD [log (25-OHD)] and PTH were analyzed together, a significant inverse relationship existed ($r = -0.42$, $r^2 = 0.18$, $p < 0.001$). For all other parameters examined, except ionized calcium, there were significant differences from the control group means. The mean (SD) daily intakes of vitamin D [121 (312) IU] and calcium [583 (3,222) mg] were below the recommended daily allowance in the community-dwelling homebound group only. For the subgroup of sunlight-deprived individuals, the mean vitamin D–binding protein level was within the normal range.

3. **Looker AC, Gunter EW.** Hypovitaminosis D in medical inpatients. N Engl J Med 1998;339:344–345; author reply 5–6.

In this correspondence, the authors state that it is difficult to compare the mean serum 25-OHD levels of the medical patients from the Thomas and Lloyd-Jones article (57% had serum 25-OHD levels ≤15 ng/mL) with the healthy patients studied in the National Health and Nutrition Examination Survey (NHANES) III. Among NHANES III patients, 9% had serum 25-OHD levels less than or equal to 15 ng/mL, less than 1% had levels greater than 8 ng/mL, and 5% had values greater than 50 ng/mL. The prevalence of vitamin D deficiency between the Boston patients and the NHANES patients likely differed in factors beyond being hospitalized, such as diet, sun exposure, age, altitude and skin pigmentation, and illness.

Questions were also raised about the difficulties in establishing a normal range for serum 25-OHD, and authors agree that using a 95% confidence interval is a flawed approach. The authors state that using parathyroid hormone (PTH) levels as a surrogate for 25-OHD levels would also be misleading because some patients with secondary hyperparathyroidism can have normal vitamin D stores when calcium intake is restricted, and others may have normal PTH levels with low vitamin D stores, such as in patients with a rapid loss of calcium from their skeletons or in patients with a high calcium intake. The authors suggest the lower limit of normal for serum 25-OHD be defined as the concentration at which the mean serum PTH concentrations begin to rise in population studies. Another proposed approach was to determine the minimal serum 5-OHD levels at which serum PTH levels no longer decrease when vitamin D and calcium are given.

4. **Zadshir A, Tareen N, Pan D,** et al. The prevalence of hypovitaminosis D among US adults: data from the NHANES III. Ethn Dis 2005;15(4 Suppl 5):S5–97–S5–101.

Data from the National Health and Nutrition Examination Survey (NHANES III) were used in this study to analyze the serum levels of 25(OH)D3 (nmol/L) among 15,390 adult participants 18 years old or older, with racial and ethnic grouping by self-identification as white, black or African American, and Hispanic. Mean levels of 25(OH)D3 were lower among the elderly (≥65 years old vs. 40–59 and 18–39) than younger participants, and were lower among females than males (71.1 vs. 78.7, $p = 0.003$). White men and women (83.0 and 76.0) had higher mean levels of vitamin D than did black men and women (52.2 and 45.3, $p = 0.0001$) and Hispanic men and women (68.3 and 56.7, $p < 0.0001$), respectively. Mild to moderate and severe deficiency of vitamin D was more prevalent among women ($p < 0.0001$) and minorities ($p < 0.0001$). Among white men, 34% were found to have low vitamin D levels.

5. **Chapuy MC, Preziosi P, Maamer M,** et al. Prevalence of vitamin D insufficiency in an adult normal population. Osteoporos Int 1997;7:439–443.

This French study evaluated vitamin D levels in 1,569 healthy, urban, French individuals between November and April from 20 French cities in nine geographical regions. 25(OH)D levels differed between regions, with the lowest concentrations in the north and the greatest values in the south, with a significant "sun" effect ($r = 0.72; p = 0.03$) and latitude effect ($r = -0.79, p = 0.01$). The 25(OH)D levels measured in the winter were less than or equal to 30 mmol/L (12 ng/mL) in 14% of the subjects, representing the lower limit (<2 SD) for a normal adult population measured in winter with the same method [radioimmunoassay (RIA) (Incstar)]. A significant negative correlation was found between serum intact parathyroid hormone (iPTH) and serum 25(OH)D concentrations ($p < 0.01$). Serum iPTH levels remained stable at 36 pg/mL when the serum 25(OH)D values were greater than 78 nmol/L (31 ng/mL), but did increase when the serum 25(OH)D levels fell below 78 nmol/L. The parathyroid hormone (PTH) values reached the upper limit of normal (55 pg/mL) in vitamin D–replete patients when the 25(OH)D levels became 11.3 nmol/L or less (4.6 ng/mL).

6. **Camacho P, Girgis M, Sapountzi P, Sinacore J.** Correlations between vitamin D, parathyroid hormone, urinary calcium excretion, markers of bone turnover and bone density of patients referred to an osteoporosis center. J Bone Miner Res 2005;20:S1–S389.

The primary aim of the study was to characterize the relationships between 25-OHD, 1–25-OHD, intact parathyroid hormone (PTH), ionized calcium, phosphorus, 24-hour urine calcium (UrCa) excretion, bone-specific alkaline phosphatase (BSAP), urinary N-telopeptide of collagen cross-links (NTX) and creatinine, and bone density. One hundred sixty-three patients (143 female, 20 male; mean age 62.5 years) evaluated for low bone mass at Loyola University Osteoporosis and Metabolic Bone Disease Center were studied. The strongest indirect relationship seen was between PTH and UrCa ($r = -0.496$, $p < 0.001$). 25-OHD showed a significant correlation with UrCa ($r = 0.420, p < 0.001$), PTH ($r = -0.215, p = 0.014$), BSAP ($r = -0.288, p = 0.010$), and a trend with spine bone mineral density (BMD) ($r = -0.156, p = 0.071$). Analysis of the subgroup with 25-OHD less than or equal to 20 ng/mL (26% of the group) showed that 25-OHD correlated significantly with PTH ($r = -0.354, p = 0.027$). The strong indirect correlation between PTH and UrCa ($r = -0.540, p = 0.021$) remained in this group. 1,25-OHD showed a trend associated with UrCa ($r = 0.459, p = 0.064$) and spine BMD ($r = -0.356, p = 0.069$). Ionized calcium, phosphorus, or NTX/creatinine did not show significant correlations with PTH or vitamin D levels. The difference between the means of PTH above and below a 25-OHD level of 30 ng/mL was significant. At 35 ng/mL, the significance was lost. The same 25-OHD level of 30 ng/mL showed significant differences in the UrCa of patients with 25-OHD above and below this threshold. This relationship was also significant at 35 ng/mL and was lost at 40 ng/mL. A level of 30 ng/mL was concluded as the cut-off of vitamin D deficiency. This was seen in 48% of the population.

7. **Silverberg SJ, Shane E, Dempster DW, Bilezikian JP.** The effects of vitamin D insufficiency in patients with primary hyperparathyroidism. Am J Med 1999;107: 561–567.

Patients ($n = 124$) with mild primary hyperparathyroidism in the United States were studied to compare biochemical, bone mineral density (BMD), and bone histomorphometric indices among patients with serum 25-OHD levels in the lowest and highest tertiles. Serum 25-OHD levels (mean ± SD) were in the low range of normal (21 ± 11 ng/mL, normal 9–52 ng/mL), with 7% (9) of patients having levels below normal and 53% (66) of patients having levels below what is suggested for vitamin D "sufficiency" (20 ng/mL). Patients with the lowest levels of 25-OHD had the highest parathyroid hormone (PTH) levels (low tertile 158 ± 66 ng/mL vs. high tertile 103 ± 2 ng/mL, $p < 0.0001$). Increased hyperparathyroidism activity in patients with low 25-OHD levels was also suggested by lower serum phosphorus levels (2.7 ± 0.4 mg/dL vs. 3.0 ± 0.4 mg/dL, $p < 0.01$), higher serum alkaline phosphatase activity (114 $\pm$ 48 U/L vs. 91 $\pm$ 35 U/L, $p < 0.03$), greater BMD at the lumbar spine (0.94 $\pm$ 0.03 g/cm^2 vs. 0.83 $\pm$ 0.03 g/cm^2, $p < 0.05$), and enhanced bone turnover on bone biopsy. No differences in vitamin D metabolism were observed between races.

8. **Painter S, Camacho P.** Metabolic bone disorders. In: Camacho P, Gharib H, Sizemore G, eds. Evidence based endocrinology, 2nd ed. Philadelphia: Lippincott Williams & Wilkins; 2006.

9. **Abrams JA, Diamond B, Rotterdam H, Green PH.** Seronegative celiac disease: increased prevalence with lesser degrees of villous atrophy. Dig Dis Sci 2004;49: 546–550.

Adults with biopsy-proven celiac disease who fulfilled strict criteria, including serologic tests at the time of diagnosis and a response to a gluten-free diet, were evaluated to determine the sensitivities of serologic testing. Of 115 patients, 71% had total villous atrophy (TVA) and 29% had partial villous atrophy (PVA). Seventy-seven percent of the TVA patients had positive endomysial antibody, while only 33% of the PVA patients were positive for the antibody ($p < 0.001$). When the type of presentation (classic vs. silent) was compared, no difference in sensitivity was observed. All antitissue transglutaminase-positive patients had TVA on biopsy. Endomysial antibody-positive and -negative patients lacked differences with respect to age at diagnosis, mode of presentation, duration of symptoms, or a family history of celiac disease.

10. **Dickey W, Hughes DF, McMillan SA.** Reliance on serum endomysial antibody testing underestimates the true prevalence of coeliac disease by one fifth. Scand J Gastroenterol 2000;35:181–183.

This study evaluated 89 patients without IgA deficiency that had biopsy-confirmed villous atrophy (VA) not primarily prompted by a positive IgA endomysial antibody (EmA) result. Serum EmA was assayed with indirect immunofluorescence, and VA was graded as partial, subtotal, or total (PVA, STVA, TVA). EmA for VA had a 78% (69 of 89) sensitivity and was similar for PVA (79%) and ST/TVA (77%). Four of the 20 EmA-negative patients had an increased serum IgA-class antigliadin antibody level measured by enzyme-linked immunosorbent assay. Clinical responses were observed in all seronegative patients who were compliant with a gluten-free diet, and histologic improvement was seen after 12 months in 67% (8 of 10) of patients who had follow-up biopsies.

11. **Jodar E, Martinez-Diaz-Guerra G, Azriel S, Hawkins F.** Bone mineral density in male patients with L-thyroxine suppressive therapy and Graves disease. Calcif Tissue Int 2001;69:84–87.

Forty-nine male patients (age 45 $\pm$ 12 years) were studied to evaluate bone mineral density (BMD), bone turnover markers (BTMs), and thyroid function in male patients who had been treated for thyroid cancer on long-term suppressive L-T4 thyroxine (TC) and in male patients with Graves disease (GD). Seventeen patients had TC [29–288 months on L-T4–suppressive therapy; free T4: 1.9 $\pm$ 0.6 ng/dL (normal $\leq$2.0); thyroid-stimulating hormone (TSH): 0.2 $\pm$ 0.3 μU/mL (normal 0.5–5.0] and 32 patients had recent onset GD [<12 weeks, free T4: 2.0 $\pm$ 1.4 ng/dL; TSH: 1.07 $\pm$ 1.8 μU/mL; TSHRAb 53 $\pm$ 45% (normal <15)]. BMD was measured by dual-energy x-ray absorptiometry (DXA, Hologic QDR1000w) at the lumbar spine (L2–L4, LS), femoral neck (FN), and Ward triangle (WT), and results were expressed as a Z-score. Bone markers measured included total alkaline phosphatase (ALP), osteocalcin (BGP), iPTH, serum phosphorus, and serum and 24-hour urine calcium. Age, weight, and body mass indices were comparable in both groups. Reduced axial BMD was observed in patients with TC and GD. No significant differences were found between the groups for BMD. Patients with GD had higher levels of the bone markers osteocalcin (BGP: 7.5 $\pm$ 3.7 vs. 4.6 $\pm$ 1.6; $p < 0.001$) and total ALP (ALP: 139 $\pm$ 76 vs. 88 $\pm$ 34, $p < 0.01$).

12. **Krakauer JC, Kleerekoper M.** Borderline-low serum thyrotropin level is correlated with increased fasting urinary hydroxyproline excretion. Arch Intern Med 1992;152:360–364.

This retrospective analysis examined 86 ambulatory patients with a limited range of diagnoses who had had thyrotropin and fasting urinary total hydroxyproline-creatinine excretion (THP-Cr) levels checked within $\pm$ 21 days. No correlation was found for thyrotropin and THP-Cr for the 47 patients with thyrotropin levels greater than 1.0 mU/L. Of the remaining 39 patients, 11 had suppressed thyrotropin levels (<0.1 mU/L) and had clearly increased levels for THP-Cr. Twenty-eight had borderline and low-normal thyrotropin levels ranging from 0.1 to 1.0 mU/L with a significantly negative correlation with THP-Cr. The THP-Cr was positively correlated with serum alkaline phosphatase levels.

13. **Kvetny J.** Subclinical hyperthyroidism in patients with nodular goiter represents a hypermetabolic state. Exp Clin Endocrinol Diabetes 2005;113:122–126.

The metabolic state was studied in 26 patients with nodular goiter, of which 13 had evidence of subclinical hyperthyroidism [SH; suppressed thyroid-stimulating hormone (TSH) values but free T4I and T3 levels within the normal reference range], and the remaining 13 were control subjects. Basal oxygen consumption (VO$_2$), bone mineral density (BMD), and the circadian variation of TSH were evaluated to determine metabolic state. Methimazole treatment was also used to lower thyroid hormone and allow for evaluation of the pituitary thyroid axis. Patients with SH were found to have significantly higher basal VO$_2$ and significantly lower BMD compared with control subjects. Also, the circadian variation of TSH in patients with SH showed an absent night surge when compared with normal individuals. VO$_2$ normalization and the re-establishment of the circadian variation of TSH occurred after restoring TSH by lowering thyroid hormone levels.

14. **Lalau JD, Sebert JL, Marie A,** et al. Effect of thyrotoxicosis and its treatment on mineral and bone metabolism. J Endocrinol Invest 1986;9:491–496.

Thirty-one hyperthyroid patients (HT) without evidence of clinical or radiographic bone disease were evaluated before and after treatment of hyperthyroidism for mineral metabolism and bone histomorphometric status. Their blood and urine biochemical values were compared with that obtained from age and sex-matched controls. Iliac bone biopsies were available from 12 untreated HT individuals, and from 6 of the 12 after treatment for analysis of trabecular bone. Mean plasma calcium was increased in HT, true hypercalcemia was found in one patient, and mean plasma iPTH was normal. Urine calcium excretion was strikingly increased, particularly in the fasting state. After treatment, biochemical markers decreased, except for continued elevated levels of serum alkaline phosphatase and increased levels in iPTH. Enhanced activities of bone formation and bone resorption were observed in the untreated group by a hyper-remodeling state. Bone mineralization was normal, and bone and mineral changes were related to serum thyroid hormone levels. Post-treatment, a continued increase was observed in the extent of formation surfaces.

15. **Lee WY, Oh KW, Rhee EJ,** et al. Relationship between subclinical thyroid dysfunction and femoral neck bone mineral density in women. Arch Med Res 2006;37:511–516.

Serum levels of thyroid-stimulating hormone (TSH), free T4, biochemical markers of bone turnover, and bone mineral density (BMD) at the lumbar and femoral neck by dual-energy x-ray absorptiometry (DXA) scan were measured in this study, which evaluated 413 women (mean age: 52.2 ± 6.6 years) with subclinical thyroid dysfunction. Both the subclinical hypothyroid and subclinical hyperthyroid groups had significantly reduced femoral neck BMD when compared with the euthyroid group (one-way ANOVA, $p < 0.001$; post hoc analysis, $p = 0.041$, $p = 0.033$). However, no differences were observed between the two groups for the lumbar spine BMD, serum alkaline phosphatase and calcium levels, urine deoxypyridinoline levels, or the urine calcium to creatinine ratio.

16. **Toh SH, Claunch BC, Brown PH.** Effect of hyperthyroidism and its treatment on bone mineral content. Arch Intern Med 1985;145:883–886.

A longitudinal prospective study using photon absorptiometry was performed to study the effects of hyperthyroidism and its treatment on bone mineral content (BMC). A significantly decreased baseline BMC was found in both young and older hyperthyroid patients compared with age- and sex-matched controls. A slight recovery of BMC in hyperthyroid individuals was observed at the 2-year interval after attaining a euthyroid state, but still with a BMC much lower than that in controls. Also, no significant restoration of BMC was found after the hyperthyroid patients had achieved a euthyroid state.

17. **Bardet S, Rohmer V, Boux de Casson F,** et al. Bone mineral density and biological markers of bone repair in patients with adrenal incidentaloma: Effect of subclinical hypercortisolism. Rev Med Interne 2002;23:508–517.

Thirty-five patients (13 men, 22 postmenopausal women, age 49–76 years) with unilateral adrenal incidentalomas were evaluated for bone mineral density (BMD) and metabolic markers of bone turnover in this study. Using dual-energy x-ray absorptiometry (DXA) scans to evaluate BMD, median values of lumbar and femoral T-score were 1.125 and – 0.920, respectively, with normal Z-score values (0.105 and 0.120, respectively). Low serum osteocalcin (BGP) levels occurred in 39% of individuals, 3% had low bone alkaline phosphatase (bALP) values, 16% had elevated urinary free deoxypyridinoline (D-Pyr)-creatinine levels, and 23% had increased urinary carboxy-telopeptide of bone type 1 collagen (CTX)-creatinine levels. A lower femoral T-score ($p < 0.02$) was found in patients who had both suppression of the contralateral adrenal on scintigraphy and an inadequate cortisol response to 1 mg dexamethasone (>50 nmol/L; $n = 14$), and also had, to a lesser extent, a lower femoral Z-score ($p = 0.11$) than other patients ($n = 21$). The first group had a greater proportion of increased values of CTX-creatinine (42% vs. 11%, $p = 0.08$) than in the second group. In terms of age, the two groups were similar, but the tumor size was larger ($p < 0.04$) and the plasma ACTH level was lower ($p < 0.02$) in patients with scintigraphic and endocrine abnormalities.

18. **Harris ST, Watts NB, Genant HK,** et al. Effects of risedronate treatment on vertebral and nonvertebral fractures in women with postmenopausal osteoporosis: A randomized controlled trial. Vertebral Efficacy With Risedronate Therapy (VERT) Study Group. JAMA 1999;282:1344–1352.

This randomized, double-blind, placebo-controlled trial enrolled 2,458 ambulatory postmenopausal women younger than 85 years with at least one vertebral fracture at baseline between December 1993 and January 1998 at 1 of 110 centers in North America. Subjects were randomly assigned to receive oral treatment for 3 years with placebo or risedronate (2.5 or 5 mg/day). All women received calcium (1,000 mg/day), and if baseline levels of 25-OHD were low, patients received vitamin D (cholecalciferol, up to 500 IU/day). New vertebral fracture incidence was detected by quantitative and semiquantitative assessments of radiographs, changes in baseline bone mineral density (BMD) were determined by dual-energy x-ray absorptiometry (DXA) scan, and the incidence of radiographically nonvertebral fractures was assessed to evaluate outcomes. The 2.5 mg/day risedronate arm was discontinued after 1 year; the 450 individuals in the placebo group and the 489 subjects in the risedronate group completed all 3 years of the trial. The cumulative incidence of new vertebral fractures was decreased by 41% (95% CI, 18%–58%) in the 5 mg/day risedronate group when compared with placebo over the 3 years (11.3% vs. 16.3%; $p = 0.003$). After the first year, a fracture reduction of 65% (95% CI, 38%–81%) was observed (2.4% vs. 6.4%, $p < 0.001$). There was a 39% reduction in cumulative incidence of nonvertebral fractures over 3 years (95% CI, 6%–61%) (5.2% vs. 8.4%, $p = 0.02$). BMD increased significantly compared with the placebo group at the femoral neck (1.6% vs. -1.2%), lumbar spine (5.4% vs. 1.1%), midshaft of radius (0.2% vs. -1.4%), and femoral trochanter (3.3% vs. -0.7%). Bone formation was histologically normal during risedronate treatment. The overall safety profile of risedronate was similar to that of the placebo, including gastrointestinal safety.

19. **Reginster J, Minne HW, Sorensen OH,** et al. Randomized trial of the effects of risedronate on vertebral fractures in women with established postmenopausal osteoporosis. Vertebral Efficacy with Risedronate Therapy (VERT) Study Group. Osteoporos Int 2000;11:83–91.

This randomized, double-blind, placebo-controlled trial investigated 1,226 postmenopausal women with evidence of two or more vertebral fractures. Subjects were assigned to receive placebo, 2.5 mg/day of risedronate, or 5 mg/day of risedronate. All women received 1,000 mg/day of elemental calcium and up to 500 IU/day of vitamin D if baseline vitamin D levels were low. The study was 3 years in duration, except the 2.5 mg group, which was discontinued by protocol amendment after 2 years. Vertebral fractures were analyzed yearly with lateral spinal radiographs, and bone mineral density (BMD) was measured at 6-month intervals using dual-energy x-ray absorptiometry (DXA) scans. The risk of new vertebral fractures was reduced by 49% over 3 years in the risedronate 5-mg group, compared with controls ($p < 0.001$). Within the first year, a significant reduction of 61% was observed ($p < 0.001$). The fracture reduction over 2 years was similar between both treatment arms of risedronate. Compared with controls, the risk of nonvertebral fractures was reduced by 33% ($p = 0.06$). BMD at the spine and hip was significantly increased within 6 months in the risedronate arm of the trial. Adverse events, including gastrointestinal side effects, were similar between the risedronate and control groups.

20. **Black DM, Cummings SR, Karpf DB,** et al. Randomised trial of effect of alendronate on risk of fracture in women with existing vertebral fractures. Fracture Intervention Trial Research Group. Lancet 1996;348:1535–1541.

    This randomized, double-blind, placebo-controlled trial investigated 2,027 women with at least one vertebral fracture at baseline, and randomly assigned subjects placebo (n = 1005) or alendronate (n = 1022) for 36 months. The alendronate dose was initially 5 mg daily, and was increased to 10 mg daily at 24 months. Baseline, 24-month, and 36-month lateral spine radiographs were performed, with new vertebral fractures as the primary end point (defined as a 20% or at least 4 mm decrease in one vertebral height). Nonspine clinical fractures were identified by radiographic reports, and new symptomatic vertebral fractures were based on self-report with radiographic confirmation. One or more new morphometric vertebral fractures occurred in 78 (8%) of women in the alendronate group compared with 145 (15%) in the placebo group [relative risk, 0.53 (95% CI, 0.41–0.68)]. Twenty-three (2.3%) alendronate patients and 50 (5.0%) in the placebo arm had clinically apparent vertebral fractures [relative hazard (RH), 0.45 (0.27–0.72)]. The main secondary endpoint was the risk of any clinical fracture any lower in the alendronate than in the placebo group [139 (13.6%) vs. 182 (18.2%)]; RH, 0.72 (0.58–0.90). Hip fracture and wrist fracture RHs were 0.49 (0.23–0.99) for the alendronate group and 0.52 (0.31–0.87) for the placebo group. No significant difference for adverse events, including upper-gastrointestinal disorders, was observed between the treatment and placebo group.

21. **Neer RM, Arnaud CD, Zanchetta JR,** et al. Effect of parathyroid hormone (1–34) on fractures and bone mineral density in postmenopausal women with osteoporosis. N Engl J Med 2001;344:1434–1441.

    Parathyroid hormone (1–34) (PTH), at doses of 20 or 40 µg subcutaneously daily, or placebo was randomly assigned to 1,637 postmenopausal women with prior vertebral fractures. Bone mineral density (BMD) was serially measured by dual-energy x-ray absorptiometry (DXA) scan, and vertebral radiographs were performed at baseline and at the end of the study (21 months was the mean duration of observation). Fourteen percent of women in the placebo group, 5% of women in the 20-µg arm, and 4% of women in the 40-µg arm developed new vertebral fractures; the relative risks of fracture in the 20- and 40-µg groups, as compared to placebo, were 0.35 and 0.31 (95% CI, 0.22–0.55 and 0.19–0.50). New nonvertebral fragility fractures occurred in 6% of patients in the placebo group and in 3% of patients in each PTH group [relative risk, 0.47 and 0.46, respectively (95% CI, 0.25–0.88 and 0.25–0.86)]. BMD increased in the 20-µg and 40-µg groups when compared with placebo by 9 and 13 more percentage points in the lumbar spine, and by 3 and 6 more percentage points in the femoral neck. BMD decreased at the shaft of the radius by more than 2 percentage points in the 40-µg group. Both PTH doses increased total-body bone mineral by 2 to 4 more percentage points than placebo. Minor side effects were observed with PTH, which included occasional nausea and headache.

22. **Wasnich RD, Miller PD.** Antifracture efficacy of antiresorptive agents are related to changes in bone density. J Clin Endocrinol Metab 2000;85:231–236.

    This metaanalysis examined the theoretical model that predicts how both short- and long-term antifracture efficacy of antiresorptive drugs will depend on the level that treatment can increase and maintain bone mineral density (BMD). Data from clinical trials of antiresorptive agents were evaluated, and the relative risk of vertebral fractures was plotted against the average change in BMD for each trial. Considerable variability in antifracture efficacy at any given level of change in BMD was observed, and confidence intervals for the individual trials were large. Overall, trials that identified larger increases in BMD tended to report greater reductions in vertebral fracture risk. Using Poisson regression, the model predicted that treatments that increase spine BMD by 8% would reduce risk by 54%; most of the total effect of treatment was explained by an 8% increase in BMD (41% risk reduction).

23. **Hochberg MC, Greenspan S, Wasnich RD,** et al. Changes in bone density and turnover explain the reductions in incidence of nonvertebral fractures that occur during treatment with antiresorptive agents. J Clin Endocrinol Metab 2002;87: 1586–1592.

    This metaanalysis examined 18 randomized, placebo-controlled trials investigating antiresorptive agents in postmenopausal women with osteoporosis [prior vertebral fracture or low bone mineral density (BMD)]. A total of 2,415 women with a history of incidental nonvertebral fractures and more than 69,369 woman-years of follow-up were enrolled in the trials. The association between BMD or bone turnover markers (BTMs) during the first year and overall reductions in risk of nonvertebral fractures (vs. the placebo group) across all trials was estimated using Poisson regression. Greater reductions in BCM and greater increases in BMD were significantly associated with larger reductions in nonvertebral fracture risk; exemplified by the observation that each 1% increase in spine BMD at 1 year was associated with an 8% reduction in nonvertebral fracture risk ($p = 0.02$). The predicted net effect on fracture risk was the same for the hip and spine, but the mean BMD changes at the hip were less than at the spine. Agents that increased hip BMD by 3% at 1 year reduced nonvertebral fracture risk by close to 46%, and agents that increased spine BMD by 3% in 1 year decreased nonvertebral fracture risk by approximately 39%. A 70% reduction in resorption BCM was predicted to reduce risk by 40%, and a 50% reduction in BCM formation would reduce risk by 44%. A separate variable for treatment was not independently significant in any model, suggesting that either BMD or BCM changes could account for the treatment effects.

24. **Garnero P, Shih WJ, Gineyts E,** et al. Comparison of new biochemical markers of bone turnover in late postmenopausal osteoporotic women in response to alendronate treatment. J Clin Endocrinol Metab 1994;79:1693–1700.

High-pressure liquid chromatography (HPLC)-fluorometric assays for urinary pyridinoline and deoxypyridinoline were used to assess bone resorption and bone formation markers in late postmenopausal (late-PMP) osteoporotic women. Eighty-five women (mean ± SD age, 63 ± 6 y) with low bone mass and all more than 5 years postmenopausal (mean ± SD y PMP, 16 ± 7 y) were compared with 46 premenopausal women (mean ± SD age, 40 ± 5 y) randomly selected from a large cohort, and all women had a normal spine bone mineral density (BMD). The late-PMP osteoporotic women were from a subset of patients enrolled in a randomized, double-blind, placebo-controlled trial comparing the effects of different doses of oral alendronate. Spinal BMD and markers of bone turnover were assessed periodically during the 2-year study. Bone resorption was measured by urinary excretion of total pyridinoline (HPLC Pyr) and deoxypyridinoline (HPLC D-Pyr) by HPLC, serum concentration of type I collagen cross-linked C-telopeptide (ICTP) by radioimmunoassay (RIA), and type I collagen cross-linked N-telopeptide and urinary free PYR (F-Pyr) by enzyme-linked immunosorbent assay (ELISA). Bone formation was assessed by bone-specific alkaline phosphatase, C-terminal propeptide of type I collagen measured by RIA, and serum and total osteocalcin. Significant increases above normal (33%–171%, $p < 0.001$) in late-PMP osteoporotic women were observed for all bone markers, except C-terminal propeptide of type I collagen, and all bone resorption markers, except ICTP. Long-term within-patient variability measured over a 15-month period in the placebo group was low and somewhat lower for serum markers (12.5%–17.4%) than for urinary markers (24%–29%). Resorption markers decreased earlier than bone formation markers in the alendronate treatment arm. Bone marker levels were reduced to the normal premenopausal range, with the exception of F-Pyr and ICTP, and this was maintained from 6 to 15 months.

25. **Prestwood KM, Pilbeam CC, Burleson JA,** et al. The short-term effects of conjugated estrogen on bone turnover in older women. J Clin Endocrinol Metab 1994;79:366–371.

This study administered conjugated estrogen (Premarin, 0.625 mg/day) for 6 weeks to 11 elderly women (mean age, 77 years) to investigate whether estrogen replacement therapy (ERT) can help reduce bone loss and fracture in women over 70 years of age. Biochemical markers of bone turnover were measured on urine and serum at baseline (two samples), after 5 and 6 weeks of ERT, and at 5 and 6 weeks post-ERT. Bone resorption markers included total and free pyridinoline and deoxypyridinoline cross-links, type 1 collagen cross-linked N-telopeptides, serum C-terminal cross-linked telopeptide, and urinary hydroxyproline. Bone formation markers were bone alkaline phosphatase, type 1 procollagen peptide, and osteocalcin. The effects of ERT on the biochemical markers were estimated using repeated measure multivariate analysis of variance. During ERT, markers of bone resorption decreased, and after ERT the bone resorption markers returned to baseline ($p < 0.05$). Bone formation markers decreased less during ERT and continued to decrease after ERT ended ($p < 0.05$).

26. **Sorensen OH, Crawford GM, Mulder H,** et al. Long-term efficacy of risedronate: A 5-year placebo-controlled clinical experience. Bone 2003;32:120–126.

A 3-year, placebo-controlled vertebral study in women with osteoporosis was extended in this study for an additional 2 years, with subjects remaining in the placebo or 5-mg risedronate group based on original randomization and with preservation of blinding. Two hundred sixty-five women (5-mg risedronate, 135; placebo, 130) entered the study extension, with 83% of subjects completing the additional 2 years. Vertebral and nonvertebral fracture assessments, bone mineral density (BMD), and biochemical markers of bone turnover were used as end points. Results for fractures were similar in the extension group as compared with the first 3 years. In years 4 and 5, the risk of vertebral fractures was significantly reduced in the risedronate group by 59% (95% CI, 19%–79%, $p = 0.01$) compared with a 49% reduction in the first 3 years. The rapid and significant decreases in bone turnover markers observed during the first 3 years continued through the next 2 years of therapy. Years 4 and 5 showed maintenance or increases in BMD of the spine and hip in the risedronate group that had occurred during the first 3 years. There was a 9.3% ($p < 0.001$) mean increase from baseline in lumbar BMD over the 5 years.

27. **Bone HG, Hosking D, Devogelaer JP,** et al. Ten years' experience with alendronate for osteoporosis in postmenopausal women. N Engl J Med 2004;350:1189–1199.

    This multinational randomized, double-blind study examined postmenopausal osteoporotic women over 10 years and the effects of alendronate compared with placebo. The study was initially 3 years long, and compared three daily doses of alendronate with placebo. The original placebo group received alendronate during years 4 and 5, and was then discharged. The original active-treatment group continued to receive alendronate during the initial extension (years 4 and 5). Women who had received 5 mg or 10 mg alendronate daily continued with the same treatment during the next two extensions (years 6 and 7, and years 8 through 10). The discontinued group received 20 mg alendronate daily for 2 years, and 5 mg daily for years 3 to 5, followed by 5 years of placebo. Blinding and randomization were maintained over the 10 years. Treatment of 10 mg alendronate daily over 10 years resulted in mean increases in bone mineral density (BMD) of 13.7% at the lumbar spine (95% CI, 12.0%–15.5%), 10.3% at the trochanter (95% CI, 8.1%–12.4%), 6.7% at the total proximal femur (95% CI, 4.4%–9.1%), and 5.4% at the femoral neck (95% CI, 3.5%–7.4%) when compared with baseline levels; smaller increases were observed in the 5-mg daily group. A gradual loss of effect was found with the discontinuation of alendronate, and was assessed by BMD and biochemical markers of bone remodeling. Prolonged treatment did not result in any loss of benefit and was analyzed by safety data, including stature and fractures.

28. **Bauer DC, Black DM, Garnero P,** et al. Change in bone turnover and hip, nonspine, and vertebral fracture in alendronate-treated women: the fracture intervention trial. J Bone Miner Res 2004;19:1250–1258.

    Data from the Fracture Intervention Trial were used to compare the relationship of bone turnover after 1 year of alendronate or placebo treatment and subsequent nonvertebral, hip, and spine fracture risk among 6,186 postmenopausal women. Biochemical markers of bone turnover and bone mineral density (BMD) of the spine and hip were measured at baseline and after 1 year of treatment. Over a mean follow-up of 3.6 years, 786 nonvertebral, 72 hip, and 336 spinal fractures were documented. Each 1 SD reduction in 1 year change of bone ALP was associated with fewer nonvertebral (RH, 0.89; CI, 0.78–1.00, $p < 0.050$), spine (odds ratio = 0.74; CI, 0.63–0.87), and hip fractures (RH, 0.61; CI, 0.46–0.78). Women treated with alendronate with at least a 30% reduction in bone ALP had a decreased risk of nonvertebral (RH, 0.72; CI, 0.55–0.92) and hip fractures (RH, 0.26; CI, 0.08–0.83) compared with those with reductions of less than 30%.

29. **Garnero P, Hausherr E, Chapuy MC,** et al. Markers of bone resorption predict hip fracture in elderly women: the EPIDOS Prospective Study. J Bone Miner Res 1996;11:1531–1538.

    This prospective cohort study examined 7,598 healthy older women to evaluate increased bone turnover as a risk factor for osteoporotic fractures. One-hundred and twenty-six women (mean age 82.5 years) who suffered a hip fracture during a mean follow-up of 22 months were age-matched with three controls that did not fracture. Prior to fracture, two bone formation markers and three urinary bone resorption markers [type I collagen cross-linked N- (NTX) or C-telopeptide (CTX) and free deoxypyridinoline (D-Pyr)] were measured at baseline. Compared with healthy premenopausal women, elderly women had increased bone formation and resorption. Patients with hip fracture had higher urinary excretion of CTX and free D-Pyr, but not other markers, compared with age-matched controls ($p = 0.02$

and 0.005, respectively). An increased hip fracture risk was associated with CTX and free D-Pyr excretion above the upper limit of the premenopausal range, with an odds ratio (95% CI) of 2.2 (1.3–3.6) and 1.9 (1.1–3.2), respectively, but bone formation markers were not associated with an increased risk of hip fracture. Increased bone resorption was observed to predict hip fracture independent of bone mass. Women at the greatest risk for hip fracture had both a femoral bone mineral density (BMD) value of at least 2.5 SD below the mean of young adults and either high CTX or high free D-Pyr levels, with an odds ratio of 4.8 and 4.1, respectively, compared with those with only low BMD or high bone resorption.

30. **Melton LJ III, Khosla S, Atkinson EJ**, et al. Relationship of bone turnover to bone density and fractures. J Bone Miner Res 1997;12:1083–1091.

An age-stratified random sample of 351 women from Rochester, Minnesota, was evaluated to measure biochemical markers of bone turnover and the risk of fracture. Serum levels of osteocalcin, bone alkaline phosphatase, and C-terminal propeptide of type I collagen (PICP), along with 24-hour urine levels of cross-linked N-telopeptides of type I collagen (NTX) and free pyridinoline (Pyd) and deoxypyridinoline (Dpd), were measured. NTX, Dpd, and PICP were negatively associated with age among the 138 premenopausal women. All biochemical markers were positively associated with age among the 213 postmenopausal women, and the prevalence of elevated turnover (>1 SD above premenopausal mean) varied from 9% (PICP) to 42% (Pyd). Most markers negatively correlated with bone mineral density (BMD) of the spine, forearm, or hip after adjustment for age [measured by dual-energy x-ray absorptiometry (DXA)], and osteoporotic women were more likely to have high bone turnover. Historical osteoporotic fractures of the spine, distal forearm, or hip were associated with reduced hip BMD and increased Pyd. Reduced bone formation as measured by osteocalcin was associated with prior osteoporotic fractures, after adjusting for lower BMD and increased bone resorption.

31. **Garnero P, Sornay-Rendu E, Duboeuf F, Delmas PD.** Markers of bone turnover predict postmenopausal forearm bone loss over 4 years: the OFELY study. J Bone Miner Res 1999;14:1614–1621.

This large population-based prospective cohort of 305 women ages 50 to 88 (mean 64 years), 1 to 38 years postmenopausal, assessed the ability of biochemical markers to predict the rate of postmenopausal bone loss. Baseline biochemical bone markers were correlated to the rate of forearm bone mineral density (BMD) [using dual-energy x-ray absorptiometry (DXA) scans] and assessed by four measurements over a 4-year period. Independent of age, higher baseline levels of bone formation (osteocalcin and serum type I collagen N-propeptide) and bone resorption markers (urinary N-telopeptides; urinary and serum C-telopeptides) were significantly associated with faster BMD loss ($r = -0.19$ to -0.30, $p < 0.001$) across the whole patient population. Among women within 5 years of menopause that have the highest rate of bone loss, the predictive value of bone markers was increased with correlation coefficients up to 0.53. Women with bone marker levels at baseline 2 SD above the premenopausal mean, indicating an abnormally high bone turnover, had a rate of bone loss two- to sixfold higher than women with a low turnover ($p = 0.01–0.0001$) according to the markers. Categorizing the population according to quartiles of bone markers at baseline showed a similar regression between increased bone marker levels and faster rates of bone loss ($p = 0.008–0.0001$). The logistic regression model showed the odds ratio of fast bone loss, defined as the rate of bone loss in the upper tertile, increased by 1.8- to 3.2-fold for biochemical marker levels in the high turnover group, compared with levels within the premenopausal range, with a limited value for identifying fast bone losers.

32. **Uebelhart D, Schlemmer A, Johansen JS**, et al. Effect of menopause and hormone replacement therapy on the urinary excretion of pyridinium cross-links. J Clin Endocrinol Metab 1991;72:367–373.

This study used a specific high-pressure liquid chromatography assay to measure 24-hour and fasting urinary pyridinoline (Pyr) and deoxypyridinoline (D-Pyr) levels to evaluate urinary excretion of Pyr and D-Pyr as sensitive markers of bone matrix degradation. Sixty early postmenopausal women and 19 age-matched premenopausal women were enrolled as subjects. Menopause caused a 62% increase in Fu Pyr (49.8 ± 18.7 vs. 30.8 ± 8.0 pmol/μmol creatinine; $p < 0.001$) and an 82% increase in Fu D-Pyr (8.2 ± 3.4 vs. 4.5 ± 1.4 pmol/μmol creatinine; $p < 0.001$). Among 20 postmenopausal women on HRT, urinary Pyr and D-Pyr returned to premenopausal levels within 6 months, whereas the placebo group experienced no changes in these levels. The 24-hour excretion of Pyr and D-Pyr was significantly less than the fasting excretion, but was similarly decreased after HRT. Urinary samples of Pyr and D-Pyr excretions from the same sample were highly correlated ($r =$ 0.85 for fasting and 0.83 for 24-hour sampling), but correlations between fasting and 24-hour levels were poor (D-Pyr, $r = 0.30$; Pyr, $r = 0.29$; $p < 0.05$ for both). Urinary cross-links and other bone turnover marker (Fu hydroxyproline/creatinine and plasma osteocalcin) correlations were significant but low (Pyr vs. osteocalcin, $r = 0.29$, $p < 0.05$; Pyr vs. hydroxyproline, $r = 0.34$; $p < 0.01$; D-Pyr vs. osteocalcin, $r = 0.39$; $p < 0.01$), except for D-Pyr vs. hydroxyproline ($r = 0.24$; $p = 0.07$), suggesting these markers may reflect different events of bone metabolism. A single measurement of the fasting excretion, but not of the 24-hour excretion, of cross-links was significantly correlated (Pyr, $r = 0.34$; $p < 0.05$; D-Pyr, $r = -0.46$, $p < 0.01$), with the following spontaneous rate of bone loss analyzed by repeated measurements of the radial bone mineral content in 37 postmenopausal women.

33. **Gertz BJ, Shao P, Hanson DA,** et al. Monitoring bone resorption in early post-menopausal women by an immunoassay for cross-linked collagen peptides in urine. J Bone Miner Res 1994;9:135–142.

This study measured urinary excretion of cross-linked N-telopeptides of type I collagen using an enzyme-linked immunosorbent assay (ELISA) approach as a measure of bone resorption. Sixty-five early postmenopausal women who participated in a placebo-controlled trial of alendronate were enrolled, and 8 blood and urine samples were analyzed over a 9-month period. Baseline cross-linked peptide excretion varied from 26 to 216 pmol BCE (bone collagen/µmol Cr). Over the 9-month period, within-subject variability (CV) for cross-linked peptide excretion was 20.2% for the placebo group, much less than that observed for other biochemical bone resorption markers: 45%, 53%, and 63% for fasting urinary calcium and hydroxyproline and 24-hour urinary lysylpridinoline (HPLC assay), respectively. Initial peptide excretion correlated inversely with lumbar spine bone mineral density (BMD) at entry ($r = -0.26$, $p < 0.05$). Baseline cross-linked peptide excretion was significantly correlated ($p < 0.001$) with baseline total urine lysylpyridinoline and serum osteocalcin, but not with other biochemical markers. Six weeks of alendronate therapy resulted in a dose-dependent suppression of cross-linked peptide excretion (0 ± 8, 29 ± 6, 56 ± 5, and $64 \pm 3\%$ for 0, 5, 20, and 40 mg, respectively, $p < 0.01$ vs. placebo for treatment effect), with a return toward pretreatment levels during follow-up.

34. **Diaz J, Agarwal M, Norton J, Camacho P.** Predicting secondary causes of osteoporosis using DXA Z scores. Endocr Pract 2006;12(Suppl 2):47–48.

This retrospective study analyzed 262 patients referred to an osteoporosis center for osteopenia or osteoporosis, to determine sensitivities and specificities of different Z-score thresholds in predicting secondary osteoporosis. Patients' histories, lab results, and dual-energy x-ray absorptiometry (DXA) T- and Z-scores of the spine and femoral neck were reviewed. To determine whether a Z-score of -1, -1.5, -2, and -2.5 was a good predictor of the presence of 1 or more secondary causes of osteoporosis, a binary logistic regression was used. The population was 11.5% male and 88.5% female, and 80% of patients were white, 3.4% were black, 1.9% were Hispanic, and 13.7% were categorized as other/not available. The mean age was 62.6 ± 14 years for the entire group, 63.4 ± 13.8 years for women, and 56.7 years ± 14.5 years for men. Mean spine Z-score was 0.54 ± 1.34, and mean spine T-score was -1.80 ± 1.33. Secondary causes of osteoporosis were identified, and prevalence per 100 was celiac disease (2.67), chronic renal failure (1.53), hypercalciuria (1.53), hypocalciuria (0.38), hypogonadism (4.2), primary hyperparathyroidism (3.82), immobilization (1.53), secondary hyperparathyroidism (16.79), organ transplant (4.58), liver disease (1.53), and vitamin D deficiency (42.37). Of the patients reviewed, 57% had at least one secondary cause of osteoporosis, 22.1% had two or more, and 5.3% had three or more. The authors proposed a DXA Z-score of -1 as a cutoff to evaluate for secondary causes of osteoporosis.

6

Secondary Causes of Osteoporosis*

Pauline M. Camacho

Hypogonadism, 82
Medications, 84
Immunosuppressants, 85
Hyperthyroidism, 86
Vitamin D Deficiency, 86
Primary Hyperparathyroidism, 88
Transplantation, 89
Gastrointestinal Diseases, 89
Hematologic Diseases, 90
Cushing Syndrome, 90
Idiopathic Hypercalciuria, 90
Screening, 91
Conclusion, 91

Current therapies for osteoporosis are efficacious in reducing fractures and improving surrogate markers [i.e., bone mineral density (BMD) and bone markers]. Correctable factors that contribute to osteoporosis are quite common (Table 6.1), and failure to identify and treat these causes can prevent osteoporosis drugs from delivering their full potential. Secondary causes of osteoporosis have been reported in up to 64% of men [1,2], more than 50% of premenopausal and perimenopausal women [1,3], and about 20% to 50% of postmenopausal women [2,4,5]. Recognition and treatment of these causes are an important part of osteoporosis management.

The vast array of secondary causes has been reported in published articles. Some of the most common causes include hypogonadism, medications, hyperthyroidism, vitamin D deficiency, primary hyperparathyroidism, solid organ transplantation, and idiopathic hypercalciuria. In men, the three most common causes are hypogonadism, corticosteroids, and alcoholism [1,6]. In premenopausal women, the most common causes are likely hypoestrogenemia and corticosteroids [3]. These two causes are also often seen in perimenopausal women, as are anticonvulsant therapy and hyperthyroidism [1].

*Adapted from **Painter S, Kleerekoper M, Camacho P.** Secondary osteoporosis: A review of recent evidence. Endocr Pract 2006;12:436–445.

Table 6.1. Common secondary causes of osteoporosis

Hypogonadism
Medications (glucocorticoids, immunosuppressants, heparin, anticonvulsants)
Vitamin D deficiency
Primary hyperparathyroidism
Alcoholism
Idiopathic hypercalciuria
Gastrointestinal disorders (celiac sprue, inflammatory bowel disease)
Endocrine disorders (hyperthyroidism, Cushing syndrome)
Hematologic disorders (multiple myeloma, MGUS, mast cell disorders)
End-organ failure and transplantation

MGUS, monoclonal gammopathy of unknown significance.

HYPOGONADISM

Hypogonadism is one of the most common causes of male osteoporosis. Testosterone and estrogen both play roles in bone metabolism. These hormones aid in bone formation and help prevent bone resorption [6–9]; interestingly, estrogen may play a bigger role in halting resorption than testosterone [8]. Indeed, 70% of gonadal effect on male BMD may be due to estrogen [8]. This contribution of estrogen is increasingly more recognized. Barrett-Connor et al. [10] found that a population of men with a known vertebral fracture had low estradiol levels even without reduced testosterone levels. Gennari et al. [11] followed 200 men over 4 years and demonstrated the decline in testosterone and bioavailable estradiol levels with age. The estradiol levels negatively correlated with changes in BMD and with bone turnover markers, which was not seen with testosterone levels. Therefore, although testosterone does play a role in achieving and sustaining BMD, estrogen is emerging as the more dominant factor in this capacity.

Besides aging, other conditions can produce a hypogonadal state. One such situation is androgen deprivation therapy (ADT) for the treatment of prostate carcinoma. A number of studies have been published that examined the relationship between this therapy and BMD decline. A small study by Mittan et al. [12] demonstrated that after 12 months of gonadotropin-releasing hormone (GnRH) therapy, a significant decrease in BMD at the hip and the ultra distal radius occurred compared with the control group. N-telopeptide (NTX) was increased at 6 and 12 months. Two other studies compared patients on GnRH agonist therapy with healthy patients and to patients with prostate cancer who were not on ADT. Both studies showed that BMD decreased significantly in those on therapy. NTX was again elevated, and alkaline phosphatase was increased in the Stoch et al. study [13]. Basaria et al. [14] also found a correlation between the length of therapy and the decrease in BMD.

More important than the decrease in BMD is the effect of ADT on fracture risk. Investigators have examined the risk of fractures in patients on

ADT. Shahinian et al. [15] assessed more than 50,000 men with prostate cancer and compared them with those who either had received ADT within the first 6 months after diagnosis or with those who had not received such therapy. In the first 5 years after diagnosis, those who were in the treatment group had significantly higher fracture rates than those who were not; 19.4% versus 12.6%, respectively. There was a positive correlation between fracture risk and the number of GnRH agonist doses. Those who had undergone orchiectomy had the highest risk of the treatment subgroups, with a relative risk for fracture of 1.54. In this study, the number needed to harm by ADT was 28 for any dose of a GnRH agonist and 16 for orchiectomy. Lopez and others [16] compared men who received LHRH agonists, with or without peripheral androgen receptor blockers, with controls over 4 to 5 years. They found that over this time, 11% of the treatment group and 4% of the control group fractured. The members of the treatment group were often older, more drank alcohol, and more had already sustained a fracture.

Hypogonadism, particularly hypoestrogenism, can be seen throughout the life cycle of women. In young women, diseases that cause low estrogen states result in decreased peak bone mass [2,5]. Two common examples are amenorrhea and anorexia nervosa (AN).

Amenorrhea can lead to osteoporosis even in young women. If a woman misses half of her menses by age 20, she can experience a decrease in BMD [5]. In addition to the severity of the disturbance in the menstrual cycle, the length of this alteration may also affect bone density [17]. In a study of amenorrheic and normal dancers and nondancers, the amenorrheic subjects had lower baseline BMD, up to 8% less than controls, and their BMDs remained lower during the 2 years of follow-up [18]. The amenorrheic subjects whose menses restarted during the study experienced an increase in BMD, but again it did not reach that of the controls. In addition, decreased spine BMD correlated with the development of stress fractures.

Anorexia is another common cause of amenorrhea in young women, and the resulting hormonal and nutritional deficiencies contribute to the decreased BMD in this situation [2,5]. Soyka et al. [17] showed that the majority of 130 anorexic women that they studied had decreased bone mineral density on dual-energy x-ray absorptiometry (DXA) scan, with more than 90% having T-scores of -1 or less and almost 40% with scores of -2.5 or below [17]. Weight, the age at first menses, and the duration of amenorrhea increased one's risk for decreased BMD. In addition to the effects of hypoestrogenemia, these women can also have secondary hyperparathyroidism from calcium and vitamin D deficiency, hypercortisolemia, and malnourishment [2,5]. Insulin-like growth factor 1 (IGF-1) may also play a role.

Investigators have explored the effect of decreased IGF-1 concentrations in anorexic women. Soyka et al. [19] found significantly decreased IGF-1 levels in those with AN compared with controls, as well as a correlation between IGF-1 levels and such reflections of nutritional status as body mass index, percent body fat, lean body mass, and leptin, but not levels of estradiol [19].

What to do when decreased BMD is found among anorexics is a topic of debate. Whether successful therapy of anorexia improves BMD is controversial [5]. A 2002 study did not demonstrate a significant increase in BMD among subjects with anorexia who gained weight after a 1-year follow-up [20]. Whether oral contraceptives (OCP) help in this setting was studied in a trial that compared 65 women with AN to 52 healthy controls [21]. Of those with anorexia, 16 had who had taken OCPs were found to have significantly higher lumbar spine BMD, although it was still lower than the BMD of the control group [21]. However, subsequent longitudinal trials did not show an increase in BMD with OCPs or hormone replacement therapy (HRT) alone [22,23].

One must remember that not all anorexics are women. Up to 5% to 10% of patients with AN are male [2]. Although osteoporosis has been reported in male anorexics, limited data are available regarding its prevalence and the effects of treatment. Further studies need to be conducted regarding this issue.

MEDICATIONS
Oral Glucocorticoids
Numerous medications have been implicated in causing bone mineral density loss. Some of the most common offenders are immunosuppressants, heparin, and anticonvulsants. Of these, corticosteroids are most often identified as a cause of osteoporosis [1,24]. They are used frequently, in 0.5% of one population examined [25]. Only a relatively small dose is needed to cause detrimental effects on BMD. One trial found less than 2.5 mg of prednisolone per day to be associated with an increased risk of fractures [26]. BMD loss begins in the first weeks to months of therapy [27,28] and the decline is most rapid during this time [29]. A loss of up to approximately one-quarter of BMD during the first 6 to 12 months of therapy has been reported [24]. The extent of this effect is broad, as up to half of patients on chronic glucocorticoids will lose bone density and develop fractures [27]. A small study of men on 50 mg of prednisolone daily for 1 to 6 months revealed a decrease in BMD by a mean of up to 4.8% [28]. Another study showed that the subjects on corticosteroids doubled their risk of hip fracture with respect to controls [29]. It has not yet been decided whether the cumulative glucocorticoid dose or the peak dose is most important. Many studies favor the cumulative dose [24]; the small study mentioned above revealed an inverse correlation between lumbar spine BMD and cumulative corticosteroid dose [28]. However, the United Kingdom General Practice Research Database (UK GPRD) [30] study demonstrated increased fracture risk with peak dose over cumulative dose.

Inhaled Glucocorticoids
Inhaled glucocorticoids have also been linked to decreases in BMD with chronic use. Israel et al. [31] studied 109 premenopausal asthmatic women on triamcinolone. They found that the bone density at the hip and the trochanter decreased by 0.00044 g/cm^2 for every puff taken per year on the

treatment. The association held after accounting for all other corticosteroids, age, and oral contraceptive pills. Wong et al. [32] showed a decrease in BMD with increased cumulative inhaled corticosteroid dose, which continued after accounting for other corticosteroids.

Glucocorticoids lower bone density by a variety of mechanisms. The main effect of glucocorticoids is on the osteoblast, causing a decrease in bone formation [24]. These bone-forming cells also have reduced function and lifespan [24,27,33]. Another effect of glucocorticoids on bone loss is increased bone resorption [24], possibly partly due to secondary hyperparathyroidism [27]. Other pathways by which corticosteroids decrease BMD include decreased calcium absorption, increased calcium excretion, and decreased sex hormone synthesis [24,27]. A decrease in the glucocorticoid dose or discontinuation of the glucocorticoid altogether can help halt this process. For instance, in the UK GPRD study, those patients who stopped taking glucocorticoids experienced a decreased risk of nonvertebral fractures [30].

Heparin

Heparin has been seen in rat models to decrease bone formation and increase bone resorption [34]. Many of the studies evaluating heparin's effects on BMD and fracture risk have investigated women on heparin during pregnancy. One such study of 184 women, on 15,000 to 30,000 IU of heparin per day for 7 to 27 weeks, revealed symptomatic vertebral fractures in approximately 2% of these women [35]. BMD decline appears to begin with a heparin dose of at least 15,000 IU daily for more than 3 months [36]. The effects of low molecular weight heparin on the skeleton have not been found to be as significant [36,37].

Anticonvulsants

Anticonvulsants have also been linked to BMD decline. One of the primary mechanisms by which they induce this damage may be by decreasing 25-hydroxylation of vitamin D and, thus, reducing calcium absorption [36]. Some of the more common culprit antiepileptic medications include phenytoin, phenobarbital, primidone, and carbamazepine [36,38]. The degree of BMD loss has been related to frequency and duration of use, with a hip BMD loss of 1.16% per year in patients on such medications continuously for several years, and a 1.7-fold increased rate of BMD decline at the hip over those not on such medications [39]. With respect to fracture risk, a study by Vestergaard and others [40] found a small but significant increase in the risk of fractures with some anticonvulsants, including carbamazepine and phenobarbital.

IMMUNOSUPPRESSANTS

Immunosuppressants, such as cyclosporine and tacrolimus, have been shown to exert negative effects on bone density in animal models [41,42], but these effects in clinical trials have been less clear. Although decreased BMD has been seen in patients taking these medications, a possible confounder may be the concomitant use of glucocorticoids in these cases [43].

Their effect on fracture risk is also uncertain; for instance, one trial did not find these medications to be significantly correlated [44].

HYPERTHYROIDISM

Hyperthyroidism can cause osteoporosis as well, decreasing BMD by 10% to 30% in women [5]. Both osteoclastic and osteoblastic activities are increased in hyperthyroidism; however, osteoclasts are amplified more [5]. Hyperthyroidism may also decrease intestinal calcium absorption [2].

The cause of the hyperthyroidism does not appear to affect the degree of bone loss. Jodar et al. [45] compared the BMDs of overtly hyperthyroid, controlled hyperthyroid, and healthy patients. They showed a lower BMD in the overtly hyperthyroid and the controlled hyperthyroid patients compared with the healthy ones. Overtly hyperthyroid patients had more bone loss than the controlled ones. No significant difference in bone density between Graves disease patients and those with toxic multinodular goiter was found. Obtaining a euthyroid state is important for increasing BMD. Kumeda et al. [46] demonstrated that patients with hyperthyroidism on drug therapy, who still had a low thyroid-stimulating hormone (TSH) despite normal thyroid hormone levels, had persistent increases in bone turnover markers. With resolution of thyroid disease, BMD increases but may not normalize [5]. Some data supporting normalization of bone density to age-expected BMD do exist, however. For instance, Karga et al. [47] compared both untreated and treated hyperthyroid patients with age-matched women without prior hyperthyroidism. They found that although BMD was lower than that of controls in untreated hyperthyroidism for up to 3 years after treatment, BMD was not significantly different from that in controls at least 3 years after therapy.

VITAMIN D DEFICIENCY

Decreased vitamin D concentrations can have deleterious effects on bone metabolism. Two important metabolic bone derangements that can result are secondary hyperparathyroidism and osteomalacia. Secondary hyperparathyroidism develops when the vitamin D concentration decreases to an insufficient and deficient level [47]. Consequently, one can see increased bone turnover [48,49] and decreased BMD [49–51]. Lips [48] suggested that vitamin D insufficiency ranges from 10 to 20 ng/mL (25–50 nmol/L). Variations do exist, as Chapuy [52] found that parathyroid hormone (PTH) increased at a higher 25(OH)D threshold, 31 ng/mL (78 nmol/L). Osteomalacia may develop after prolonged vitamin D deficiency [48,50]. According to Lips [48], this can be found at 25(OH)D levels of less than 5 ng/mL (<12.5 nmol/L). Various trials have further substantiated these theories, confirming an inverse correlation between PTH and 25(OH)D [4,48,52]. In addition, the presence of increased bone turnover can be inferred by the inverse relationship between bone turnover markers and vitamin D levels [49,53]. Interestingly, a study reported a stronger inverse correlation between 24-hour urinary calcium excretion and PTH than 25-OHD and PTH level [4].

The gold standard in diagnosing osteomalacia is bone biopsy. This is not always readily available, however. Frequently, the diagnosis can be inferred from the presence of high total or bone-specific alkaline phosphatase, in the setting of a low vitamin D level, hypocalciuria, and secondary hyperparathyroidism. These individuals complain of bone pain (deep aching hip or pelvic pain), motor weakness, and recurrent fractures.

The loss of bone density among vitamin D–deficient individuals has been demonstrated in various trials. For instance, Mezquita-Raya et al. [51] showed a positive correlation between 25(OH)D concentrations and BMD. Elsewhere, a 4% lower trochanter BMD has been demonstrated with 25(OH)D levels less than 10 ng/mL (25 nmol/L) [49]. In addition, Sahota et al. [53] reported a significant decrease in BMD at the hip with 25(OH)D concentrations between 6.1 and 12 ng/mL (15.25 to 30 nmol/L) [53]. One might further reason that decreased vitamin D is linked to an increase in risk of fracture. These data are not as firm, but there have been reports of an association [48,54].

The effect of this deficiency on bone density can also be illustrated by changes that occur after vitamin D is supplemented. With such replacement, PTH concentration decreases, bone turnover calms, and BMD improves [48,55]. In addition, the incidence of fractures decreases. For instance, Adams et al. [55] showed a 4% to 5% increase in BMD at the lumbar spine and the femoral neck per year with vitamin D repletion. Also, Dawson-Hughes et al. [56] demonstrated a significant increase in BMD and a significant decrease in nonvertebral fractures with calcium and vitamin D supplementation over 3 years. A metaanalysis showed that vitamin D reduced the incidence of vertebral fractures [relative risk (RR) 0.63, 95% confidence interval (CI) 0.45–0.88, $p < 0.01$] and showed a trend toward reduced incidence of nonvertebral fractures (RR 0.77, 95% CI 0.57–1.04, $p = 0.09$) [57].

Vitamin D deficiency is increasingly being recognized as a contributing factor to osteoporosis. In fact, Favus [58] has postulated that it is possibly the most common etiology [58]. Numerous studies assessing its prevalence have been performed. The Multiple Outcomes of Raloxifene Evaluation clinical trial found 4% of their subjects with a 25(OH)D of less than 10 ng/mL (<25 nmol/L) and almost one-quarter with a level of 10 to 20 ng/mL (25–50 nmol/L) [49]. Holick et al. [59] found that half of the women that he evaluated, postmenopausal women in North America on osteoporosis treatment, had a 25(OH)D level of less than 30 ng/mL (75 nmol/L). Chapuy et al. [52] saw a 25(OH)D concentration of 12 ng/mL (30 nmol/L) or less in 14% of the French women they studied. In addition, 75% of their subjects had a 25(OH)D level of less than 31 ng/mL (78 nmol/L). In a study of 104 patients at least 98 years old, 99 had an undetectable concentration of 25(OH)D [60]. Although this deficiency can be seen among ambulatory patients, it is more common in hospitalized patients, those living in nursing homes, and patients who have sustained hip fractures [48,54]. For instance, a study of hospitalized general medicine patients revealed that 57% had a 25(OH)D level of less than 15 ng/mL (37.5 nmol/L). Seventy-seven of the patients in this study were younger than 65 years old and were without known risks for vitamin D deficiency; 42% of this subgroup was deficient [61]. Although not as common, decreased concentrations of vitamin D are also seen in the younger population. For example, Tangpricha et al. [62] found that 36% of the patients aged 18 to 29 years in their study had 25(OH)D levels less than

20 ng/mL (50 nmol/L) at the end of winter; this decreased to less than 10% at summer's end.

Several reasons exist for the increased prevalence of vitamin D deficiency among the elderly. These include less sun exposure [48,54,58,63], decreased ability to synthesize vitamin D_3 [48,58,63], inadequate vitamin D intake [48,52,58,63], and decreased intestinal responsiveness to vitamin D [64]. In addition, dysfunction of the liver or the kidney can contribute to the deficiency [54,58], as can the ingestion of medications that increase vitamin D clearance [58].

Since much of one's vitamin D supply comes from sun exposure, it seems logical that concentrations may fluctuate with the seasons and with location. Multiple studies have confirmed this seasonal variation, with lower levels in the winter than in the summer [49,62,65]. This has also been shown with respect to the inverse relationships of 25(OH)D with PTH [48,54,62] and with bone turnover markers [48]. In addition, Chapuy et al. [52] found a location difference in 25(OH)D concentrations, with a significant decrease in the north in comparison to the south of France.

PRIMARY HYPERPARATHYROIDISM

Primary hyperparathyroidism can cause decreased BMD and increased risk of fractures. This occurs mainly due to an increase in bone resorption [50]. Parathyroid hormone is likely catabolic in cortical bone, such as in the distal radius, and anabolic in cancellous bone, such as in the lumbar spine [66–68]. Thus, usually more cortical bone is lost than cancellous bone [51,68], although decreased density of cancellous bone has been seen [66–68]. The correlation between parathyroid hormone and BMD has been shown in such studies as that by Sitges-Serra et al. [69], who found a significantly increased PTH concentration in osteoporotic patients. Although it seems that this decreased bone density would correlate with an increase in fractures, results are not consistent. Khosla et al. [70] compared the fracture risk in more than 400 patients with mild primary hyperparathyroidism to that in the general population. They found a significant risk of vertebral and pelvic fractures. Other trials have not found an increased risk of fractures, however [66,67].

Effects of primary hyperparathyroidism can also be seen by assessing bone density and fractures after parathyroidectomy. Several studies have investigated these changes, and they have demonstrated an increased bone mineral density and a decreased fracture risk after surgery. A study by Silverberg et al. [71] followed 121 patients with primary hyperparathyroidism for 10 years. They noted that the patients who underwent parathyroidectomy experienced an increase in BMD—8% at the lumbar spine and 6% at the femoral neck after the first year, then 12% at the lumbar spine and 14% at the femoral neck after 10 years. Sitges-Serra et al. [69] compared the DXA scans of 28 hyperparathyroid patients taken before and 1 year after parathyroidectomy. They demonstrated a significant increase in BMD at the femoral neck and the proximal femur, especially in the osteoporotic patients. Rao et al. [72] studied 53 patients with mild primary hyperparathyroidism and randomized these subjects to surgery or no surgery. Small but significant yearly increases in BMD were seen at the femoral neck and at the total hip after parathyroidectomy. Finally, Vestergaard and Mosekilde [73] showed a 31% decreased risk of fracture after parathyroidectomy.

TRANSPLANTATION

Multiple factors contribute to the decline in BMD in patients with solid organ failure, as well as those who have received transplants. The disease itself, risk factors that develop because of the disease, and medications, including loop diuretics and glucocorticoids, all contribute to the decreased BMD. Many of the patients with end-organ failure are older, immobile, malnourished, Caucasian, vitamin D–deficient, hypogonadal, tobacco users, or alcohol consumers [5,42,74]. After transplantation, many of these risks still exist. In addition, of prime importance are the immunosuppressants that are used in the post-transplant period [5,42].

Osteoporosis has been documented in these patients before and after transplant. In pretransplant patients, it has been reported in up to 19% of those with heart failure [74], 29% to 61% with lung disease [42,75,76], and 26% to 52% with liver failure [42,77]. Fractures have also been reported in these patients; for instance, 25% to 29% of end-stage lung disease patients were found to have suffered a vertebral fracture in one study [75]. After transplant, much of the density loss occurs in the first several months [5,42]. Shane et al. [78] showed that cardiac transplant patients lost a mean of 7% to 11% of the density in their lumbar spine and femoral necks in the first year; most of this occurred in the first 6 months in the lumbar spine [78]. This is similar to other reported data [42]. Postliver transplant patients may lose up to one-quarter of their BMD in the spine in the first year, although this is controversial [42]. Bone density in liver transplant patients may improve as early as 6 months after transplant, at times increasing to pretransplant density [5,42,79,80]. After lung transplant, 2% to 5% of bone density is lost in the first year [42]. An increased risk of fracture after transplant has also been reported. In the first year, up to two-thirds of patients can fracture [81]. Leidig-Bruckner et al. [82] found that after two years, about one-fourth of the heart transplant patients and about one-fifth of the liver transplant patients suffered a vertebral fracture [82].

GASTROINTESTINAL DISEASES

Various gastrointestinal diseases have been linked to osteoporosis, particularly inflammatory bowel disease (IBD) and celiac sprue. Up to three-quarters of IBD patients may have decreased BMD [83]. One study assessing 51 patients with Crohn disease (CD) and 40 patients with ulcerative colitis (UC) found that 55% of the CD patients and 67% of those with UC had osteopenia, and 37% of the CD and 18% of the UC patients had osteoporosis [84]. Although this study did not have such findings, many other studies have found that the decline in BMD is more pronounced with Crohn disease than with ulcerative colitis [83]. With this BMD decline, an increase in fracture risk over that of the general population has been seen, but the actual risk is likely still small [83,85,86]. Aspects of the disease and its treatment contribute to this loss, particularly glucocorticoid use, malabsorption, vitamin D deficiency, undernutrition, and cytokines [83,86].

Celiac sprue has also emerged as a disease frequently discovered during osteoporosis evaluation. The primary pathogenesis is malabsorption and subsequent decreased calcium and vitamin D and secondary hyperparathyroidism
[87,88]. Osteoporosis has been seen in one-quarter to one-third of the patients
with this disease [89]. Stenson and others [90] found sprue to be more common in osteoporotic patients than in those without osteoporosis. They diagnosed sprue in 3.4% of the 266 osteoporotic patients, compared with 0.2% of
the 574 nonosteoporotic subjects. With respect to fracture risk, the findings
are conflicting. For instance, one study found the risk to be 3½ times higher in
these patients [87], whereas another did not find an increase [91]. Part of the
explanation for this may be the relatively younger age of these patients.

The diagnosis of celiac sprue is suggested by positive antigliadin, antien-
domysial, or transglutaminase antibodies. Antibody levels can be low when
patients are on a gluten-free diet or can be negative when patients have mild
disease. The gold standard is demonstration of atrophic villi on an upper gastrointestinal tract biopsy.

HEMATOLOGIC DISEASES

A number of hematologic diseases, such as multiple myeloma, systemic mastocytosis, leukemia, and lymphoma, have been associated with bone loss [2].
Of these, one of the most studied is multiple myeloma. The main mechanism
for the bone loss in multiple myeloma is plasma cell synthesis of cytokines
and other local factors, such as receptor activator nuclear κ (RANK)-ligand,
that activate osteoclasts. Up to one-quarter of those with multiple myeloma
can have low bone mass [2]. Abrahamsen et al. [92] found an increased
prevalence of multiple myeloma and monoclonal gammopathy of undetermined significance (MGUS) in osteoporotic patients when they compared
these patients to others without osteoporosis [92]. Either multiple myeloma
or MGUS existed in about 5% of those with osteoporosis. On the other hand,
no patients without osteoporosis had multiple myeloma, and only 2% had
MGUS. A study done at the Mayo Clinic revealed an increased risk of fracture in patients with multiple myeloma of about two times [93].

CUSHING SYNDROME

Elevated cortisol concentrations resulting from exogenous sources and endogenous production can adversely affect BMD [2]. Numerous studies have
evaluated the effect of endogenous hypercortisolism on the human skeleton.
Normal patients have exhibited a positive correlation between cortisol concentrations and the rate of bone loss [94,95]. Decreased BMD has been seen
in those with subclinical hypercortisolism [96]. In those with Cushing syndrome, a negative association between cortisol concentrations and BMD has
also been shown. BMD decreases of approximately 21% at the lumbar spine
and 18% at the femoral neck in these patients have been observed [97]. The
degree of BMD loss may be more severe in those with Cushing syndrome of
adrenal origin than those with Cushing disease [98].

IDIOPATHIC HYPERCALCIURIA

Idiopathic hypercalciuria (IH) is found in more than one-half of patients
with recurrent renal stones [99]. In addition to causing stones, IH is also

associated with decreased BMD [100–102]. Studies have reported a decrease of up to 20% [99–100]. Idiopathic hypercalciuria causes bone loss by many mechanisms. First, there is increased bone resorption, likely stimulated by cytokines. Misael da Silva et al. [102] studied 40 patients with recurrent renal stones, separated into hypercalciuric and normocalciuric groups, as well as 10 patients without nephrolithiasis. They found that the hypercalciuric patients had more bone erosion and osteoclasts; this was even more pronounced in the hypercalciuric patients who were osteopenic. In addition, IL-6 and TNF were elevated in the osteopenic hypercalciuric group with respect to the normocalciuric group. Another process by which bone density may be lost is through increased prostaglandin E_2 synthesis [100]. Finally, less calcium is reabsorbed by the kidney, causing a relative hypocalcemic state [100].

These changes result in low bone mass. One study demonstrating this is by Garcia-Nieto and others [100]. They assessed 80 patients with idiopathic hypercalciuria. In addition to T-scores of at least less than -1 in more than 60% of the adult women, a Z-score of less than -1 at the lumbar spine or the femoral neck was seen in about 48% of them. The Z-score was significantly lower at the lumbar spine with respect to controls [100].

SCREENING

Various recommendations exist regarding when to search for secondary causes. According to Stein and Shane, all women who have not entered menopause and all men who experience fragility fractures or have a Z-score of less than -1 should undergo further evaluation [5]. Several approaches to this investigation have been proposed. For instance, the authors just named have suggested that all patients with osteoporosis have a complete blood count (CBC), complete metabolic panel, erythrocyte sedimentation rate (ESR) or C-reactive protein (CRP), thyroid function tests, and a 24-hour urine for calcium and creatinine checked; also, men should have testosterone, luteinizing hormone (LH), and follicle-stimulating hormone (FSH) levels drawn [5]. Favus [58] suggested a fasting calcium, creatinine, 25(OH) vitamin D, creatinine clearance, and 24-hour urine for calcium; a PTH should then be drawn if the calcium is abnormal or the creatinine clearance is decreased. One study looked at the necessity of checking for secondary causes of osteoporosis in healthy postmenopausal women with osteoporosis. They found that checking a serum calcium, PTH, and 24-hour urine for calcium, as well as a TSH level if the patient is on thyroid therapy, diagnosed secondary causes in 47 of 55 patients with such disorders, and cost $75 per patient [103]. The presence of a secondary cause in a patient should at least prompt a DXA scan. Further studies need to be done to guide clinicians in determining the extent of work-up for secondary causes and the threshold at which this needs to be done, perhaps based on DXA Z-scores and other parameters.

CONCLUSION

Secondary osteoporosis is a common disease, affecting patients who have not typically been considered at high risk for decreased BMD, namely men and premenopausal women. It also contributes to low BMD in postmenopausal women, in whom, historically, classic primary osteoporosis is prominent. The causes of this disease are broad. A few of the more common ones that have been discussed recently in the literature have been presented here. Heightened awareness of the possibility of secondary osteoporosis and increased vigilance for its detection are essential in improving bone health in these patients.

REFERENCES
Annotations by Alexandra Reiher

1. **NIH Consensus Development Panel on Osteoporosis Prevention, Diagnosis, and Therapy.** Osteoporosis prevention, diagnosis, and therapy. JAMA 2001;285: 785–795.

   This article reviews the consensus reached by an expert panel regarding osteoporosis. It was concluded that osteoporosis occurs in all populations and all ages, but is most prevalent in white postmenopausal women. Risk factors for osteoporosis and for fracture overlap but are not exactly the same. Individuals with risk factors for secondary osteoporosis should be carefully monitored. Calcium and vitamin D are important supplements for the development of adequate bone mass and for preservation of bone mass. It is important to recognize gonadal steroids as a determinant of peak and lifetime bone mass in all persons. Regular exercise, particularly resistance, may reduce the risk of falls in the elderly and also contribute to the development of peak bone mass. When evaluating individuals for osteoporosis, it is important to assess bone mass, identify fracture risks, and determine whether or not to treat. The primary treatment goal for patients with osteoporosis is fracture prevention. Any adult with a distal forearm, hip, vertebral, or rib fracture should be evaluated for osteoporosis and treated appropriately.

2. **Harper K, Weber T.** Secondary osteoporosis diagnostic considerations. Endocrinol Metab Clin North Am 1998;27:325–348.

   This article reviews major causes of secondary osteoporosis that significantly impact bone loss and also increase fracture risk. Hypogonadism, endogenous and exogenous thyroxine excess, hyperparathyroidism, malignancies, medications, connective tissue disorders, and gastrointestinal diseases are some of the major causes.

3. **Kulak C, Schussheim D, McMahon D,** et al. Osteoporosis and low bone mass in premenopausal and perimenopausal women. Endocr Pract 2000;6:296–304.

   Risk factors for osteoporosis were evaluated in 111 young women (<55 years old) who were referred for evaluation of osteoporosis or low bone mineral density (BMD). Sixty-six percent had identifiable causes of bone loss, the most common causes being estrogen deficiency (premenopausal estrogen deficiency, menopause) and conditions associated with estrogen deficiency (anorexia nervosa, cancer chemotherapy). The second most common cause was prolonged steroid use. Of those with no identifiable cause, 21 were premenopausal (mean age, 38 ± 10 years) and 17 were perimenopausal (mean age, 50 ± 3 years). Mean lumbar T-score was −2.51 ± 0.6 in the perimenopausal women and −2.18 ± 1.0 in the premenopausal women. Forty-two percent of premenopausal and 57% of perimenopausal women had a history of a nontraumatic fracture. A family history of osteoporosis was present for 71% of the premenopausal and 47% of the perimenopausal women.

4. **Camacho P, Girgis M, Sapountzi P, Sinacore J.** Correlations between vitamin D, parathyroid hormone, urinary calcium excretion, markers of bone turnover, and bone density of patients referred to an osteoporosis center. J Bone Miner Res 2005; 20(Suppl 1):S389.

   The primary aim of the study was to characterize the relationships between 25-OHD, 1-25-OHD, intact parathyroid hormone (PTH), ionized calcium, phosphorus, 24-hour urine calcium excretion (UrCa), bone-specific alkaline phosphatase, urinary N-telopeptide (NTX)/creatinine and bone density; 163 patients (143 female, 20 male; mean age 62.5 years) evaluated for low bone mass at Loyola University Osteoporosis and Metabolic Bone Disease Center were studied. The strongest indirect relationship seen was between PTH and UrCa ($r = -0.496$, $p \leq 0.001$). Hydroxyvitamin D showed a significant correlation with UrCa ($r = 0.420$, $p \leq 0.001$), PTH ($r = -0.215$, $p = 0.014$), bone-specific alkaline phosphatase (BSAP) ($r = -0.288$, $p = 0.010$), and a trend with spine bone mineral density (BMD) ($r = -0.156$, $p = 0.071$). Analysis of the subgroup with 25-OHD less than or equal to 20 ng/mL (26% of the group) showed that 25-OHD correlated significantly with parathyroid hormone (PTH; $r = -0.354$, $p = 0.027$). The strong indirect correlation between PTH and UrCa ($r = -0.540$, $p = 0.021$) remained in this group. 1,25-OHD showed a trend associated with UrCa ($r = 0.459$, $p = 0.064$) and spine BMD ($r = -0.356$, $p = 0.069$). Ionized calcium, phosphorus, or N-telopeptide (NTX)/creatinine did not show significant correlations with PTH or Vit D levels. The difference between the means of PTH above and below a 25-OHD level of 30 ng/mL was significant. At 35 ng/mL, the significance was lost. The same 25-OHD level of 30 ng/mL showed significant differences in the UrCa of patients with 25-OHD above and below this threshold. This relationship was also significant at 35 ng/mL and was lost at 40 ng/mL. A level of 30 ng/mL was concluded as the cutoff of vitamin D deficiency. This was seen in 48% of the population.

5. **Stein E, Shane E.** Secondary osteoporosis. Endocrinol Metab Clin North Am 2003;32:115–134.

    This article describes the major causes of secondary osteoporosis and the steps to take in a diagnostic work-up of patients suspected of having secondary osteoporosis.

6. **Meunier P.** Prevention of hip fractures by correcting calcium and vitamin D insufficiencies in elderly people. Scand J Rheumatol Suppl 1996; 103:75–78.

7. **Khosla S, Bilezikian J.** The role of estrogens in men and androgens in women. Endocrinol Metab Clin North Am 2003;32:195–218.

    This article discusses the roles sex steroids have on bone formation in both genders. *In vivo* human data suggests that estrogen is more potent than testosterone in inhibiting bone resorption. Both testosterone and estrogen are important for bone formation, and both enhance bone size, most likely through effects on periosteal bone formation.

8. **Falahati-Nini A, Riggs B, Atkinson E,** et al. Relative contributions of testosterone and estrogen in regulating bone resorption and formation in normal elderly men. J Clin Invest 2000;106:1553–1560.

    This study evaluated which sex steroid deficiency, estrogen (E) or testosterone (T), played a more important role in contributing to increased bone resorption and decreased bone formation leading to bone loss. Endogenous T and E production was directly eliminated in 59 older men (mean age, 68 years), and were then studied by giving physiologic T and E replacement. The impact on bone turnover was then assessed by withdrawing both sex steroids, withdrawing only T or only E, or continuing both. In the absence of both hormones, bone resorption markers increased significantly, but the markers were unchanged in men receiving both hormones. Estrogen played the major role in preventing an increase in bone resorption markers, while testosterone had no effect. Serum osteocalcin decreased in the absence of both hormones, but was maintained in the presence of both hormones.

9. **Leder B, LeBlanc K, Schoenfeld D,** et al. Differential effects of androgens and estrogens on bone turnover in normal men. J Clin Endocrinol Metab 2003;88:204–210.

    This randomized study evaluated the role of androgens and estrogen in the maintenance of normal bone turnover in men. Men ages 20 to 44 years old received one of three regimens. Group 1 received a gonadotropin-releasing hormone (GnRH) analog (goserelin acetate) alone for 12 weeks; Group 2 received goserelin plus transdermal testosterone (Androderm); and Group 3 received goserelin plus testosterone plus an aromatase inhibitor (anastrozole). Bone resorption markers increased in both the hypogonadal group (Group 1) and in the group with selective estrogen deficiency (Group 3). Urinary deoxypyridinoline excretion increased significantly more in Group 1 than in Group 3 ($p = 0.023$), suggesting a significant effect of androgens on bone resorption. Serum N-telopeptide levels increased significantly more in Group 3 than in Group 2 ($p = 0.037$), suggesting a significant effect of estrogen on bone resorption. Bone formation markers declined in all groups initially, and then increased in Groups 1 and 3. Between-group comparisons were consistent for all formation markers. Bone formation markers increased more in Group 1 than in Group 2 ($p = 0.001$, 0.037, 0.005 for osteocalcin; C-terminal propeptide of type I procollagen; and A-terminal propeptide of type I procollagen, respectively). Bone formation markers also increased more in Group 1 than in Group 3 but these differences were not statistically significant. These results suggest that both androgens and estrogens have independent and important roles in controlling bone resorption in men.

10. **Barrett-Connor E, Mueller J, Von Muhlen D,** et al. Low levels of estradiol are associated with vertebral fractures in older men, but not women: the Rancho Bernardo Study. J Clin Endocrinol Metab 2000;85:219–223.

    This was a longitudinal study evaluating the relationship between sex hormone levels and occurence of vertebral fractures in postmenopausal women without estrogen use (mean age, 72 years) and men (mean age, 66 years). At least one vertebral fracture was found in 21% of women and 8% of men. Age-adjusted hormone levels among men differed by fracture status only for total ($p = 0.012$) and bioavailable ($p = 0.008$) estradiol. A graded association between higher concentrations of total and bioavailable estradiol and lower fracture prevalence was present (trend $p < 0.01$ for both hormones). Men with levels of total testosterone congruent with hypogonadism (<7 nmol/L) were not more likely to have vertebral fractures. In women, none of the measured sex hormones were associated with vertebral fractures. In women with estradiol levels below the assay sensitivity (<11 pmol/L), there was no increased prevalence of fractures.

11. **Gennari L, Merlotti D, Martini G,** et al. Longitudinal association between sex hormone levels, bone loss, and bone turnover in elderly men. J Clin Endocrinol Metab 2003;88:5327–5333.

    Over four years, hormone levels, bone turnover markers, bone mineral density (BMD), and rate of bone loss were evaluated in 200 elderly men. Sex hormone–binding globulin (SHBG) levels increased significantly in the total population, and serum testosterone (T), calculated bioavailable estradiol, free androgen index (FAI), and free estrogen index (FEI) [but not serum estradiol (E[2])] decreased significantly with age. Men with FEI, c-bioE(2), and E(2) levels below the median had higher rates of bone loss at the lumbar spine and the femoral neck, as well as higher speed-of-sounds decreases at the calcaneus with respect to men with these levels above the median. Serum bone alkaline phosphatase and urinary crosslaps were significantly higher in men with FEI, c-bioE(2), and E(2) in the lower quartile than in men with these levels in the higher quartile. No statistically significant differences were observed in relation to T, c-bioT, or FAI levels. The ratio between E(2) and T, an indirect measure for aromatase activity, increased significantly with age and was higher in normal individuals than in osteoporotic subjects. Based on these results, estrogen and the ability to aromatize testosterone to estradiol play important roles in the regulation of bone loss and bone metabolism in elderly men.

12. **Mittan D, Lee S, Miller E,** et al. Bone loss following hypogonadism in men with prostate cancer treated with GnRH analogs. J Clin Endocrinol Metab 2002;87: 3656–3661.

    This study investigated the effects of gonadotropin-releasing hormone (GnRH) analog treatment on bone loss and bone resorption in men with prostate cancer. After 1 year of GnRH treatment, the total hip and distal radius bone mineral density (BMD) decreased significantly ($p < 0.001$) in men with prostate cancer compared with controls. The mean bone loss was 3.3% and 5.3%, respectively. Reductions in BMD at the spine (2.8%) and the femoral neck (2.3%) were not statistically significant. The control group did not have significant bone loss. The concentration of urine N-telopeptide was significantly increased from baseline and from controls at 6 and 12 months in patients treated with GnRH therapy compared with controls ($p < 0.05$). The concentration of bone-specific alkaline phosphatase was not significantly different from baseline or from controls at 6 and 12 months. The decreased total hip and ultra distal radius BMD and increased urinary N-telopeptide concentration after testosterone withdrawal demonstrates an increase in trabecular bone loss and enhanced bone resorption.

13. **Stoch S, Parker R, Chen L,** et al. Bone loss in men with prostate cancer treated with gonadotropin-releasing hormone agonists. J Clin Endocrinol Metab 2001;86: 2787–2791.

    This study investigated whether or not gonadotropin-releasing hormone (GnRH) agonists would have a negative impact on bone mass. Sixty men with prostate cancer, 19 of whom were treated with GnRH therapy and 41 of whom were eugonadal, were compared with 197 age-matched healthy controls.

    Men receiving GnRH therapy had significantly lower bone mineral density (BMD) at the lateral spine (0.69 ± 0.17 vs. 0.83 ± 0.20 g/cm^2; $p \le 0.01$), total hip (0.94 ± 0.14 vs. 1.05 ± 0.16 g/cm^2; $p \le 0.05$), and forearm (0.67 ± 0.11 vs. 0.78 ± 0.07 g/cm^2; $p < 0.01$) compared with the eugonadal men with prostate cancer. Significant differences were also seen at the total body, finger, and calcaneus (all $p < 0.01$). BMD values in eugonadal men with prostate cancer and healthy controls were found to be similar. Markers of bone resorption (urinary N-telopeptide) and bone formation (bone-specific alkaline phosphatase) were increased in men receiving GnRH therapy compared with those in eugonadal men with prostate cancer. Men receiving GnRH agonists had a higher percent total body fat ($p < 0.01$) and lower percent lean body weight ($p < 0.01$) compared with eugonadal men with prostate cancer. These results suggest men with prostate cancer receiving androgen deprivation therapy have an increased risk of fracture.

14. **Basaria S, Lieb J, Tang A,** et al. Long-term effects of androgen deprivation therapy in prostate cancer patients. Clin Endocrinol 2002;56:779–786.

   The effects of androgen deprivation therapy (ADT) on men with prostate cancer were investigated in this cross-sectional study. The following individuals were enrolled: 20 men with prostate cancer (PCa) who were undergoing medical castration with gonadotropin-releasing hormone (GnRH) agonists for at least 12 months prior to the onset of the study (ADT group), 18 age-matched men with nonmetastatic PCa who were post prostatectomy and/or radiotherapy but had not yet undergone ADT (non-ADT group), and 20 age-matched normal men who were healthy and ambulatory (control group) were enrolled. Men on ADT had castrate levels of serum total testosterone ($p < 0.0001$), free testosterone ($p < 0.0001$), and estradiol ($p < 0.0001$), which were significantly lower than in the other groups. Total body ($p = 0.03$) and lumbar spine ($p < 0.0001$) bone mineral density (BMD) was significantly lower in patients on ADT compared with other groups and was associated with higher levels of urinary N-telopeptide ($p = 0.02$). Compared with the other groups, the ADT group had higher fat mass ($p = 0.0001$) and significantly decreased upper body strength ($p = 0.001$) when compared with non-ADT patients. The ADT group had lower overall scores on Watts Sexual Function Questionnaire compared with other groups ($p = 0.0001$), especially decreased desire, arousal, and frequency of spontaneous early-morning erections. The ADT group also had lower overall quality of life scores, resulting in significant limitation of physical function ($p = 0.001$), role limitation ($p = 0.02$), and perception of physical health ($p = 0.004$).

15. **Shahinian V, Kuo Y, Freeman J, Goodwin J.** Risk of fracture after androgen deprivation for prostate cancer. N Engl J Med 2005;352:154–164.

   This retrospective study investigated the risk of fracture after androgen deprivation therapy (ADT). Of those who survived at least 5 years after diagnosis, 19.4% of men who received ADT had a fracture, as compared with 12.6% of those not receiving ADT ($p < 0.001$). In the Cox proportional-hazards analyses, adjusted for characteristics of the patient and the tumor, there was a statistically significant relationship between the number of doses of gonadotropin-releasing hormone (GnRH) received during the 12 months after diagnosis and the subsequent risk of fracture. This study found ADT increased the risk of fracture.

16. **Lopez A, Pena M, Hernandez R, Val F**. Fracture risk in patients with prostate cancer on androgen deprivation therapy. Osteoporos Int 2005;16:707–711.

   The clinical significance of loss of bone mass in men treated with androgen deprivation therapy (ADT) [luteinizing hormone–releasing hormone (LHRH) agonists] for prostate cancer was investigated in this retrospective cohort study. The incidence rates of peripheral and vertebral fractures in the group of men on ADT were 1.9 and 0.8 per 100 patient-years, respectively. Incidence rates in the control group were 0.5 and 0.2, respectively. The number of patients with at least one fracture was significantly higher in the ADT group when compared with controls ($p = 0.001$ by the log-rank test). The unadjusted risk ratio was 4.2 (CI, 2.0–8.9). A similar value (risk ratio, 3.6; CI, 1.6–7.7, $p = 0.001$) was found after it was adjusted for other factors, such as age or prior fractures.

17. **Grinspoon S, Thomas E, Pitts S,** et al. Prevalence and predictive factors for regional osteopenia in women with anorexia nervosa. Ann Intern Med 2000;133: 790–794.

   This prospective cohort analysis investigated the prevalence and predictive factors for regional bone loss in women with anorexia nervosa. The prevalence of osteopenia and osteoporosis was 50% and 13% for the anterior-posterior spine, 57% and 24% for the lateral spine, and 47% and 16% for the total hip, respectively. Bone mineral density (BMD) was reduced by at least 1.0 SD at one or more skeletal sites in 92% of patients and by at least 2.5 SD in 38% of patients. The most consistent predictor of BMD was weight. Of the 130 women studied, 23% were current estrogen users and 58% were previous estrogen users. BMD did not differ by history of estrogen use at any site. These results suggest that weight, but not estrogen use, is a significant predictor of BMD in these individuals at all skeletal sites.

18. **Warren M, Brooks-Gunn J, Fox R,** et al. Osteopenia in exercise-associated amenorrhea using ballet dancers as a model: A longitudinal study. J Clin Endocrinol Metab 2002;87:3162–3168.

    The effects of amenorrhea (with and without exercise) on bone mineral density (BMD) in young women were studied in this 2-year comparison of 54 dancers and 57 nondancers. Reduced BMD in the wrist, foot, and spine were found in both hypothalamic amenorrheic groups, and their BMD was far below that of the normal dancers and nondancers throughout the 2 years. Only amenorrheic dancers showed significant changes in spine BMD (12%, $p < 0.05$) but still remained below controls, and within this subgroup, only those with delayed menarche showed a significant increase. The amenorrheic subjects who resumed menses during the study showed an increase in spine and wrist BMD (17%; $p < 0.001$) without achieving normalization. Delayed menarche was the only variable that predicted stress fractures ($p < 0.005$). The amenorrheic women had a higher incidence of dieting behavior, as manifested by higher Eating Attitudes Test scores ($p < 0.05$) and higher fiber intakes ($p < 0.001$).

19. **Soyka L, Grinspoon S, Levitsky L,** et al. The effects of anorexia nervosa on bone metabolism in female adolescents. J Clin Endocrinol Metab 1999;84:4489–4496.

    To evaluate bone metabolism in anorexic girls, osteopenia, bone formation, and bone resorption were evaluated. Nineteen adolescent girls with anorexia nervosa (AN) were studied, and the mean duration of AN was 19 ± 5 months. Lumbar anteroposterior bone mineral density (BMD) was more than 1 SD below the mean in 42% of patients, and lateral spine BMD was more than 1 SD below the mean in 63% of patients, compared with controls. Lean body mass significantly predicted lumbar bone mineral content ($r = 0.75$; $p < 0.0001$) in controls only. The most significant predictor of spinal BMD in AN was duration of illness (lumbar: $r = -0.44$; $p = 0.06$; lateral: $r = -0.59$; $p = 0.008$). AN adolescents with mature BA (15-y and greater) were hypogonadal, although dehydroepiandrosterone sulfate and urinary free cortisol levels did not differ. Leptin levels were reduced in AN ($p < 0.0001$). Insulin-like growth factor I (IGF-I) was reduced in AN to 50% of control levels ($p < 0.0001$) and correlated with all measures of nutritional status, especially leptin ($p = 0.80$; $p < 0.0001$). Surrogate markers of bone formation, serum osteocalcin (OC) and bone-specific alkaline phosphatase (BSAP), were significantly ($p = 0.02$) reduced in AN compared with controls. Most of the variation in bone formation in AN was due to IGF-I levels (OC, $r^2 = 0.72$; $p = 0.002$; BSAP, $r^2 = 0.53$; $p = 0.01$) in stepwise regression analyses. Bone resorption was similar in AN individuals and controls.

20. **Soyka L, Misra M, Frenchman A,** et al. Abnormal bone mineral accrual in adolescent girls with anorexia nervosa. J Clin Endocrinol Metab 2002;87:4177–4185.

    This prospective study followed 19 adolescent girls with anorexia nervosa (AN) more than 1 year, and evaluated the impact of their nutritional state on their bone mineral density (BMD) and body composition. Nutritional status in subjects with AN improved (mean percentage increase in BMI from baseline, 9.2 ± 1.9% and 15.2 ± 2.6% at 6 and 12 months, respectively), with 11 subjects having recovered weight at 12 months. Despite this, lumbar BMD at 12 months (AN, 0.88 ± 0.02 g/cm², vs. control, 0.98 ± 0.03 g/cm²; $p = 0.008$) remained significantly reduced in AN compared with controls, even in those who recovered. These results were due to significant increases in lumbar BMD in controls while there were no changes in AN subjects over the year ($p = 0.04$). At 12 months, the most significant determinant of change in lumbar BMD was change in lean body mass in both AN ($r = 0.62$; $p = 0.008$) and control ($r = 0.80$; $p = 0.0006$) groups. There were significant increases in bone turnover markers in AN individuals compared with controls as assessed by osteocalcin ($p = 0.0007$), bone-specific alkaline phosphatase ($p = 0.002$), deoxypyridinoline ($p = 0.005$), and N-telopeptide ($p = 0.01$). Changes in IGF-I levels over the year were highly correlated with changes in bone turnover over the same period in AN (osteocalcin, $r = 0.77$; $p = 0.001$; deoxypyridinoline, $r = 0.66$; $p = 0.01$). A rise in N-telopeptide over the year was correlated with an increase in all bone mineral measures, including lumbar bone mineral content ($r = 0.58$; $p = 0.03$) and BMD ($r = 0.53$; $p = 0.05$) and total bone mineral content ($r = 0.69$; $p = 0.006$) and BMD ($r = 0.69$; $p = 0.006$) in the AN group. These results show that even with recovery over 12 months, poor BMD persists in young girls with AN when compared with the rapidly increasing BMD of healthy girls.

21. **Seeman E, Szmukler G, Formica C,** et al. Osteoporosis in anorexia nervosa: The influence of peak bone density, bone loss, oral contraceptive use, and exercise. J Bone Miner Res 1992;7:1467–1474.

This study investigated whether oral contraceptives or exercise have a protective effect against osteoporosis in 65 young women with anorexia nervosa (AN). Compared with controls, the patients with AN had significantly lower bone mineral density (BMD), weight, fat mass, and fat-free mass (all $p < 0.001$), even after adjusting for age and height differences. Lumbar spine and femoral neck BMD was reduced more in the 12 patients with primary amenorrhea when compared with the 37 women with secondary amenorrhea ($p = 0.001$ and $p = 0.04$, respectively). BMD at the lumbar spine in the 16 patients with 31.8 ± 8.3 months of contraceptive exposure was greater than in the 49 patients with no history of contraceptive use (1.14 ± 0.05 vs. 1.02 ± 0.02, $p < 0.02$) but was lower than in controls ($p < 0.01$). No protective effect of contraceptive exposure was observed at the femoral neck. The 19 patients who exercised vigorously had higher BMD at the proximal femoral sites than sedentary patients.

22. **Gordon C, Grace E, Emans S,** et al. Effects of oral dehydroepiandrosterone on bone density in young women with anorexia nervosa: A randomized trial. J Clin Endocrinol Metab 2002;87:4935–4941.

This randomized, prospective study enrolled 61 young women with anorexia nervosa (AN) and compared the effects of oral dehydroepiandrosterone (DHEA) treatment (50 mg/day) versus conventional hormone replacement therapy (HRT) (20 µg ethinyl estradiol/0.1 mg levonorgestrel) over 1 year. Total hip bone mineral density (BMD) in both groups increased comparably and significantly (+1.7%). Hip BMD increases were positively correlated with increases in insulin-like growth factor-I (IGF-I) ($r = 0.44$; $p = 0.030$). Bone-specific alkaline phosphatase increased significantly only in the DHEA treatment group ($p = 0.003$). There was significant weight gain in both groups over the year, and after controlling for weight gain, no treatment effect was found. No significant change in lumbar BMD was observed in either group. Both bone-specific alkaline phosphatase and osteocalcin increased transiently at 6 to 9 months in subjects receiving DHEA compared with the HRT group ($p < 0.05$). Both DHEA and HRT significantly reduced levels of the bone resorption marker, urinary N-telopeptides ($p < 0.05$). A positive correlation was observed between changes in IGF-I and changes in weight, body fat determined by DXA, and estradiol for both groups. Using three validated psychological instruments, an improvement was found in patients receiving DHEA treatment. Both DHEA and HRT had similar effects on hip and spinal BMD. No significant increase in hip or spinal BMD was found after accounting for weight gain, but there was maintenance of both hip and spinal BMD over the year. Bone resorption was significantly decreased in both the DHEA and HRT groups. Based on the significant increases in bone formation markers, the positive correlation between increases in hip BMD and IGF-1, DHEA appears to have more anabolic effects than HRT.

23. **Grinspoon S, Thomas L, Miller K,** et al. Effects of recombinant human IGF-1 and oral contraceptive administration on bone density in anorexia nervosa. J Clin Endocrinol Metab 2002;87:2883–2891.

The effects of recombinant human insulin-like growth factor-I (rhIGF-I) alone or in combination with oral contraceptives (OCP) on bone mineral density (BMD) in women with anorexia nervosa (AN) was investigated in this randomized, placebo controlled, single-blinded study. Sixty osteopenic women with AN were randomized to one of four treatment groups [rhIGF-I (30 µg/kg sc twice daily) and a daily oral contraceptive (Ovcon 35, 35 µg ethinyl estradiol and 0.4 mg norethindrone)], rhIGF-I alone (30 µg/kg sc twice daily), oral contraceptive alone, or neither treatment for 9 months. All subjects received supplemental calcium and vitamin D. The rhIGF-I was titrated to maintain IGF-I levels within the age-adjusted normal range for each patient and was well tolerated. Anteroposterior spinal BMD significantly increased in response to rhIGF-I ($p = 0.05$ for all rhIGF-I vs. all placebo treated). However, OCP did not increase BMD ($p = 0.21$, all OCP vs. all non-OCP treated). BMD increased the most in the combined treatment group (rhIGF-I and OCP), compared with control patients receiving no active therapy ($p < 0.05$ for rhIGF-I and OCP vs. no active therapy). These results support the use of rhIGF-I treatment in osteopenic women with AN, and demonstrate that OCP use alone is not enough to increase BMD in AN patients.

24. **Saag K.** Glucocorticoid-induced osteoporosis. Endocrinol Metab Clin North Am 2003; 32:135–157.

This article discusses the pathogenesis and epidemiology of glucocorticoid-induced osteoporosis (GIOP), proper diagnosis, and how to prevent GIOP using evidence-based medicine.

25. **Walsh L, Wong C, Pringle M,** et al. Use of oral corticosteroids in the community and the prevention of secondary osteoporosis: A cross sectional study. BMJ. 1996;313:344–346.

This cross-sectional study investigated the use of oral steroids in the general population of the United Kingdom, and the occurrence of osteoporosis prevention among these individuals taking oral steroids. Of the 65,786 individuals studied, 303 (0.5%) individuals were currently taking at least three months of continuous oral steroid treatment. This number included 65% of women ages 12 to 94 years, and 1.4% of patients 55 years or older. Prednisolone was the most commonly prescribed; the mean dose was 8.0 mg/day, and the median duration of oral steroid treatment determined in 149 patients was 3 years. Rheumatoid arthritis (23%), polymyalgia rheumatica (22%), and asthma or COPD (19%) were the most common reasons for continuous oral steroid treatment. Only 14% of patients taking oral steroids had received preventative osteoporosis treatment over the previous 4 years.

26. **van Staa T, Leufkens H, Abenhaim L,** et al. Use of oral corticosteroids and risk of fractures. J Bone Miner Res 2000;15:993–1000.

This retrospective, cohort study in the United Kingdom examined the risk of fracture in patients taking oral steroids, and the reversibility of this risk after discontinuing steroid treatment. Respiratory disease was the most common reason for treatment (40%), and the average age of patients taking steroids was 57.1 years. During oral steroid treatment, the relative rate of nonvertebral fracture was 1.33 (95% CI, 1.29–1.38), hip fracture was 1.61 (1.47–1.76), forearm fracture 1.09 (1.01–1.17), and that of vertebral fracture 2.60 (2.31–2.92). There was a dose dependence of fracture risk. With a standardized daily dose of less than 2.5 mg prednisolone, hip fracture risk was 0.99 (0.82–1.20) relative to control, and increased to 1.77 (1.55–2.02) at daily doses of 2.5–7.5 mg, and 2.27 (1.94–2.66) at doses of 7.5 mg or greater. For vertebral fracture, the relative rates were 1.55 (1.20–2.01), 2.59 (2.16–3.10), and 5.18 (4.25–6.31), respectively. After cessation of oral corticosteroids, there was a rapid decline in fracture risk toward baseline.

27. **Lukert B, Raisz L.** Glucocorticoid-induced osteoporosis: pathogenesis and management. Ann Intern Med 1990;112:352–364.

This article reviewed studies published after 1970 regarding glucocorticoid-induced osteoporosis. From the studies reviewed, it was concluded that osteoporosis occurs in approximately 50% of individuals receiving long-term glucocorticoid treatment. Physical activity, adequate calcium and vitamin D intake, gonadal hormone replacement, and the lowest dose of steroids possible are some of the recommendations which may decrease glucocorticoid-induced osteoporosis. For refractory cases, calcitonin, bisphosphonates, anabolic steroids, or sodium fluoride may be beneficial.

28. **Pearce G, Tabensky A, Delmas P,** et al. Corticosteroid-induced bone loss in men. J Clin Endocrinol Metab 1998;83:801–806.

This prospective, controlled study investigated the pathophysiology of corticosteroid-related bone loss. Biochemical and hormonal determinants of bone turnover, as well as bone mineral density (BMD), were measured in 9 men treated with prednisolone to decrease antisperm antibodies, and compared with 10 age-matched controls. At baseline, BMD was similar between groups. The men received 50 mg prednisolone daily for 3.7 ± 0.6 months. BMD decreased by $4.6 \pm 0.8\%$ at the lumbar spine ($p = 0.0007$), by $2.6 \pm 0.6\%$ at the trochanter ($p = 0.004$), and by $4.8 \pm 1.9\%$ at the Ward triangle ($p < 0.04$). There was a correlation between the decrease in lumbar spine BMD and the total dose of corticosteroids ($r = -0.49; p = 0.03$). Serum osteocalcin and bone alkaline phosphatase decreased by $28.5 \pm 15.5\%$ ($p = 0.08$) and $24.2 \pm 8.6\%$ ($p < 0.03$), respectively. The decrease in lumbar spine BMD correlated with the decrease in osteocalcin ($r = -0.48; p < 0.02$). Serum testosterone and sex hormone–binding globulin decreased by $28.6 \pm 4.4\%$ ($p < 0.003$) and $28.5 \pm 8.3\%$ ($p < 0.007$), respectively. There was no change in the testosterone/sex hormone-binding globulin ratio. The decrease in total testosterone correlated with the decrease in osteocalcin ($r = -0.40; p = 0.05$). No detectable change in urinary C-telopeptide, serum PTH, or serum calcium was found. Estradiol decreased by $23.5 \pm 11.4\%$ ($p < 0.003$).

29. **Cooper C, Coupland C, Mitchell M.** Rheumatoid arthritis, corticosteroid therapy and hip fracture. Ann Rheum Dis 1995;54:49–52.

Patients with rheumatoid arthritis or receiving corticosteroids were evaluated in this population-based case-control body to determine the risk of hip fracture in these individuals as compared with sex-matched controls. An increased risk of hip fracture was observed in patients with rheumatoid arthritis [odds ratio (OR), 2.1; 95% CI, 1.0–4.7] and those receiving corticosteroids (OR, 2.7; 95% CI, 1.2–5.8). After adjusting for functional impairment, there was a large reduction in risk due to rheumatoid arthritis. However, the risk attributable to steroid use was unchanged after adjusting for body mass index, smoking, alcohol, and functional status. These results show a risk of hip fracture that is doubled among patients with rheumatoid arthritis or individuals taking steroids.

30. **van Staa T, Leufkens H, Abenhaim L,** et al. Oral corticosteroids and fracture risk: Relationship to daily and cumulative doses. Rheumatology 2000;39:1383–1389.

This study reviewed medical records of 244,235 corticosteroid users and 244,235 controls to evaluate the risk of fracture in patients taking corticosteroids. Compared with individuals taking 2.5 mg or less of prednisolone daily, patients taking at least 7.5 mg daily of prednisolone had significantly increased risks of nonvertebral fracture (RR = 1.44, 95% CI, 1.34–1.54), hip fracture (RR = 2.21, 95% CI, 1.85–2.64), and vertebral fracture (RR = 2.83, 95% CI, 2.35–2.40). Individuals exposed to higher total doses of oral corticosteroids appeared to have an elevated fracture risk, but this risk normalized after adjusting for age, gender, and daily dose. Based on these results, the risk of developing fracture increases quickly in patients taking oral steroids, and there is a dose-dependent relationship. Also, total steroid exposure does not appear to be a major player in the risk of developing fractures.

31. **Israel E, Banerjee T, Fitzmaurice G,** et al. Effects of inhaled glucocorticoids on bone density in premenopausal women. N Engl J Med 2001;345:941–947.

The effect of inhaled glucocorticoids on bone mass was investigated in this 3-year, prospective study on premenopausal women who had asthma and were taking inhaled triamcinolone acetonide. A dose-related decrease in bone mineral density (BMD) was observed for inhaled steroids at the total hip and the trochanter of 0.00044 g/cm^2 per puff per year ($p = 0.01$ and $p = 0.005$, respectively). There was no dose-related effect at the spine or femoral neck. The association between number of puffs per year and reduced BMD existed even after exclusion of all women who had received parenteral or oral steroids at any time during the study. Serum and urinary markers of bone turnover and adrenal function were measured, but did not estimate the extent of bone loss.

32. **Wong C, Walsh L, Smith C,** et al. Inhaled corticosteroid use and bone-mineral density in patients with asthma. Lancet 2000;355:1399–1403.

To determine if a relationship existed between the dose of inhaled corticosteroids given and bone mineral density (BMD), women with asthma who took inhaled corticosteroids were evaluated. The median cumulative dose of inhaled steroids was 876 mg, and the median duration of treatment was 6 years (range, 0.5–24). Using multiple regression analysis, a negative association was found between cumulative dose of inhaled steroids and BMD at the lumbar spine, Ward triangle, trochanter, and femoral neck. This association was found both before and after adjusting for age and sex. Doubling the dose of inhaled steroids resulted in a decrease in BMD at the lumbar spine of 0.16 SD (95% CI, 0.04–0.28), with similar decreases occurring at the trochanter, femoral neck, and Ward triangle. This association remained after adjusting for potential confounding factors.

33. **O'Brien C, Jia D, Plotkin L,** et al. Glucocorticoids act directly on osteoblasts and osteocytes to induce their apoptosis and reduce bone formation and strength. Endocrinology 2004;145:1835–1841.

This was the first study to demonstrate that excess glucocorticoids directly affect bone forming cells *in vivo*. Glucocorticoid action on osteoblastic/osteocyctic cells *in vivo* was blocked by transgenic expression of 11 beta-hydroxysteroid dehydrogenase type 2 (an enzyme that inactivates glucocorticoids). The transgene did not affect normal bone development or turnover. Excess glucocorticoid administration caused equivalent bone loss in transgenic mice and wild-type mice. Cancellous osteoclasts were unaffected by the transgene. Osteoblasts, osteoid area, and bone formation were significantly greater in the glucocorticoid-treated transgenic mice when compared with glucocorticoid-treated wild-type mice. Glucocorticoid-induced osteocyte apoptosis was prevented in transgenic mice. Although both groups had equivalent bone loss, the decrease in vertebral compression strength seen in the steroid-treated wild-type mice was prevented in the transgenic mice.

34. **Muir J, Andrew M, Hirsh J,** et al. Histomorphometric analysis of the effects of standard heparin on trabecular bone in vivo. Blood 1996;88:1314–1320.

To investigate the mechanism by which heparin induces osteoporosis, rats were given once daily subcutaneous injections of heparin or saline for up to 32 days. Heparin caused both a time- and dose-dependent decrease in trabecular bone volume in the distal third of the right femur proximal to the epiphyseal growth plate, as determined by histomorphometric analysis. Most of the decrease was observed within the first 8 days of treatment. Heparin doses of 1.0 IU/g/d caused a 32% trabecular bone loss, a 37% decrease in osteoblast surface, and a 75% reduction in osteoid surface. The osteoclast surface was 43% higher in heparin-treated rats when compared with control rats, providing evidence that heparin does increase the rate of bone resorption. Heparin was also found to produce a dose-dependent reduction in serum alkaline phosphatase, and also caused a temporary increase in urinary type 1 collagen cross-linked pyridinoline.

35. **Dahlman T.** Osteoporotic fractures and the recurrence of thromboembolism during pregnancy and the puerperium in 184 women undergoing thromboprophylaxis with heparin. Am J Obstet Gynecol 1993;168:1265–1270.

    This study investigated the occurrence of osteoporotic fractures in 184 women being treated with long-term subcutaneous heparin during gestation. The average duration of treatment was 25 weeks, and the mean heparin dose was 13,000 to 40,000 IU over 24 hours. Four women experienced symptomatic osteoporotic spinal fractures postpartum (2.2%), with a mean duration of treatment 7 to 27 weeks (mean 17 weeks), and a mean dose of 15,000 to 30,000 IU heparin in 24 hours. Five women had thromboembolic complications (2.7%) despite heparin prophylaxis and were later found to either have a subtherapeutic concentration of heparin or were diagnosed with a coagulation disorder.

36. **Tannirandorn P, Epstein S.** Drug-induced bone loss. Osteoporos Int 2000;11: 637–659.

    This article reviews the mechanisms of drug-induced bone loss, the pathophysiology behind it, and appropriate treatments for drug-induced bone loss.

37. **Carlin A, Farquharson R, Quenby S,** et al. Prospective observational study of bone mineral density during pregnancy: low molecular weight heparin versus control. Hum Reprod 2004;19:1211–1214.

    This ethically approved prospective observational study examined the effects of long-term low molecular weight heparin (LMWH) on bone mineral density (BMD) during pregnancy. Fifty-five women with recurrent miscarriage and known antiphospholipid syndrome were treated with LMWH and aspirin during pregnancy and through 6 weeks postpartum, and were compared with 20 pregnant controls with a history of miscarriage that did not require any treatment. The two groups did not have significantly different characteristics. Lumbar spine BMD loss during pregnancy was comparable in the treatment (4.17%) and control (3.56%) groups, and was not statistically significant ($p = 0.88$). No patient in either group experienced a vertebral fracture during the study. These results suggest LMWH does not affect a woman's risk of bone loss during pregnancy.

38. **Farhat G, Yamout B, Mikati M,** et al. Effect of antiepileptic drugs on bone density in ambulatory patients. Neurology 2002;58:1348–1353.

    This cross-sectional study evaluated ambulatory patients on anticonvulsant drugs (AED) to determine the effects of AED on vitamin D levels and bone mineral density (BMD), and to determine if the risk of bone loss differed between enzyme-inducing and enzyme noninducing AED or between single versus multiple therapy. Of 42 adults and 29 children and adolescents on AED, more than 50% had low vitamin D levels, but this did not correlate with BMD. Adults taking AED had decreased BMD. Significant determinants of BMD, particularly at sites rich in cortical bone, included duration of epilepsy, generalized seizures, and polypharmacy. Patients taking enzyme-inducing drugs tended to have reduced BMD when compared with patients on noninducers.

39. **Ensrud K, Walczak T, Blackwell T,** et al. Antiepileptic drug use increases rates of bone loss in older women. Neurology 2004;62:2051–2057.

    The effects of antiepileptic drug (AED) use on bone mineral density (BMD) in a population of elderly community-dwelling women was examined in this prospective study. The average rate of decrease in total hip BMD steadily increased from -0.70% per year in nonusers to -0.87% per year in partial AED users to -1.16% per year in continuous AED users (p value for trend $= 0.015$). Increased rates of bone loss were observed at subregions of the hip and at the calcaneus in continuous AED users. A significant increased rate of loss was observed in continuous phenytoin users, with an adjusted 1.8-fold greater mean rate of loss at the calcaneus compared with nonusers (−2.68 vs. −1.46%/year; $p < 0.001$) and an adjusted 1.7-fold greater mean rate of loss at the total hip compared with nonusers (−1.16 vs. −0.70%/year; $p = 0.069$). The risk of hip fracture among continuous AED users is estimated to increase by 29% over a 5-year period.

40. **Vestergaard P, Rejnmark L, Mosekilde L.** Fracture risk associated with use of antiepileptic drugs. Epilepsia 2004;45:1330–1337.

This case-control study investigated the effects of newer antiepileptic drugs (AEDs) on bone mineral density (BMD). All AEDs were associated with an increased risk of fracture in an unadjusted analysis. After adjusting for prior fracture, any use of corticosteroids, social variables, comorbidities, and a diagnosis of epilepsy, carbamazepine (OR, 1.18; 95% CI, 1.10–1.26), oxcarbazepine (1.14, 1.03–1.26), clonazepam (1.27, 1.15–1.41), phenobarbital (1.79, 1.64–1.95), and valproate (1.15, 1.05–1.26) had a statistically significant association with risk of any fracture. No significant difference was found for risk of fracture after adjusting for confounding variables with ethosuximide, lamotrigine, phenytoin, primidone, tiagabine, vigabatrin, or topiramate. The observed increased risk was comparable for both the significant and nonsignificant results. A dose-response relationship was observed for carbamazepine, phenobarbital, oxycarbazepine, and valproate. An increased risk of fracture was observed with liver-inducing AEDs (OR, 1.38; 95% CI, 1.31–1.45) than with non-inducing AEDs (1.19; 95% CI, 1.11–1.27).

41. **Maalouf N, Shane E.** Osteoporosis after solid organ transplantation. J Clin Endocrinol Metab 2005;90:2456–2465.

This article reviews transplantation-related osteoporosis, including the epidemiology, contributing factors, preventative measures, and treatment options available.

42. **Cohen A, Shane E.** Osteoporosis after solid organ and bone marrow transplantation. Osteoporos Int 2003;14:617–630.

This review article discusses transplant-associated osteoporosis, including the pathophysiology of post-transplant bone loss, prevention, and proper treatment.

43. **Monegal A, Navasa M, Guanabens N,** et al. Bone mass and mineral metabolism in liver transplant patients treated with FK506 or cyclosporine A. Calcif Tissue Int 2001;68:83–86.

This prospective study evaluated the effects of cyclosporine A and FK506 on bone mineral density (BMD) in 25 liver transplant patients. Lumbar BMD decreased 5.2 ± 1.2% ($p = 0.0005$) and 2.9 ± 2.1% (not significant) in CyA and FK506 groups, respectively, at 6 months. Baseline values for lumbar BMD were reached at 1 year in the FK506 group and at 2 years after liver transplantation in the cyclosporine A group. Significant intergroup differences in femoral neck BMD changes after 2 years of transplant were observed (CyA: −5.2 ± 1.97 vs. FK506: +1.55 ± 2.2%; $p = 0.039$). Both groups had large increases in parathyroid hormone (PTH) and vitamin D levels at the first year post-transplant. A negative correlation existed between BMD changes at the lumbar spine and the mean cumulative dose of glucocorticoids ($p = 0.022$). Patients in the cyclosporine A treatment group received a higher cumulative dose of steroids, which could explain the greater bone loss in this group.

44. **Patel S, Kwan J, McCloskey E,** et al. Prevalence and causes of low bone density and fractures in kidney transplant patients. J Bone Miner Res 2001;16:1863–1870.

This study investigated bone loss in kidney transplant patients to determine its prevalence and which kidney transplant patients are most at risk for bone loss. Of the 70 female participants, 40 were postmenopausal, compared with one hypogonadal male among 85 men. A significant reduction was observed in bone mineral density (BMD) at the radius and femoral neck, but the lumbar spine was normal. At all skeletal sites, BMD was lower in women than men. Osteopenia was found in 35% to 50% and osteoporosis in 10% to 44% of women. An inverse relationship was observed between BMD and time since transplantation, as well as cumulative prednisolone dose. There was a history of a low trauma fracture or vertebral deformities in 16% of patients post-transplant. Of those with a fracture, 37% were men and 63% were women. Fourteen of the women with a fracture were postmenopausal. Similar results were observed for cumulative doses of tacrolimus and cyclosporine. Characteristics of fracture patients included older age, a longer period of renal failure, transplantation, dialysis, larger total steroid dose, and increased bone resorption markers.

A significant increase in fracture risk was found for duration of dialysis and time since transplantation, with an odds ratio for each year of dialysis or transplantation being 1.21 (CI, 1.00–1.48) and 1.14 (CI, 1.05–1.23), respectively.

45. **Jodar E, Munoz-Torres M, Escobar-Jimenez F,** et al. Bone loss in hyperthyroid patients and in former hyperthyroid patients controlled on medical therapy: Influence of aetiology and menopause. Clin Endocrinol 1997;47:279–285.

This study examined hyperthyroid patients to determine how whether bone mineral density (BMD) loss is reversible after treatment, and whether the etiology of hyperthyroidism affected BMD loss. BMD in hyperthyroid patients with active disease or treated disease was reviewed, as well as the BMD for patients with Graves disease and toxic nodular goiter. A generalized decrease in axial BMD was observed in patients with active hyperthyroidism when compared with controls, whereas former hyperthyroid patients had a partial recovery of BMD at the lumbar spine and Ward triangle.

Mean Z-scores at lumbar spine, femoral neck, and Ward triangle were -0.92, -0.79, and -0.89 in patients with active hyperthyroidism; -0.74, -0.23, and -0.44 in former hyperthyroid patients; and 0.18, 0.09, and 0.36 in controls, respectively. After adjusting for age and sex, no significant differences were found in BMD between patients with Graves disease and in patients with toxic nodular goiter, or between pre- and postmenopausal women.

46. **Kumeda Y, Inaba M, Tahara H,** et al. Persistent increase in bone turnover in Graves' patients with subclinical hyperthyroidism. J Clin Endocrinol Metab 2000;85:4157–4161.

This study investigated bone metabolism in thyroid-stimulating hormone (TSH)–suppressed premenopausal Graves disease patients with normal FT3 and FT4 levels after antithyroid treatment compared with TSH-normal premenopausal Graves disease patients. The relationship between biochemical markers of bone metabolism and serum TSH receptor antibody was also examined. No difference was found between the two groups in serum Ca, phosphorus, intact PTH, or in urinary Ca excretion. Markers of bone resorption were significantly higher in the TSH-suppression group than in the TSH-normal group [bone alkaline phosphatase (B-ALP), $p < 0.05$; urine pyridinoline, $p < 0.001$; urine deoxypyridinoline, $p < 0.001$]. For all Graves disease patients enrolled in this study, TSH had a significant negative correlation with alkaline phosphatase ($r = -0.300$; $p < 0.05$), urine pyridinoline ($r = -0.389$; $p < 0.05$), and urine deoxypyridinoline ($r = -0.446$; $p < 0.05$), but FT3 and FT4 lacked a significant correlation. The TSH receptor Ab had a significantly positive correlation with B-ALP ($r = 0.566$; $p < 0.0001$), U-PYD ($r = 0.491$; $p < 0.001$), and U-DPD ($r = 0.549$; $p < 0.0001$) for all Graves disease patients and was still significantly positive in Graves disease patients with a normal serum TSH [B-ALP ($r = 0.638$; $p < 0.001$), U-PYD ($r = 0.638$; $p < 0.001$), and U-DPD ($r = 0.641$; $p < 0.001$)].

47. **Karga H, Papapetrou P, Korakovouni A,** et al. Bone mineral density in hyperthyroidism. Clin Endocrinol 2004;61:466–472.

This cross-sectional study evaluated women with untreated or previously treated symptomatic hyperthyroidism 0 to 31 years ago to determine if previous hyperthyroidism results in permanent secondary osteoporosis. Women diagnosed with hyperthyroidism at a younger age (13 to 30 years) had a significantly greater bone mineral density (BMD) loss when examined in the first 3 years after diagnosis (regardless of treatment status) than after the first 3 years of treatment. After at least 3 years from the first episode of hyperthyroidism, there was no difference in mean Z-score from controls. This pattern was also seen in older women (ages 51–70 years), but significant differences were not found. Middle-aged women (31–50 years) had the lowest loss of BMD during the first three years. No significant difference was found for relative risk of osteoporosis between older women with hyperthyroidism and age-matched controls, but this study lacked enough power for valuable relative risk results. The results of this study suggest that symptomatic hyperthyroidism causes transient loss in BMD initially, but this loss resolves after treatment. Also, age at diagnosis is not a factor in determining whether a patient with hyperthyroidism develops osteoporosis.

48. **Lips P.** Vitamin D deficiency and secondary hyperparathyroidism in the elderly: consequences for bone loss and fractures and therapeutic implications. Endocr Rev 2001;22:477–501.

This review article discusses vitamin D deficiency in the elderly, and the importance of vitamin D_3 supplementation in housebound elderly patients to reduce the risk of hip fracture in this population.

49. **Lips P, Duong T, Oleksik A,** et al. A global study of vitamin D status and parathyroid function in postmenopausal women with osteoporosis: baseline data from the Multiple Outcomes of Raloxifene Evaluation clinical trial. J Clin Endocrinol Metab 2001;86:1212–1221.

The international Multiple Outcomes of Raloxifene Evaluation study was a large, prospective intervention trial in postmenopausal osteoporotic women, and the data were used in this study to compare vitamin D status and parathyroid function. Serum 25-OHD was less than 25 nmol/L in 4% of the women, and this was found to be associated with a 30% higher serum parathyroid hormone (PTH). A serum 25-OHD between 25 and 50 nmol/L, which occurred in 24% of patients, was associated with a 15% higher serum PTH when compared with women who had a serum OHD higher than 50 nmol/L. Low vitamin D levels were also associated with a decreased bone mineral density (BMD) of the trochanter and an increased alkaline phosphatase. A significant increase in serum 25-OHD and decrease in serum PTH occurred after treatment with vitamin D_3 and calcium, and this effect was the most pronounced in those with the lowest baseline serum 25-OHD.

50. **Kleerekoper M, Edelson G.** Biochemical studies in the evaluation and management of osteoporosis: current status and future prospects. Endocr Pract 1996;2: 13–19.

This article reviews the bone remodeling cycle, including hormonal control of bone remodeling, as well as the biochemical markers of bone formation and bone resorption, and their use in the clinical setting.

51. **Mezquita-Raya P, Munoz-Torres M, de Dios Luna J,** et al. Relation between vitamin D insufficiency, bone density, and bone metabolism in healthy postmenopausal women. J Bone Miner Res 2001;16:1408–1415.

The role of vitamin D insufficiency as a risk factor for osteoporosis and fracture in healthy postmenopausal women with osteoporosis was examined in this study. Vitamin D insufficiency was found in 39.1% of subjects, and was significantly lower in women with osteoporosis (15.7 ± 5.3 ng/mL vs. 21.8 ± 9.7 ng/mL; $p < 0.001$). Lumbar spine bone mineral density (BMD) was significantly associated with vitamin D levels, body mass index (BMI), and years after menopause (YSM; $R^2 = 0.253$; $p < 0.001$), after adjusting for all other variables. Significant independent predictors for femoral neck BMD included YSM, BMI, intact PTH (iPTH), and vitamin D ($R^2 = 0.368$; $p < 0.001$). After adjusting for YSM, BMI, iPTH, and dietary calcium intake, patients with vitamin D insufficiency had the highest probability of meeting osteoporosis BMD criteria [odds ratio (OR), 4.17, 1.83–9.48].

52. **Chapuy M, Preziosi P, Maamer M,** et al. Prevalence of vitamin D insufficiency in an adult normal population. Osteoporos Int 1997;7:439–443.

The vitamin D status of a general adult population living in 20 different urban cities in France was estimated between the months of November and April. Individuals living in northern regions had the lowest vitamin D levels, and the highest levels were observed in southern regions. A significant "sun" effect ($r = 0.72$; $p = 0.03$) and latitude effect ($r = -0.79$; $p = 0.01$) was observed. Fourteen percent of individuals had 25-OHD levels less than or equal to 30 nmol/L (12 ng/mL), which is the lower limit (<2 SD) for a normal adult population measured in winter. Serum intact PTH (iPTH) had a significantly negative correlation with serum 25-OHD levels ($p < 0$ <0.01). Serum iPTH remained stable when serum 25-OHD values were greater than 78 nmol/L (31 ng/mL), but increased when serum 25-OHD values fell below this level. Serum iPTH values reached the upper limit of normal (55 pg/mL) when serum 25-OHD levels dropped to 113 nmol/L (4.6 ng/mL) or lower.

53. **Sahota O, Masud T, San P, Hosking D.** Vitamin D insufficiency increases bone turnover markers and enhances bone loss at the hip in patients with established vertebral osteoporosis. Clin Endocrinol 1999;51:217–221.

The relationship between bone turnover markers and bone mineral density (BMD) in vitamin D insufficient and vitamin D sufficient patients with established vertebral osteoporosis was examined in this study. A significant correlation was observed between parathyroid hormone (PTH) and 25-OHD ($r = -0.42$, $p < 0.01$). Vitamin D insufficiency was present in 26.9% of subjects (25-OHD ≥6.1 and ≤12 μg/L), resulting in a statistically significant increase in bone turnover markers compared with the vitamin D sufficient group (bone alkaline phosphatase, $p < 0.05$; osteocalcin, $p < 0.01$; hydroxyproline, $p < 0.05$; free deoxypyridinoline, $p < 0.05$; and lower BMD at the total hip, $p < 0.01$).

54. **Mosekilde L.** Vitamin D and the elderly. Clin Endocrinol 2005;62:265–281.

This article reviews vitamin D status in the elderly, including the definition and prevalence of vitamin D insufficiency and deficiency, the relationship between vitamin D status and diseases common in the elderly, and the utility of treatment with vitamin D and calcium.

55. **Adams J, Kantorovich V, Wu C,** et al. Resolution of vitamin D insufficiency in osteopenic patients results in rapid recovery of bone mineral density. J Clin Endocrinol Metab 1999;84:2729–2730.

This prospective study investigated vitamin D status in 118 community-dwelling individuals with osteopenia or osteoporosis over 2 years, and the role of vitamin D supplementation in reversal of bone loss. Low serum 25-OHD levels (≤14 ng/mL) were found in 18 subjects, and of those, 12 consented to receive replacement with 50,000 IU vitamin D_2 twice weekly for 5 weeks. Treatment resulted in significant increases in 25-OHD (+24.3 ± 16.9 ng/mL; $p < 0.001$) and the fasting urinary calcium or creatinine excretion ratio (+0.06 ± 0.004; $p = 0.01$), and significant decreases in serum parathyroid hormone (PTH) (−32.9 ± 36.9 pg/mL; $p < 0.001$) and osteocalcin (−4.9 ± 2.4 ng/mL; $p < 0.001$). Both the lumbar spine ($p < 0.001$) and femoral neck ($p = 0.03$) bone mineral density (BMD) significantly increased 4% to 5% annually after vitamin D repletion.

56. **Dawson-Hughes B, Harris S, Krall E, Dallal G.** Effect of calcium and vitamin D supplementation on bone density in men and women 65 years of age or older. N Engl J Med 1997;337:670–676.

This prospective, placebo-controlled trial evaluated the use of vitamin D and calcium supplementation in 389 community-dwelling adults older than 65 years to evaluate its efficacy in reducing the incidence of nonvertebral fractures. There were significantly fewer nonvertebral fractures in the calcium–vitamin D group over the 3 years studied compared with subjects receiving placebo ($p = 0.02$). Patients receiving calcium–vitamin D (cholecalciferol) had significantly greater increases in bone mineral density (BMD) at all skeletal sites after 1 year compared with placebo [femoral neck, +0.5 ± 4.80% and −0.70 ± 5.03%, respectively ($p = 0.02$); spine, +2.12 ± 4.06 and +1.22 ± 4.25% ($p = 0.04$); and total body, +0.06 ± 1.83 and −1.09 ± 1.71% ($p < 0.001$)], but only total-body BMD was significantly greater in the treatment group during the second and third years.

57. **Papadimitropoulos E, Wells G, Shea B,** et al., for the Osteoporosis Methodology Group and the Osteoporosis Research Advisory Group. Meta-analyses of therapies for postmenopausal osteoporosis. VIII: Meta-analysis of the efficacy of vitamin D treatment in preventing osteoporosis in postmenopausal women. Endocr Rev 2002; 23:560–569.

58. **Favus M.** Postmenopausal osteoporosis and the detection of so-called secondary causes of low bone density. J Clin Endocrinol Metab 2005;90:3800–3801.

This editorial discusses the importance of measuring 25-OHD levels in patients with low bone mineral density (BMD) before initiating treatment in postmenopausal women with osteoporosis. Secondary causes of osteoporosis are reviewed, as well as a suggested complete work-up, including measuring fasting serum calcium, creatinine, 25-OHD, calculated or direct measurement of creatinine clearance, and 24-hour urine calcium excretion prior to beginning treatment with bisphosphonates.

59. **Holick M, Siris E, Binkley N,** et al. Prevalence of vitamin D inadequacy among postmenopausal North American women receiving osteoporosis therapy. J Clin Endocrinol Metab 2005;90:3215–3224.

Risk factors for suboptimal (<30 ng/mL) 25-OHD were evaluated in 1,536 community-dwelling postmenopausal North American women. The mean age of the women studied was 72, and 92% were Caucasian. Mean serum 25-OHD was 30.4 ng/mL, 18% had a serum 25-OHD level of less than 20 ng/mL, 36% had a level of less than 25 ng/mL, and 52% had a level of less than 30 ng/mL. There was a significantly higher prevalence of suboptimal 25-OHD in subjects who took less than 400 IU/day of vitamin D when compared with subjects taking 400 IU/day or more. A significantly negative correlation was observed between serum parathyroid hormone (PTH) and 25-OHD. Vitamin D insufficiency risk factors included age, BMI, race, medications known to affect vitamin D metabolism, exercise, vitamin D supplementation, education, and physical counseling regarding vitamin D.

60. **Passeri G, Pini G, Troiano L,** et al. Low vitamin D status, high bone turnover, and bone fractures in centenarians. J Clin Endocrinol Metab 2003;88:5109–5115.

Bone status and metabolism were assessed in 104 healthy individuals over 98 years of age (90 women, 14 men). Thirty-eight subjects had sustained a total of 55 fractures throughout their lives, and 75% of these were fragility fractures. The proximal femur was involved in 28 of the fractures, 14 of which occurred after age 94. Serum 25-OHD was undetectable in 99 of the 104 patients. Parathyroid hormone (PTH) and serum C-terminal collagen type 1 were high in 64% and 90% of patients, respectively, with a trend toward hypocalcemia. Serum interleukin-6 (IL-6) was elevated in 81% of subjects, and was positively correlated with PTH and negatively correlated with serum calcium. Bone alkaline phosphatase was close to the upper limit of normal. Using bone ultrasonography, most centenarians had low values, and ultrasonographic parameters correlated with resorption markers. The authors postulate that extreme decades of life are marked by a pathophysiologic sequence of events that link low serum calcium, vitamin D deficiency, and secondary hyperparathyroidism with an increase in bone resorption and severe osteopenia.

61. **Thomas M, Lloyd-Jones D, Thadhani R,** et al. Hypovitaminosis D in medical inpatients. N Engl J Med 1998;338:777–783.

This study assessed vitamin D deficiency and associated risk factors among 290 patients hospitalized on a general medical service. Vitamin D deficiency (serum 25-OHD ≤15 ng/mL) was found in 57% of patients; of those patients, 22% were found to have severe vitamin D deficiency (25-OHD <8 ng/mL). An inverse relationship was observed between serum 25-OHD and parathyroid hormone (PTH). Significant univariate predictors of hypovitaminosis D included lower vitamin D intake, less exposure to ultraviolet light, anticonvulsant-drug therapy, renal dialysis, nephrotic syndrome, hypertension, diabetes mellitus, winter season, higher serum concentrations of PTH and alkaline phosphatase, and lower serum concentrations of ionized calcium and albumin. Vitamin D deficiency occurred in 69% of patients who consumed less than the recommended daily allowance of vitamin D and 43% of patients with vitamin D intakes above the recommended daily allowance. Using a multivariate model, winter season, housebound status, and inadequate vitamin D intake were independent predictors of hypovitaminosis D. Among a subgroup of patients less than 65 years of age without known risk factors for hypovitaminosis D, 42% had a vitamin D deficiency.

62. **Tangpricha V, Pearce E, Chen T, Holick M.** Vitamin D insufficiency among free-living healthy young adults. Am J Med 2002;112:659–662.

63. **Bell N, Jackson G.** Role of vitamin D in the pathogenesis and treatment of osteoporosis. Endocr Pract 1995;1(1):44–47.

This article reviews vitamin D metabolism, changes in vitamin D metabolism that occur with aging and menopause, and its role in senile osteoporosis.

64. **Ebeling P, Sandgren M, DiMagno E,** et al. Evidence of an age-related decrease in intestinal responsiveness to vitamin D: Relationship between serum 1,25-dihydroxyvitamin D_3 and intestinal vitamin D receptor concentrations in normal women. J Clin Endocrinol Metab 1992;75:176–182.

This study investigated the relationship between serum 1,25-dihydroxyvitamin D_3 [1,25-$(OH)_2D_3$], calcium absorption, and intestinal vitamin D receptor (VDR) among 44 healthy, ambulatory women ages 20 to 87 years. VDR concentrations were measured from biopsy specimens taken from the second part of the duodenum during esophagogastroduodenoscopy (EGD) in 35 of the women. Despite an age-related increase in serum PTH ($r = 0.48$; $p < 0.001$) and in serum 1,25-$(OH)_2D_3$ concentration ($r = 0.32$; $p < 0.05$), there was a decrease in intestinal VDR concentration ($r = -0.38$; $p = 0.03$), and fractional calcium absorption did not change with age. Based on these findings, the authors postulate impaired intestinal responsiveness to 1,25-$(OH)_2D_3$ action contributes to the lack of an increase in serum 1,25-$(OH)_2D_3$ concentration late in life.

65. **Levis S, Gomez A, Jimenez C,** et al. Vitamin D deficiency and seasonal variation in an adult south Florida population. J Clin Endocrinol Metab 2005;90:1557–1562.

The prevalence of vitamin D deficiency in adults living in south Florida was investigated to determine if seasonal variation occurs in regions of year-round sunny weather. The mean winter 25(OH)D concentration was 24.9 ± 8.7 ng/mL (62.3 ± 21.8 nmol/L) in men and 22.4 ± 8.2 ng/mL (56.0 ± 20.5 nmol/L) in women. The prevalence of hypovitaminosis D [25(OH)D <20 ng/mL or <50 nmol/L] in winter was 38% in men and 40% in women. Ninety-nine of the 212 subjects returned for the end of summer visit, and the mean 25(OH)D concentration was 31.0 ± 11.0 ng/mL (77.5 ± 27.5 nmol/L) in men and 25.0 ± 9.4 ng/mL (62.5 ± 23.5 nmol/L) in women. A statistically significant increase of 14% in men and 13% in women for 25(OH)D concentrations in the summer was observed.

66. **Syed Z, Khan A.** Skeletal effects of primary hyperparathyroidism. Endocr Pract 2000;6:385–388.

This was a metaanalysis study examining the effect of primary hyperparathyroidism on bone mass and fracture risk. Bone density was well preserved at cancellous bone sites. Fracture incidence in patients with primary hyperparathyroidism is not clear, as retrospective and case-control studies have found conflicting results. Parathyroidectomy does help improve bone mineral density (BMD) at both the femoral neck and lumbar spine. Hormone replacement therapy in postmenopausal women with primary hyperparathyroidism is effective in improving BMD and decreasing bone turnover. Early studies with alendronate show improved BMD. Calcimimetic agents may become a useful treatment option in the medical management of primary hyperparathyroidism.

67. **Khan A, Bilezikian J.** Primary hyperparathyroidism: Pathophysiology and impact on bone. CMAJ 2000;163:184–187.

This article reviews the pathophysiology of primary hyperparathyroidism and the effectiveness of the various treatment modalities.

68. **Bilezikian J, Potts J, Fuleihan G, et al.** Summary statement from a workshop on asymptomatic primary hyperparathyroidism: A perspective for the 21st century. J Clin Endocrinol Metab 2002;87:5353–5361.

69. **Sitges-Serra A, Girvent M, Pereira J, et al.** Bone mineral density in menopausal women with primary hyperparathyroidism before and after parathyroidectomy. World J Surg 2004;28:1148–1152.

This prospective, observational study examined the prevalence of reduced bone mineral density (BMD) in women with primary hyperparathyroidism (pHPT). The prevalence of reduced BMD was 80% to 100%, depending on the site. PTH was higher among patients with osteoporosis (319 ± 181 pg/mL) than in those with osteopenia (230 ± 83 pg/mL) or normal BMD (148 ± 81 pg/mL; $p < 0.04$). Of 28 patients who had a parathyroidectomy, BMD significantly improved at all sites after one year, especially for patients with osteoporosis. Age correlated inversely with BMD increases at the femoral sites ($r = -0.47$; $p = 0.02$) but not at the lumbar spine; 25-OHD$_3$ levels correlated inversely with BMD increases at proximal femur ($r = -0.76$; $p < 0.0001$). One year post-parathyroidectomy, significant increases in BMD, most pronounced at femoral sites, were observed in younger patients, in patients with preoperative osteoporosis, and in those with lower serum levels on 25-OHD$_3$.

70. **Khosla S, Melton L, Wermers R, et al.** Primary hyperparathyroidism and the risk of fracture: a population-based study. J Bone Miner Res 1999;14:1700–1707.

This large, population-based inception cohort of 407 cases of primary HPT investigated whether or not mild, asymptomatic primary hyperparathyroidism (HPT) increases fracture risk. The subjects with primary HPT enrolled mostly had mild disease (mean serum calcium, 10.9 ± 0.6 mg/dL). Overall fracture risk was significantly increased in patients with primary HPT [standardized incidence ratio (SIR) 1.3, 95% CI,1.1–1.5]. Primary hyperparathyroidism was associated with an increased risk of vertebral, distal forearm, rib, and pelvic fractures, with only a marginal increase in risk of proximal femur fracture. Significant predictors of fracture risk by univariate analysis were increased age and female gender. Higher serum calcium levels were also associated with increased fracture risk, and parathyroidectomy may have had a protective effect. Using multivariate analysis, only age (RH per 10-year increase, 1.6; 95% CI, 1.4–1.9) and female gender (RH, 2.3; 95% CI, 1.2–4.1) remained significant independent predictors of fracture risk.

71. **Silverberg S, Shane E, Jacobs T, et al.** A 10-year prospective study of primary hyperparathyroidism with or without parathyroid surgery. N Engl J Med 1999;341: 1249–1255.

This 10-year prospective study evaluated the clinical course of 121 individuals with primary hyperthyroidism, 83% of whom were asymptomatic. Fifty percent of patients underwent parathyroidectomy during the study, and this led to normalization of serum calcium concentrations and a mean increase in lumbar spine bone mineral density (BMD) of 8 ±

2% after 1 year ($p = 0.005$) and 12 ± 3% after 10 years ($p = 0.003$). Femoral neck BMD increased 6 ± 1% after 1 year ($p = 0.002$) and 14 ± 4% after 10 years ($p = 0.002$). No significant change was observed for BMD of the radius. Of the 52 asymptomatic patients who did not undergo surgery, there were no changes in serum calcium, urinary calcium, or BMD. However, 27% of these patients had progression of disease, which was defined as the development of at least one new indication for parathyroidectomy.

72. **Rao D, Phillips E, Divine G, Talpos G.** Randomized controlled clinical trial of surgery versus no surgery in patients with mild asymptomatic primary hyperparathyroidism. J Clin Endocrinol Metab 2004;89:5415–5422.

This randomized, prospective, controlled clinical trial examined the benefits and risks associated with parathyroidectomy in treating mild, asymptomatic primary hyperparathyroidism. Patients were randomly assigned to receive either parathyroidectomy ($n = 25$) or regular follow-up ($n = 28$). After parathyroidectomy, bone mineral density (BMD) increased at the spine (1.2%/y, $p < 0.001$), femoral neck (0.4%/y, $p = 0.031$), total hip (0.3%/y, $p = 0.07$), and forearm (0.4%/y, $p < 0.001$), and a decrease was observed for serum total and ionized calcium, serum parathyroid hormone (PTH), and urine calcium ($p < 0.001$ for all). Patients who did not undergo parathyroidectomy experienced a decrease in BMD at the femoral neck (-0.4%/y, $p = 0.117$) and total hip (-0.6%/y, $p = 0.007$), but had increased BMD at the spine (0.5%/y; $p =$ ns) and forearm (0.2%/y, $p = 0.047$), with no significant changes in biochemical measurements of disease. Therefore, parathyroidectomy significantly affected BMD only at the femoral neck (group difference of 0.8%/y; $p = 0.01$) and total hip (group difference of 1.0%/y; $p = 0.001$) but not at the forearm (group difference of 0.2%/y) or spine (group difference of 0.6%/y). Using a 36-item short-form health survey to determine quality of life, parathyroidectomy was associated with a modest measurable benefit in social and emotional role function ($p = 0.007$ and 0.012, respectively). Using a revised symptom checklist, parathyroidectomy was associated with a significant decrease in anxiety ($p = 0.003$) and phobia ($p = 0.024$).

73. **Vestergaard P, Mosekilde L.** Cohort study on effects of parathyroid surgery on multiple outcomes in primary hyperparathyroidism. BMJ 2003;327:530–534.

This cohort study of 3,213 patients with primary hyperparathyroidism investigated the effects of surgery compared with conservative treatment. Sixty percent of patients underwent parathyroidectomy. At the time of diagnosis of primary HPT, patients who ultimately underwent surgery had a lower prevalence of previous fracture (OR, 0.64; 95% CI, 0.51–0.80), acute myocardial infarction (0.59, 0.42–0.83), stroke (0.57, 0.37–0.88), psychiatric disorders (0.54, 0.31–0.94), and painful muscle disorders (0.44, 0.26–0.76), whereas kidney stones (2.49, 1.93–3.23) and acute pancreatitis (2.77, 1.33–5.76) were more prevalent. After diagnosis, patients treated surgically had lower risks of fracture (hazard ratio 0.69, 0.56–0.84) and gastric ulcers (0.59, 0.41–0.84) than those treated conservatively. Patients treated surgically had a higher prevalence of events involving kidney or urinary tract stones than nonsurgical patients (1.87, 1.30–2.68). Mortality was lower among surgical patients (0.65, 0.57–0.73).

74. **Shane E, Mancini D, Aaronson K,** et al. Bone mass, vitamin D deficiency, and hyperparathyroidism in congestive heart failure. Am J Med 1997;103:197–207.

Patients with severe congestive heart failure (CHF; NYHA Class III or IV) who were being considered for heart transplant were evaluated to investigate the prevalence of osteoporosis in this cross-sectional study. Osteoporosis was present in 7% of patients at the lumbar spine, 6% at the total hip, and 19% at the femoral neck. Osteopenia was present in 43% at the lumbar spine, 47% at the total hip, and 42% at the femoral neck. Women were more severely affected ($p = 0.007$). Extremely low serum 25-OHD (≤ 9 pg/mL) and 1,25$(OH)_2$D (≤ 15 pg/mL) levels were found in 17% and 26% of the patients, respectively, and 30% of patients had high serum PTH (>65 pg/mL) levels. Low serum 1,25$(OH)_2$D and elevated serum PTH were both associated with prerenal azotemia. Bone mineral density (BMD) was not associated with vitamin D or PTH status. Patients with more severe CHF had significantly decreased levels of vitamin D metabolites and increased bone turnover, while elevated PTH was associated with improved left ventricular ejection fraction (LVEF) (21 ± 1 vs. 18 ± 1%; $p = 0.05$) and correlated positively with resting cardiac output (CO) ($r = 0.220$; $p = 0.04$).

75. **Shane E, Silverberg S, Donovan D,** et al. Osteoporosis in lung transplantation candidates with end-stage pulmonary disease. Am J Med 1996;101:262–269.

This study investigated the association between patients with end-stage pulmonary disease who were awaiting lung transplantation and the prevalence of osteoporosis. Patients enrolled included 28 with chronic obstructive pulmonary disease (COPD), 11 with cystic fibrosis, idiopathic pulmonary fibrosis, and 31 with other lung diseases (Other). Osteoporosis was present in 30% of all patients at the lumbar spine and 49% of all patients at the femoral neck. Of all patients, osteopenia was present in an additional 35% of patients at the lumbar spine and 31% at the femoral neck. For patients with COPD, cystic fibrosis, and idiopathic pulmonary fibrosis, the average lumbar spine T-score was in the osteopenic range. Patients with COPD and cystic fibrosis had significantly lower bone mineral density (BMD) at the femoral neck than patients in the other lung disease category ($p < 0.001$). Vertebral fractures were present in 29% of COPD patients and 25% of cystic fibrosis patients. Low BMD in cystic fibrosis patients confirmed that their low BMD was not due to smaller body size. Vitamin D deficiency was present in 36% of cystic fibrosis patients and 20% of patients with COPD and other lung diseases. Patients with a history of treatment with glucocorticoids had significantly more vertebral fractures ($p < 0.05$), and the length of exposure was negatively correlated with lumbar spine BMD ($r = -0.398$; $p = 0.008$). COPD and Other patients not treated with steroids had mild osteopenia at the lumbar spine (0.972 ± 0.06 g/cm^2; $T = -1.2 \pm 0.6$). Also, only a minority of patients on steroids were on a regimen to prevent osteoporosis.

76. **Trombetti A, Gerbase M, Spiliopoulos A,** et al. Bone mineral density in lung-transplant recipients before and after graft: prevention of lumbar spine post-transplantation-accelerated bone loss by pamidronate. J Heart Lung Transplant 2000; 19:736–743.

    This prospective study evaluated bone mineral density (BMD) in patients before and after receiving lung transplantation, and compared different treatment modalities of osteoporosis in this population. After adjusting for gender and mean age, lumbar spine and femoral neck BMD was significantly decreased before transplantation (-0.6 ± 0.2, $p < 0.01$, and -1.5 ± 0.2, $p < 0.001$, respectively). Prior to transplantation, 29% were osteoporotic (T-score < -2.5), whereas 55% had a T-score below -1.0. Pamidronate decreased the rate of lumbar spinal bone loss during the first 5 months, and at 1 year resulted in a significant increase of BMD compared with the calcium–vitamin D group ($p < 0.002$), and also at the femoral neck (but not significantly). Twenty-five percent (3 out of 12) patients receiving calcium–vitamin D experienced a clinically evident fracture, whereas only 5% (1 out of 20) from the pamidronate group suffered a fracture.

77. **Ninkovic M, Love S, Tom B,** et al. High prevalence of osteoporosis in patients with chronic liver disease prior to liver transplantation. Calcif Tissue Int 2001;69: 321–326.

    This study investigated bone mineral density (BMD) in adults with chronic liver disease awaiting liver transplantation. Osteoporosis at either the lumbar spine or femoral neck was present in 36.6%, osteopenia in 48.1%, and normal BMD in only 15.2% of patients. There was no difference in prevalence of osteoporosis between genders. Among women, those with osteoporosis were close to 10 years older than those with normal BMD ($p = 0.002$). On average, patients with osteoporosis had lower body weight than those with normal BMD ($p = 0.003$). T-scores in patients with cholestatic liver disease were lower than in patients with noncholestatic disease, and were the lowest in patients with cystic fibrosis. Using logistic regression, significant independent risk factors for osteoporosis in women were increasing age ($p = 0.004$; OR = 1.12; CI, 1.04–1.21) and lower body weight ($p = 0.01$; OR = 0.95; CI, 0.91–0.99), but menopause and presence or absence of cholestasis were not significant. No independent risk factors were found in men.

78. **Shane E, Rivas M, McMahon D,** et al. Bone loss and turnover after cardiac transplantation. J Clin Endocrinol Metab 1997;82:1497–1506.

    This 3-year prospective study investigated the causes and patterns of bone loss after cardiac transplantation. Seventy patients were enrolled, and patients received daily calcium and vitamin D supplementation. The mean rate of bone loss during the first year was $7.3 \pm 0.9\%$ at the lumbar spine and $10.5 \pm 1.1\%$ at the femoral neck. Compared with the first year, the rate of bone loss slowed ($p < 0.001$) at both sites ($0.9 \pm 0.9\%$ and $0.1 \pm 1.0\%$, respectively) during the second year. Although bone mineral density (BMD) at the femoral neck did not change during the third year, lumbar spine BMD increased at a rate of $2.4 \pm 0.8\%$/y ($p < 0.02$ compared with year 2). The mean lumbar spine BMD decreased rapidly during the first 6 months of the first year, after which there was no further decline. The femoral neck continued to fall at an annual rate of $8.2 \pm 1.3\%$ during the second half of the first year, however. Rates of bone loss were not different between men and women. At 1 and

3 months after transplantation, decreases in serum testosterone and osteocalcin and increases in all bone resorption markers occurred. Levels returned to baseline at six months. Increased exposure to prednisone, lower serum concentrations of vitamin D metabolites, increased suppression of osteocalcin, elevated bone resorption marker levels, and lower serum testosterone concentrations in men, were associated with higher rates of bone loss.

79. **Floreani A, Fries W, Luisetto G,** et al. Bone metabolism in orthotopic liver transplantation: A prospective study. Liver Transpl Surg 1998;4:311–319.

Fifty-four patients with end-stage liver disease who subsequently underwent orthotopic liver transplantation (OLT) were enrolled in this study to evaluate bone mineral density (BMD) and mineral metabolism in OLT patients. Prior to transplantation, 40.7% of patients had BMD below the fracture threshold. BMD was significantly ($p < 0.001$) affected by age, PTH level, and serum creatinine level, but not by liver function tests or the presence or absence of cholestasis. After OLT, a 1.4% decrease ($p < 0.006$) was observed in BMD at 3 months post-transplant. After 3 months, BMD returned to pretransplant values. At 6 ($p < 0.02$) and 12 months ($p < 0.001$) after OLT, serum BGP significantly increased, indicating metabolic activation of osteoblasts. PTH levels increased gradually at 3 ($p < 0.02$), 6 ($p < 0.001$), and 12 ($p < 0.0001$) months after OLT, but did not appear to be caused by cyclosporine-induced nephropathy.

80. **Hussaini S, Oldroyd B, Stewart S,** et al. Regional bone mineral density after orthotopic liver transplantation. Eur J Gastroenterol Hepatol 1999;11:157–163.

This retrospective analysis examined bone mineral density (BMD) in patients before and up to 2 years after liver transplantation. Osteoporosis was found in 23% of patients pre-transplant. No change in total BMD was observed before and after transplantation. At 1 month after transplantation, however, there was a fall in lumbar spine BMD (1.04 ± 0.03 to 1.02 ± 0.03 g/cm^2; $p < 0.04$). This decrease in lumbar spine BMD was observed up to 12 months, with BMD at months 18 to 24 being comparable to pre-transplant values. Femoral neck BMD fell after 6 to 9 months (0.96 ± 0.06 to 0.83 ± 0.04 g/cm^2; $p < 0.03$), and subsequently remained below pre-transplant levels until the end of the follow-up period. These results suggest that total BMD does not decrease after transplantation, but regional lumbar spine and femoral neck BMD does fall with a risk of femoral neck fracture for up to 2 years post-transplant.

81. **Rodino M, Shane E.** Osteoporosis after organ transplantation. Am J Med 1998; 104:459–469.

This article reviews osteoporosis in patients receiving organ transplantation, and the need for early preventative treatment in transplant patients. The use of steroids and drugs that inhibit calcineurin-calmodulin plays a role in the rapid bone loss seen in patients after transplantation. The incidence of fracture during the first year after transplantation is anywhere from 8% to 65%, with fracture rates being the lowest in renal transplant recipients and highest in patients receiving a liver for primary biliary cirrhosis. The first 6 to 12 months after transplantation appear to be associated with the highest rates of bone loss and fracture. Hypogonadal men and postmenopausal women are at increased risk of osteoporosis and fractures among transplant recipients. The rapid bone loss within the first 3 to 6 months is multifactorial, with uncoupling of bone formation from resorption playing a possible role.

82. **Leidig-Bruckner G, Hosch S, Dodidou P,** et al. Frequency and predictors of osteoporotic fractures after cardiac or liver transplantation: A follow-up study. Lancet 2001;357:342–347.

This prospective study evaluated the prevalence of osteoporotic fractures in patients after cardiac or liver transplantation, and assessed risk factors for fractures in this population. Patients who had heart transplants experienced more vertebral fractures in the first and second year (Kaplan-Meier estimates, first year, 21%; second year, 27%) than those receiving liver transplants (first year, 14%; second year, 21%). One-third of patients from both groups experienced one or more vertebral fractures during the third and fourth years. Seven percent of patients experienced nonvertebral fractures after liver transplantation, and 3% of cardiac transplantation patients had a vascular necrosis of the hip head. No dose-dependent effect of immunosuppressive therapy on fracture risk was identified in either group. Using multivariate analysis, independent predictors were age (hazard ratio increase of 5 years: 1.71; 95% CI, 1.1–2.7) and lumbar bone mineral density (BMD) (decrease of 1 SD T-score, 1.97; 95% CI, 1.2–3.2) in cardiac transplantation patients, and vertebral fractures before transplantation (6.07; 95% CI, 1.7–21.7) for liver transplantation patients.

83. **Harpavat M, Keljo D, Regueiro M.** Metabolic bone disease in inflammatory bowel disease. J Clin Gastroenterol 2004;38:218–224.

   This article reviews the risk of osteoporosis among patients with inflammatory bowel disease, including specific risk factors and treatment options for these patients.

84. **Ardizzone S, Bollani S, Bettica P,** et al. Altered bone metabolism in inflammatory bowel disease: There is a difference between Crohn's disease and ulcerative colitis. J Intern Med 2000;247:63–70.

   This cross-sectional study evaluated bone metabolism in patients with inflammatory bowel disease, and also examined differences in the mechanisms of bone loss in patients with Crohn disease (CD) versus ulcerative colitis (UC). Normal bone mineral density (BMD) was found in only 8% of CD patients and 15% UC patients, while osteopenia was present in 55% CD and 67% UC patients, and osteoporosis in 37% CD and 18% UC patients. Compared with control subjects, 1,25-OHD$_3$ levels were significantly lower in both CD and UC patients ($p < 0.05$). No significant differences were found for levels of PTH or 25-OHD$_3$ concentrations between CD and UC patients and controls. Bone turnover was significantly increased in UC patients compared with CD patients for both osteocalcin (OC; CD = 7.77 ± 5.06, UC = 10.03 ± 6.24, C = 6.58 ± 2.87, $p < 0.05$ vs. C) and type 1 collagen C-terminal telopeptide (CD = 5.74 ± 3.94, UC = 10.2 ± 8.47, C = 3.48 ± 0.95, $p < 0.05$ vs. CD and C). In CD patients, the femur T-score was significantly inversely related to disease duration ($r^2 = 0.125$, $F = 6.06$). In UC patients, the spine T-score was inversely related to age ($r^2 = 0.107$, $F = 5.49$) and significantly related to sex (more negative in males: $r^2 = 0.3$, $F = 16.1$); the femur T-score was significantly related to sex (more negative in males) and inversely related to the cumulative prednisolone dose ($r^2 = 0.283$, $F = 7.3$).

85. **Bernstein C, Blanchard J, Leslie W,** et al. The incidence of fracture among patients with inflammatory bowel disease. Ann Intern Med 2000;133:795–799.

   The incidence of fractures among individuals with inflammatory bowel disease was assessed in this population-based matched cohort study. A significantly increased incidence of fractures occurred among individuals with IBD at the spine [incidence rate ratio (IRR), 1.74 (95% CI, 1.34–2.24); $p < 0.001$], wrist or forearm [IRR, 1.33 (CI, 1.11–1.58); $p = 0.001$], hip [IRR, 1.59 (CI, 1.27–2.00); $p < 0.001$], and rib [IRR, 1.25 (CI, 1.02–1.52); $p = 0.03$] and of any of these fractures [IRR, 1.41 (CI, 1.27–1.56); $p < 0.001$]. These results show an incidence of fracture among IBD patients that is 40% higher than that of the general population.

86. **Silvennoinen J, Niemela S, Lehtola J,** et al. A controlled study of bone mineral density in patients with inflammatory bowel disease. Gut 1995;37:71–76.

   Bone mineral density was assessed among patients with inflammatory bowel disease to determine the prevalence and risk factors for low bone mineral density (BMD) in this population. BMD was significantly lower in patients with IBD than control patients at the lumbar spine (1.177 vs. 1.228, p 0.034), femoral neck (0.948 vs. 1.001, $p = 0.009$), and the trochanter (0.838 vs. 0.888, $p = 0.012$). There was no significant effect on BMD based on the type or extent of IBD or in patients with a history of a previous small bowel resection. There was a small, but statistically significant, negative correlation between BMD and total lifetime corticosteroid dose (lumbar spine $r = -0.164$, $p = 0.04$; femoral neck $r = -0.185$, $p = 0.02$; Ward triangle $r = -0.167$, $p = 0.04$; trochanter $r = -0.237$, $p = 0.003$). Patients who had taken more than 10 g of steroids over their lifetime had a particularly low BMD compared with patients who had taken 5 g or less for their lifetime steroid intake ($p < 0.05$).

87. **Vazquez H, Mazure R, Gonzalez D,** et al. Risk of fractures in celiac disease patients: a cross-sectional, case-control study. Am J Gastroenterol 2000;95:183–189.

   This cross-sectional, retrospective review assessed the prevalence of fractures in patients with celiac disease. There were significantly more nonvertebral fractures among patients with celiacs (25%) when compared with controls (8%; odds ratio, 3.5; 95% CI, 1.8–7.2; $p < 0.0001$). Spinal radiographs showed evidence of lumbar spine deformities in only two patients, but using lateral films, nine lumbar spine vertebral deformities (as well as five peripheral fractures) were detected in celiac patients compared with four in the control subjects. Fractures were detected in 80% of patients before the diagnosis of celiac disease or in patients noncompliant with the gluten-free diet. After starting treatment, only 7% of patients suffered fractures. Patients with fractures were diagnosed later ($p < 0.06$) and remained without a diagnosis for a longer period of time ($p < 0.05$).

88. **Selby P, Davies M, Adams J, Mawer E.** Bone loss in celiac disease is related to secondary hyperparathyroidism. J Bone Miner Res 1999;14:652–657.

This study investigated the relationship between low bone mineral density (BMD) at peripheral sites in celiac disease and parathyroid hormone (PTH) levels. Thirty-five patients with celiac disease on an established gluten-free diet were enrolled. At all sites, BMD was below normal for the patient's age and gender. The most pronounced bone loss was at the distal forearm, where the BMD was 1.40 SD below expected ($p < 0.001$). There was a negative relationship between BMD and PTH levels at the forearm ($r = -0.49$, $p = 0.009$), confirming the presence of secondary parathyroidism. A negative relationship between 1,25-OH-$_2$D and BMD occurred at the forearm and lumbar spine. There was no relationship between BMD and 25-hydroxyvitamin D at any skeletal sites.

89. **Meyer D, Stavropolous S, Diamond B,** et al. Osteoporosis in a North American adult population with celiac disease. Am J Gastroenterol 2001;96:112–119.

The presence of osteoporosis among 123 patients with celiac disease who lived in the United States was determined. Osteoporosis was present in 34% of patients at the lumbar spine, 27% at the femoral neck, and 36% at the radius. Osteopenia was present in 38% at the lumbar spine, 44% at the femoral neck, and 32% at the radius. Compared with age-matched controls, men were affected more severely than women. No differences were found in bone mineral density (BMD) regarding the use of a gluten-free diet. After measuring BMD 16 months after 5 patients started a gluten-free diet, however, BMD did increase by 7.5% at the femoral neck ($p < 0.02$). Sixteen patients who had followed a gluten-free diet for an average of 12 years were found to have stable BMD over 2 years of additional observation.

90. **Stenson W, Newberry R, Lorenz R,** et al. Increased prevalence of celiac disease and need for routine screening among patients with osteoporosis. Arch Intern Med 2005;165:393–399.

This study evaluated 840 individuals, 266 with and 574 without osteoporosis, to determine the prevalence of celiac disease among osteoporotic patients. Celiac disease was diagnosed using serologic screening in 4.5% of patients with osteoporosis and 1.0% of patients without osteoporosis. Biopsy-proven celiac disease was present in 3.4% of the osteoporotic patients and 0.2% of the nonosteoporotic patients. Antitissue transglutaminase levels correlated with the severity of osteoporosis. After treating patients with celiac disease with a gluten-free diet, there was a noticeable improvement in T-scores.

91. **Vestergaard P, Mosekilde L.** Fracture risk in patients with celiac disease, Crohn's disease, and ulcerative colitis: A nationwide follow-up study of 16,416 patients in Denmark. Am J Epidemiol 2002;156:1–10.

Fracture risk among 16,416 Danish patients with celiac disease, Crohn disease, or ulcerative colitis was evaluated. There was no increase in fracture risk for celiac disease patients before or after diagnosis. Among patients with Crohn disease, the overall fracture risk was increased before diagnosis (incidence rate ratio = 1.15; 95% CI, 1.00–1.32) and after diagnosis (incidence rate ratio = 1.19; 95% CI, 1.06, 1.33). There was a small increase in fracture risk at the time of diagnosis in patients with ulcerative colitis, but overall fracture risk was not increased. Crohn disease was associated with a small increase in overall fracture risk, while celiac disease and ulcerative colitis were not.

92. **Abrahamsen B, Andersen I, Christensen S,** et al. Utility of testing for monoclonal bands in serum of patients with suspected osteoporosis: Retrospective, cross sectional study. BMJ 2005;330:818.

This retrospective, cross-sectional, observational study evaluated the utility of measuring monoclonal bands (M component) in the serum of patients referred to osteoporosis clinics. The M component was found in the serum of 4.9% of patients with osteoporosis and 2.2% of patients without osteoporosis ($\chi^2 = 3.66$, $p = 0.04$). Three patients with osteoporosis were diagnosed with multiple myeloma (absolute risk, 0.8%; 95% CI, 0.11%–1.7%). The relative risk of multiple myeloma in patients with osteoporosis was 75 (10 to 160). The M component in serum had a specificity of 95.0% and a positive predictive value of 17.6% as a diagnostic test for multiple myeloma in patients with osteoporosis. All patients diagnosed with multiple myeloma had a history of fragility fractures. Monoclonal gammopathy of undetermined significance was diagnosed in 3.6% of patients with osteoporosis and in 2.0% of patients with normal bone mineral density (BMD) or osteopenia.

93. **Melton L, Kyle R, Achenbach S,** et al. Fracture risk with multiple myeloma: A population based study. J Bone Miner Res 2005;20:487–493.

This population-based, retrospective cohort study investigated the risk of pathologic versus osteoporotic fractures among patients with multiple myeloma. Sixteen times more fractures were observed than expected in the year prior to diagnosis, most of which were pathologic fractures of the ribs and vertebrae. After diagnosis, there was a ninefold increase in fracture risk. Of these, 69% were pathologic and another 11% were found incidentally. Excluding those two groups, subsequent fracture risk was increased threefold, with a twofold increase in the risk of developing an osteoporotic fracture. Using multivariate analyses, overall fracture risk predictors were elevated serum calcium levels and oral corticosteroid use, while pathologic fractures were additionally predicted by chemotherapy use.

94. **Dennison E, Hindmarsh P, Fall C,** et al. Profiles of endogenous circulating cortisol and bone mineral density in healthy elderly men. J Clin Endocrinol Metab 1999; 84:3058–3063.

This study investigated whether endogenous circulating cortisol concentrations play a role in bone mass among healthy male adults. A small negative association between integrated cortisol concentrations and lumbar spine bone mineral density (BMD) ($r = -0.37$; $p < 0.05$) was observed, with similar results at three of five proximal femoral sites ($p < 0.05$). Over the four years of follow-up, a significantly positive association was found between the trough cortisol concentration and bone loss rate at the lumbar spine ($r = 0.38$; $p < 0.05$), femoral neck ($r = 0.47$; $p < 0.001$), and the trochanter ($r = 0.41$; $p = 0.02$). The influence of cortisol concentration on bone loss remained significant after adjusting for cigarette smoking, adiposity, dietary calcium intake, alcohol consumption, serum testosterone and estradiol levels, and physical activity.

95. **Reynolds R, Dennison E, Walker B,** et al. Cortisol secretion and rate of bone loss in a population-based cohort of elderly men and women. Calcif Tissue Int 2005;77: 134–138.

This study evaluated whether or not endogenous glucocorticoids influence skeletal mass in 247 healthy adults ages 61 to 73. In men, an elevated peak plasma cortisol was associated with an accelerated loss of bone mineral density (BMD) at the lumbar spine ($r = 0.16$, $p = 0.05$). This remained significant after adjusting for testosterone, estradiol, 25-hydroxyvitamin D, and PTH levels ($r = 0.22$, $p = 0.01$), and after an additional adjustment for age, activity, cigarette and alcohol consumption, and Kellgren-Lawrence score ($r = 0.19$, $p = 0.03$). In women, elevated peak plasma cortisol was associated with lower baseline BMD at the femoral neck ($r = -0.23$, $p = 0.03$) and greater femoral neck loss rate ($r = 0.24$, $p = 0.02$). No associations were found between plasma cortisol concentrations after dexamethasone or urinary total cortisol metabolite excretion and BMD or bone loss at any site.

96. **Hadjidakis D, Tsagarakis S, Roboti C,** et al. Does subclinical hypercortisolism adversely affect the bone mineral density of patients with adrenal incidentalomas? Clin Endocrinol 2003;58:72–77.

This large cohort study evaluated bone mineral density (BMD) in 42 postmenopausal women with adrenal incidentalomas. Eighteen of the women were found to have subclinical hypercortisolism (SH); 24 did not. Postmenopausal women with SH had a small but significantly lower absolute and age-adjusted BMD compared with non-SH women at the femoral neck ($p < 0.05$) and trochanter ($p < 0.01$). BMDs were lower at Ward triangle in patients with SH, but results were not significant. BMD at the lumbar vertebra was not different between women with and without SH. Few patients had BMD in the osteoporotic ranges, and no significant differences were observed between the two groups. The frequency of osteopenia in women with SH was significantly higher than in women without SH at the trochanter and Ward triangle. Women with SH had significantly lower levels of serum osteocalcin compared with women without SH (18.6 ± 8.6 vs. 26.2 ± 8.1 ng/mL, $p < 0.01$). No differences were found between groups for parathyroid hormone (PTH) concentrations.

97. **Cortet B, Cortet C, Blanckaert F,** et al. Quantitative ultrasound of bone and markers of bone turnover in Cushing's syndrome. Osteoporos Int 2001;12:117–123.

The use of quantitative ultrasound (QUS) and markers of bone turnover as part of the evaluation of bone loss in patients with Cushing syndrome was investigated in this study. Both BUA (broadband ultrasound attenuation) and SI (Stiffness Index) at the heel were decreased in patients with Cushing syndrome ($p < 0.01$), but the speed of sound (SOS) was not ($p = 0.08$). Bone mineral density (BMD) was markedly decreased in Cushing syndrome at both the femoral neck and lumbar spine ($p < 0.005$). Patients with Cushing syndrome had significantly lower levels of osteocalcin ($p < 0.001$) and urinary type 1 collagen C-telopeptide breakdown products (CTX) ($p < 0.05$) compared with age- and sex-matched controls. The areas under the receiving operating characteristic curve (AUC) were 0.72 (BUA), 0.73 (SI), 0.90 (BMD at lumbar spine), 0.81 (BMD at femoral neck), 0.83 (osteocalcin), and 0.64 (CTX), respectively. AUC was significantly greater for BMD at the lumbar spine than for both BUA and SI ($p < 0.05$). AUC was higher for osteocalcin than for other bone turnover markers. AUC was not significantly different for BMD at the femoral neck when compared with BUA or SI.

98. **Minetto M, Reimondo G, Osella G,** et al. Bone loss is more severe in primary adrenal than in pituitary-dependent Cushing's syndrome. Osteoporos Int 2004;15: 855–861.

This retrospective study investigated osteopenia induced by Cushing disease (CD) due to a pituitary adrenocorticotrophic hormone (ACTH)–producing adenoma ($n = 26$) versus osteopenia due to an adrenal-dependent Cushing syndrome (ACS) ($n = 12$). Patients with ACD had a significantly larger reduction in lumbar bone mineral density (BMD) than patients with CD ($p = 0.04$). Patients with CD and ACS had greater reductions in femoral BMD than controls, but results were not significantly different between the two groups. There was a significant decrease in dehydroepiandrosterone sulfate (DHEA-S) Z-score levels among patients with ACS compared with patients with CD ($p = 0.0001$). There was a significant correlation between DHEA-S Z-scores and lumbar BMD ($r = 0.41$, $p = 0.02$) and femoral BMD ($r = 0.43$, $p = 0.01$). DHEA-S Z-scores were also significantly correlated with osteocalcin levels ($r = 0.45$, $p = 0.01$). Overall, these data suggest that patients with ACS have greater bone loss than patients with CD, but the results need to be confirmed by a study with more power.

99. **Levy F, Adams-Huet B, Pak C.** Ambulatory evaluation of nephrolithiasis: an update of a 1980 protocol. Am J Med 1995;98:50–59.

This study evaluated 1,270 ambulatory patients with recurrent nephrolithiasis to review classifications of nephrolithiasis. The most common diagnosis was hypercalciuric calcium nephrolithiasis (60.9% of patients). Six variants were found: absorptive hypercalciuria Type I and II, renal hypercalciuria, primary hyperparathyroidism, and unclassified hypercalciuria (renal phosphate leak and fasting hypercalciuria). Ten percent of patients had gouty diathesis (GD) and 35.8% of patients were diagnosed with hyperuricosuria calcium nephrolithiasis (HUCN). Patients with HUCN had hyperuricosuria and normal urinary pH, whereas GD patients had normal urinary acid and low urinary pH (< -5.5). Hyperoxaluric Ca nephrolithiasis was found in 8.1% of patients, and was subdivided into enteric, primary, and dietary variants. Hypomagnesiuric Ca nephrolithiasis (6.8%), infection stones (5.9%), and cystinuria (0.9%) were uncommon. Hypocitraturic Ca nephrolithiasis, in its idiopathic variant, affected 28% of patients. Hypocitraturia due to renal tubular acidosis or chronic diarrheal syndrome affected 3.3% of patients. The acquired problem of low urine volume (< -1 L/day) was found in 15.3% of patients.

100. **Garcia-Nieto V, Navarro J, Monge M, Garcia-Rodriguez V.** Bone mineral density in girls and their mothers with idiopathic hypercalciuria. Nephron Clin Pract 2003;94:c89–c93.

This study evaluated bone mineral density (BMD) in girls with idiopathic hypercalciuria (IH) and their mothers with IH to assess the role genetics has on bone mass in patients with IH. A Z-score of less than -1 at the lumbar spine was observed in 42.5% of the girls, while a Z-score less than -1 at the lumbar spine or femoral neck was found in 47.5% of the mothers and a T-score of less than -1 in 62.5%. The Z-score at the lumbar spine was significantly lower in girls and their mothers compared with controls, but this did not apply for the femoral neck Z-score in the mothers. The daughters of mothers with osteopenia had significantly lower Z-scores than the daughters of mothers with normal BMD. The Z-score of the girls was significantly associated with the T-score at the lumbar spine in the mothers ($r = 0.32$, $p < 0.05$). The authors suggest evaluating BMD during the third or fourth decades of life in individuals with nephrolithiasis or in children diagnosed with IH.

101. **Tasca A, Cacciola A, Ferrarese P,** et al. Bone alterations in patients with idiopathic hypercalciuria and calcium nephrolithiasis. Urology 2002;59:865–869.

Seventy patients with calcium nephrolithiasis and hypercalciuria were divided into a fasting hypercalciuria (FH, $n = 39$) and absorptive hypercalciuria (AH, $n = 31$) group to assess changes in bone mineral density (BMD) and bone turnover in these groups. Only patients with FH had a lower lumbar spine BMD than controls ($p < 0.001$), and also had elevated bone alkaline phosphatase and urinary hydroxyproline levels compared with control subjects ($p < 0.005$ and $p < 0.015$, respectively). Hypercalciuric patients had lower blood pH levels, although within the normal range, than control subjects ($p < 0.01$). Urinary hydroxyproline levels were negatively correlated with lumbar spine and femoral neck BMD in FH patients ($p < 0.001$ and $p < 0.005$, respectively), and blood pH correlated positively with lumbar spine BMD.

102. **Misael da Silva A, dos Reis L, Pereira R,** et al. Bone involvement in idiopathic hypercalciuria. Clin Nephrol 2002;57:183–191.

This study investigated bone mass in patients with idiopathic hypercalciuria. Patients with hypercalciuria (Hca) were found to have inadequate nutrition with high protein (80.9% of the patients), carbohydrate (76.2%), and sodium (90%) intake. Calcium intake was low in normocalciuric patients (Nca) (83%) and Hca (57%) patients. No differences were observed for interleukin-6 (IL-6) and tumor necrosis factor (TNF) levels between the Hca and Nca groups, but these levels were higher in the Hca patients with osteopenia compared with normocalciuric patients. IL-1 beta levels were significantly high in both Hca and Nca patients when compared with controls. Femoral neck (BMD) was lower in Hca osteopenic patients compared with Hca nonosteopenic patients and Nca patients. Serum parathyroid hormone (PTH) was negatively correlated with trabecular bone volume and positively correlated with eroded surface in Hca osteopenic patients. $1,25\text{-OHD}_3$ levels were positively correlated with osteoblastic surface. Calcium intake was positively correlated with trabecular bone volume and inversely with eroded surface. IL-6 levels were negatively correlated with Z-score of the femoral neck.

103. **Tannenbaum C, Clark J, Schwartzman K,** et al. Yield of laboratory testing to identify secondary contributors to osteoporosis in otherwise healthy women. J Clin Endocrinol Metab 2002;87:4431–4437.

This cross-sectional study investigated appropriate and cost-effective screening tests for detection of disorders of bone and mineral metabolism in postmenopausal osteoporotic women. Previously undiagnosed disorders of bone and mineral metabolism were discovered in 32% of the 173 women who met the inclusion criteria for the study. The most frequent diagnoses were disorders of calcium metabolism and hyperparathyroidism. A suggested testing strategy involved measuring 24-hour urine calcium, serum calcium, and serum PTH for all women, and serum TSH for women on thyroid replacement therapy. This approach would have diagnosed 85% of these women, at an estimated cost of $75 per patient screened.

7

Acquired Vitamin D Deficiency

Pauline M. Camacho

Epidemiology, 115
Definition, 115
Vitamin D Metabolism, 116
Effects of Vitamin D Deficiency on Calcium Homeostasis, 117
Pleotropic Effects of Vitamin D, 117
Clinical Conditions That Cause Vitamin D Deficiency, 117
Vitamin D Deficiency and Fractures, 118
Biochemical Evaluation, 119
Osteomalacia, 119
Treatment, 120

EPIDEMIOLOGY

This chapter focuses on acquired vitamin D deficiency among adults. The prevalence of this condition has been reported to be as high as 30% to 54% among homebound elderly patients [1], 57% among inpatients [2], and 14% among the general population [3]. There is a seasonal variation, and latitude plays a role in the prevalence of the disease [4], with a higher prevalence in colder countries. However, it appears that even in sunny countries, it is still highly prevalent [5]. In populations of ambulatory patients referred to bone centers, the prevalence of vitamin D deficiency was not particularly higher than described in other populations, 54% when less than 30 ng/mL is used as cutoff, and 39% in another study that used less than 15 ng/mL [6,7].

DEFINITION

The definition of vitamin D has evolved in the past few years, as the assays for 25-OHD have advanced. Vitamin D adequacy is defined as 25-OHD level above 30 ng/mL. This level was found to be the critical level, below which secondary hyperparathyroidism develops [3]. Various groups have proposed nomenclatures for stratifying patients based on 25-OHD levels. Individuals with levels below 30 but above 20 ng/mL are considered to have vitamin D inadequacy or mild vitamin D deficiency. Below 20 ng/mL but above 10 ng/mL is moderate vitamin D deficiency, and below 10 ng/mL is severe vitamin D deficiency. It is important to consider the possibility of osteomalacia among those with moderate and severe vitamin D deficiency, as these individuals should not be candidates for antiresorptive or anabolic therapy. Severe vitamin D deficiency is usually associated with secondary hyperparathyroidism, hypocalcemia, hypophosphatemia, and in cases of osteomalacia, elevation in bone or total alkaline phosphatase. Patients with mild vitamin D deficiency, particularly those with levels in the mid or high 20s, may have normal parathyroid hormone (PTH) levels.

VITAMIN D METABOLISM

Vitamin D refers to either D_2 or D_3, two forms of the vitamin that are utilized by the human body. Vitamin D_2 comes from plants and yeasts, whereas vitamin D_3 is synthesized in the skin through the action of sunlight and is found in food sources such as fish and cod liver oil. The potency of vitamin D_2 is approximately one-third that of vitamin D_3 [8].

Synthesis of vitamin D starts with the conversion of cutaneous 7-dehydrocholesterol (provitamin D_3) to previtamin D_3 through exposure to sunlight (Fig. 7.1). Previtamin D_3 is then rapidly isomerized to vitamin D_3, which then travels in the circulation, bound to vitamin D–binding protein (DBP). This is transported to the liver where it undergoes 25-hydroxylation to form 25-hydroxyvitamin D (25-OHD). This is the major circulating and storage form of vitamin D in the body. An increase in the vitamin D precursors (such as with increased oral intake or sunlight exposure) quickly manifests as an

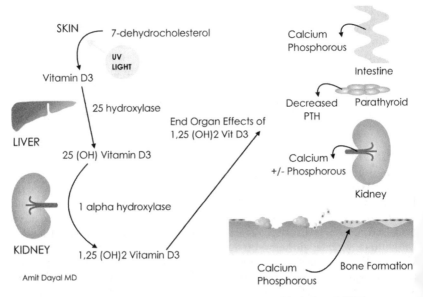

Figure 7.1. Vitamin D metabolism and effects. (Courtesy of Amit Dayal, MD.)

increase in 25-OHD; thus measurement of its concentration is the ideal test for vitamin D adequacy.

After hydroxylation in the liver, 25-OHD is then transported to the kidneys where 1α-hydroxylase converts 25-OHD to the final, and active, form, 1-25 dihydroxyvitamin D (1-25-OHD). This appears to be the major vitamin D metabolite that exerts effects on bone and calcium homeostasis.

EFFECTS OF VITAMIN D DEFICIENCY ON CALCIUM HOMEOSTASIS

When vitamin D is deficient, gut absorption of calcium decreases, leading to diminished total body calcium stores and subsequent increase in PTH secretion. PTH increases the activity of 1α-hydroxylase, which drives the activation of 25-OHD to 1-25-OHD. Therefore, in states of vitamin D deficiency, 1-25-OHD concentrations can be low, normal, or high. With mild-to-moderate deficiency and in the absence of renal insufficiency, 1-25-OHD is high. Increased 1-25-OHD improves absorption of calcium in the gut, and to a much smaller degree, increases osteoclastic activity. This effect on intestinal calcium absorption, in conjunction with the activation of osteoclastic activity by PTH, restores calcium equilibrium. The mechanism is tightly regulated, and is the reason why only in severe states of vitamin D deficiency do we see low serum total or ionized calcium levels. Serum calcium is often normal in mild-to-moderate vitamin D deficiency. Decreased urinary calcium is one of the earlier compensatory mechanisms, and thus hypocalciuria is often seen.

PLEOTROPIC EFFECTS OF VITAMIN D

The effects of vitamin D extend beyond the skeletal system. Vitamin D receptors are found in most organ systems, such as the heart, muscles, nervous system, breast, pancreas, colon, and gonads. A correlation between vitamin D and various disease states such as autoimmune diseases—multiple sclerosis, type 1 diabetes, psoriasis, rheumatoid arthritis, inflammatory bowel disease—has been reported. In addition, vitamin D appears to influence blood pressure control through its effects on the renin-angiotensin system. Reports of correlations between vitamin D and myocardial function have also been published. The antiproliferative effects of 1-25-OHD are well known and utilized in the treatment of psoriasis.

CLINICAL CONDITIONS THAT CAUSE VITAMIN D DEFICIENCY

Malabsorption

Various conditions, such as inflammatory bowel disease, celiac sprue, pancreatic insufficiency, biliary disease, and short bowel syndrome, can lead to decreased absorption of both calcium and vitamin D from the gastrointestinal tract. The biochemical manifestations include a low serum 25-OHD, high PTH, low urinary calcium excretion, low phosphorus, and in severe cases low ionized or total calcium. When the condition is not treated, osteomalacia may result (see following discussion) and an elevation of bone-specific and total alkaline phosphatase can be seen.

Renal Insufficiency

As kidney function declines, there is decreased production of 1-25-OHD. Phosphate levels are usually in the high or high-normal range due to diminished urinary excretion. Both of these lead to secondary hyperparathyroidism. Biochemically, 25-OHD and 1-25-OHD levels are usually low, intact PTH levels high, phosphate high, and in severe cases, ionized and total calcium levels low.

Medication Use

Antiseizure medications increase the hepatic catabolism of both 25-OHD and 1-25-OHD, leading to low 25-OHD, high PTH, and sometimes biochemical evidence of osteomalacia. Glucocorticoids and rifampin affect vitamin D metabolism in a similar way.

VITAMIN D DEFICIENCY AND FRACTURES

In the postfracture population, numerous studies from all over the world have documented high rates of vitamin D deficiency, ranging from 50% to as high as 90% [9–15]. Mean vitamin D levels have been consistently lower in the fracture patients in these studies. The effects of vitamin D on calcium and bone metabolism have been discussed here, but in addition, vitamin D deficiency leads to muscle weakness, which increases the risk of falls. In one study, muscle biopsies were done on individuals who suffered hip fractures. The patients were divided into two groups, vitamin D–deficient group (25-OHD >-39 nmol/L) and normal group. The mean type II fiber diameter in the deficient group (15.4 ± 4.2 μm) was significantly smaller than that in the sufficient group (38.7 ± 8.1 μm) ($p < 0.0001$). A significant correlation between the mean type II fiber diameter with the serum 25-OHD concentration ($r = 0.714$, $p = 0.0011$) was seen [16]. It is possible that both inactivity and vitamin D deficiency led to the severe atrophy seen in the vitamin D–deficient group.

After a comprehensive review of calcium/vitamin D trials in the literature, one paper concluded that vitamin D alone was not able to prevent vertebral and nonvertebral fractures, but a marginal effect on fracture risk was seen on hip fractures (seven trials, 10,376 participants; RR, 0.81; 95% CI, 0.68–0.96), and nonvertebral fractures (seven trials, 10,376 participants; RR, 0.87; 95% CI, 0.78–0.97); but there was no evidence showing a significant reduction in vertebral fractures with vitamin D and calcium [17]. A metaanalysis, however, showed more robust fracture reduction, a reduction of 36% in the incidence of vertebral fractures (RR, 0.63; 95% CI, 0.45–0.88; $p < 0.01$) and a trend toward reduced incidence of nonvertebral fractures (RR, 0.77; 95% CI, 0.57–1.04; $p = 0.09$) [18].

In another study conducted in Italy, in which women older than 65 years were given 400,000 IU oral vitamin D_2 during the winter months of 2000 through 2002, the age-adjusted risk reduction of hip fracture during 2001 and 2002 decreased by 17% ($p = 0.056$) and 25% ($p = 0.005$), respectively [19]. A study conducted in the United States offered 1,000 mg of elemental calcium as calcium carbonate and 400 IU (10 μg) of vitamin D_3 to a total of 4,957 participants (with 50% participation). A 16% reduction in fracture incidence rate (RR, 0.84; CI, 0.72–0.98; $p < 0.025$) was seen [20].

The common element among these trials is that only a small-to-moderate dose of vitamin D was administered, and it is unclear whether these amounts actually corrected the deficiency. Furthermore, we suspect that when moderate-to-severe vitamin D deficiency is treated with therapeutic doses of vitamin D, such that the 25-OHD levels are brought up to the goal of 30 ng/mL, secondary hyperparathyroidism resolves, and any baseline hypocalciuria is corrected, the effect on fracture risk will be much higher than what has been reported.

BIOCHEMICAL EVALUATION

As mentioned previously, the best way to assess for vitamin D adequacy is by measuring the concentration of 25-OHD. 1-25-OHD may be normal or even high due to the increased 1α-hydroxylation being driven by increased PTH secretion. Ionized or total calcium, phosphorus, intact PTH, serum creatinine, and alanine aminotransferase (ALT), as well as 24-hour urine calcium and creatinine, must be obtained. Screening tests for malabsorption, particularly celiac sprue, should be done when there is clinical suspicion. In general, relatively younger patients who are found to be vitamin D—deficient should have testing for celiac antibodies, and a serious consideration should be given to confirming the presence of villous atrophy. An increasing number of asymptomatic celiac disease patients are being diagnosed in bone centers. The workup for malabsorption for older osteoporotic patients with mild or moderate vitamin D deficiency does not have to be as extensive; however, for those who appear to be exhibiting signs of osteomalacia, or have hypocalcemia, and severe secondary hyperparathyroidism, malabsorption work-up should be considered, as well.

Vitamin D deficiency is frequently associated with hypocalciuria, and when dealing with the elderly population, an estimated glomerular filtration rate (GFR) must be known.

OSTEOMALACIA

Osteomalacia refers to defective mineralization of bone leading to predisposition to fractures. This is usually seen in children with nutritional or congenital vitamin D deficiency, but is increasingly being seen among adults with severe and prolonged vitamin D deficiency.

Classically, the symptoms include deep aching bone pain particularly in the hips, bone tenderness on palpation, proximal muscle weakness; manifesting as difficulty with gait, the classic "waddling gait," or difficulty arising from a sitting position. Patients may suffer from spontaneous or low trauma fractures in vertebral or nonvertebral sites, such as the pelvis. On examination, patients may have signs of hypocalcemia, such as Chvostek sign (contraction of the facial nerve when it is tapped at the parotid area), Trosseau sign (carpal spasm when a blood pressure cuff is wrapped around the arm and inflated between systolic and diastolic for around 2 to 3 minutes), and hyperactive deep tendon reflexes.

Histologically, bone biopsies show an increase in unmineralized osteoid. Dual-energy x-ray absorptiometry (DXA) scan will confirm decreased bone mineral density (BMD), but it is important to remember that not all patients with decreased BMD have osteoporosis. DXA scans merely measure bone density but will not distinguish osteomalacia from osteoporosis. This distinction is made by the physician using clinical, biochemical parameters and, if necessary, through bone biopsy.

Treatment of severe vitamin D deficiency will be covered in the next section, but it is imperative to know that antiresorptive and anabolic therapies for osteoporosis are contraindicated.

TREATMENT

Various vitamin D analogues are available, but the most commonly used agents are ergocalciferol (vitamin D_2), cholecalciferol (vitamin D_3), and calcitriol (1-25-OHD). Although cholecalciferol is three times more potent than ergocalciferol, the latter is more readily available in the United States.

Several treatment protocols have been published, but no study has compared these protocols with fractures or BMD as endpoints. Common treatment protocols are as follows:

- Ergocalciferol 50,000 IU (or cholecalciferol 15,000 IU) once weekly for 6 to 9 weeks, followed by a maintenance of 50,000 IU once monthly
- Ergocalciferol 50,000 IU once weekly for 6 to 9 weeks, followed by a maintenance dose of 1,000 to 1,200 IU daily
- Ergocalciferol 50,000 IU once weekly, indefinitely

Situations that require the use of the active vitamin D analogue, calcitriol, include renal insufficiency or renal failure, malabsorption, and the presence of hypocalcemia. Correction of secondary hyperparathyroidism is much faster with calcitriol, it being a direct suppressant of PTH. The onset of action and thus subsequent relief of symptoms also occurs much more quickly with calcitriol than with ergocalciferol or cholecalciferol. In our practice, patients who have severe elevations in PTH (>150 pg/mL) or have evidence of osteomalacia are treated with calcitriol as first-line therapy. The initial dose can be started at 0.25 or 0.5 µg every day, depending on the severity. It is important to monitor urinary and serum calcium closely when calcitriol is used. The question of whether there is an added benefit to replenishing 25-OHD as well, owing to its various pleotropic effects, has been raised and can be a focus of future research.

Individuals who are vitamin D–deficient are also frequently calcium-deficient. They must be advised to take 1,200 to 1,500 mg of elemental calcium daily in divided doses. Those who have hypocalcemia at baseline may require much higher doses of calcium. Phosphorus supplementation is rarely necessary because hypophosphatemia corrects easily with vitamin D therapy.

Patients with stage 4 or 5 kidney disease may develop hypercalcemia when calcitriol is used to treat both vitamin D deficiency and secondary hyperparathyroidism. In such cases, newer vitamin D analogues, pericalcitol (19-nor-1,25-$(OH)_2D_2$) and doxercalciferol (1α-$(OH)_2D_2$), may be preferable, as they are able to lower PTH more effectively with a lower incidence of hypercalcemia than calcitriol. The disadvantage, however, is that these agents are less effective in increasing gut calcium absorption, and if this is the effect that is desired, such as in hypocalcemic patients or those with osteomalacia, calcitriol would be the preferred agent.

Monitoring of Therapy

Within a few weeks of starting therapy, patients will usually report an improvement in clinical symptoms; alleviation of bone pain, improvement in muscle strength, and possibly increased sense of well-being.

Biochemically, the goals of therapy are as follows:

- 25-OHD levels to more than 30 ng/mL
- Intact PTH levels in the mid-to-normal range
- Urinary calcium excretion between 150 and 300 mg/24 hours in patients with normal renal function, and lower goals for those with renal insufficiency
- Normal serum calcium and phosphorus levels
- When osteomalacia is present, normalization of bone-specific alkaline phosphatase or total serum alkaline phosphatase.

There may be an improvement in BMD in the spine and hip even within just 1 year of treatment. Fracture risk reduction has been shown in several prospective studies discussed previously.

In certain situations, PTH may remain high, despite normalization of 25-OHD concentrations. Detailed questioning about compliance with both vitamin D therapy and calcium supplementation must be undertaken. Another scenario that can lead to this situation is the presence of renal insufficiency, which results in inadequate activation of 25-OHD.

REFERENCES

1. **Gloth FM III, Gundberg CM, Hollis BW**. Vitamin D deficiency in homebound elderly persons. JAMA 1995;274:1683–1686.
   A cohort study of 244 subjects at least 65 years old; 116 subjects (85 women and 31 men) who had been confined indoors for at least 6 months and 128 healthy ambulatory subjects. In the sunlight-deprived group, the mean 25-OHD level was 30 nmol/L (12 ng/mL) [range, <10–77 nmol/L (<4–31 ng/mL)] and the mean 1,25-OHD level was 52 pmol/L (20 pg/mL) [range, 18–122 pmol/L (7–47 pg/mL)]. In the sunlight-deprived subjects, 54% of community dwellers and 38% of nursing home residents had serum levels of 25-OHD below 25 nmol/L (10 ng/mL) [normal range, 25–137 nmol/L (10–55 ng/mL)]; 25-OHD was inversely related to parathyroid hormone (PTH) $(r = -0.42; r^2 = 0.18; p < 0.001)$.

2. **Thomas MK, Lloyd-Jones DM, Thadhani RI,** et al. Hypovitaminosis D in medical inpatients. N Engl J Med 1998;338:777–783.
   Vitamin D intake, ultraviolet-light exposure, risk factors for hypovitaminosis D, serum 25-OHD, intact parathyroid hormone (iPTH), and ionized calcium were measured in 290 consecutive patients on a general medical ward. Fifty-seven percent of the patients were vitamin D–deficient (25-OHD $\leq$15 ng/mL), and 22% were considered severely vitamin D–deficient (25-OHD <8 ng/mL). An inverse correlation was seen between 25-OHD and PTH. Lower vitamin D intake, less exposure to ultraviolet light, anticonvulsant drug therapy, renal dialysis, nephrotic syndrome, hypertension, diabetes mellitus, winter season,

higher serum concentrations of parathyroid hormone and alkaline phosphatase, and lower serum concentrations of ionized calcium and albumin were significant univariate predictors of vitamin D deficiency. Sixty-nine percent of the patients who consumed less than the recommended daily allowance of vitamin D and 43% of the patients with vitamin D intakes above the recommended daily allowance were vitamin D–deficient. In a multivariate analysis, inadequate vitamin D intake, winter season, and housebound status were independent predictors of vitamin D deficiency. Even in the subgroup without known risk factors for hypovitaminosis D, the prevalence of vitamin D deficiency was 42%.

3. **Chapuy MC, Preziosi P, Maamer M,** et al. Prevalence of vitamin D insufficiency in an adult normal population. Osteoporos Int 1997;7:439–443.

    This study aimed to determine the vitamin D status of a general adult urban population in 20 French cities located between 43 degrees and 51 degrees N latitude. Major differences in 25-hydroxyvitamin D (25-OHD) concentration were found between regions, the lowest values being seen in the north and the greatest in the south, with a significant "sun" effect ($r = 0.72; p = 0.03$) and latitude effect ($r = -0.79; p = 0.01$). Of 1,569 subjects who had their blood drawn between November and April, 14% of subjects had 25-OHD values less than or equal to 30 nmol/L (12 ng/mL). A significant negative correlation was found between intact parathyroid hormone (PTH) and serum 25-OHD values ($p < 0.01$). PTH held a stable plateau level at 36 pg/mL at 25-OHD levels above 78 nmol/L (31 ng/mL), but increased when the 25-OHD value fell below this.

4. **McKenna MJ.** Differences in vitamin D status between countries in young adults and the elderly. Am J Med 1992;93:69–77.

    Vitamin D studies from various geographic regions published between 1971 and 1990 were reviewed. Vitamin D status varies with the season in young adults and in the elderly, and is lower during the winter in Europe than in both North America and Scandinavia. Vitamin D intake is lower in Europe than in both North America and Scandinavia. Vitamin D deficiency is most common in elderly residents in Europe but is reported in all elderly populations. The study recommended that all countries should adopt a fortification policy, particularly for the elderly population.

5. **Hochwald O, Harman-Boehm I, Castel H.** Hypovitaminosis D among inpatients in a sunny country. Isr Med Assoc J 2004;6:82–87.

    This study aimed to determine the prevalence and determinants of vitamin D deficiency among patients in internal medicine wards in a sunny country (Israel). In the study, 296 internal medicine inpatients admitted consecutively to the Soroka University Medical Center, vitamin D deficiency (serum 25-OHD < 15 ng/mL) was found in 77 inpatients (26.27%). The amount of sunlight exposure, serum albumin concentration, being housebound or resident of a nursing home, vitamin D intake, ethnic group, cerebrovascular accident, and glucocorticoid therapy were all significantly associated with vitamin D deficiency. Multivariate analysis showed a significant association between vitamin D deficiency and Bedouin origin, sun exposure, vitamin D intake, and stroke. Parathyroid hormone (PTH) levels were significantly higher in patients with 25-OHD levels lower than 15 ng/mL.

6. **Mezquita-Raya P, Munoz-Torres M, Luna JD,** et al. Relation between vitamin D insufficiency, bone density, and bone metabolism in healthy postmenopausal women. J Bone Miner Res 2001;16:1408–1415.

    Of 161 consecutive ambulatory women with osteoporosis referred to a bone metabolic unit, the prevalence of vitamin D insufficiency (25-OHD ≤ 15 ng/mL) was 39.1%. 25-OHD was lower in the osteoporotic subjects (15.7 ± 5.3 ng/mL vs. 21.8 ± 9.7 ng/mL; $p < 0.001$). After controlling for all other variables, lumbar spine BMD was found to be significantly associated with 25(OH)D, body mass index (BMI), and years after menopause (YSM) ($r^2 = 0.253$; $p < 0.001$). For femoral neck (FN), significant independent predictors of BMD were YSM, BMI, intact parathyroid hormone (iPTH), and 25(OH)D ($r^2 = 0.368; p < 0.001$).

7. **Camacho P, Girgis M, Sapountzi P, Sinacore J.** Correlations between vitamin D, parathyroid hormone, urinary calcium excretion, markers of bone turnover and bone density of patients referred to an osteoporosis center. J Bone Miner Res 2005:S1: S389.

    The primary aim of the study was to characterize the relationships between 25-OHD, 1-25-OHD, intact parathyroid hormone (iPTH), ionized calcium, phosphorus, 24-hour urine calcium excretion, bone-specific alkaline phosphatase (BSAP), urinary N-telopeptide (NTX) or creatinine, and bone density. One hundred sixty-three patients (143 female, 20 male; mean age, 62.5 years) evaluated for low bone mass at Loyola University Osteoporosis and Metabolic Bone Disease Center were studied. The strongest indirect relationship seen was between PTH and 24-hour urinary calcium excretion (UrCa) ($r = -0.496$, $p < 0.001$). 25-OHD showed a significant correlation with UrCa ($r = 0.420$, $p < 0.001$), PTH ($r = -0.215$, $p = 0.014$), BSAP ($r = -0.288$, $p = 0.010$), and a trend with spine BMD ($r = -0.156$, $p = 0.071$). Analysis of the subgroup with 25-OHD less than or equal to 20 ng/mL (26% of the group) showed that 25-OHD correlated significantly with PTH ($r = -0.354$, $p = 0.027$). The strong indirect correlation between PTH and UrCa ($r = -0.540$, $p = 0.021$) remained in this group. 1,25-OHD showed a trend associated with UrCa ($r = 0.459$, $p = 0.064$) and spine BMD ($r = -0.356$, $p = 0.069$). Ionized calcium, phosphorus, or NTX or creatinine did not show significant correlations with PTH or vitamin D levels. The difference between the means of PTH above and below a 25-OHD level of 30 ng/mL was significant. At 35 ng/mL, the significance was lost. The same 25-OHD level of 30 ng/mL showed significant differences in the UrCa of patients with 25-OHD above and below this threshold. This relationship was also significant at 35 ng/mL and was lost at 40 ng/mL. A level of 30 ng/mL was concluded as the cutoff for vitamin D deficiency. This was seen in 48% of the population.

8. **Armas LA, Hollis BW, Heaney RP.** Vitamin D_2 is much less effective than vitamin D_3 in humans. J Clin Endocrinol Metab 2004;89:5387–5391.

To compare the relative potencies of vitamins D_2 and D_3, single doses of 50,000 IU of the respective calciferols were given to 20 healthy male volunteers. Serum 25-OHD levels were measured over a 28-day period. Vitamin D_2 and D_3 produced similar rises in serum concentration of the administered vitamin, indicating equivalent absorption. Both produced similar initial rises in serum 25-OHD over the first 3 days, but 25-OHD continued to rise in the D_3-treated subjects, peaking at 14 days, whereas serum 25-OHD fell rapidly in the D_2-treated subjects and was not different from baseline at 14 days. Area under the curve (AUC) to day 28 was 60.2 ng/day/mL (150.5 nmol/day/L) for vitamin D_2 and 204.7 (511.8) for vitamin D_3 ($p < 0.002$). Calculated AUC (infinity) indicated an even greater differential, with the relative potencies for D_3:D_2 being 9.5:1. Vitamin D_2 potency is less than one-third that of vitamin D_3.

9. **Elliott ME, Binkley NC, Carnes M,** et al. Fracture risks for women in long-term care: High prevalence of calcaneal osteoporosis and hypovitaminosis D. Pharmacotherapy 2003;23:702–710.

Nine women aged 68 to 100 years in a skilled nursing facility had bilateral calcaneal BMDs measured as well as serum 25-OHD by radioimmunoassay. Fifty-nine percent of these women (95% CI, 44–74%) were found to have calcaneal osteoporosis (T-score < −2.5). Osteoporosis was documented in the records of 17%, or 23, of these women. Sixty percent had 25-OHD levels of 20 ng/mL or less, which is associated with secondary hyperparathyroidism; only 4% of women had levels higher than 30 ng/mL. Vitamin D status was suboptimal, even in most women taking multivitamins.

10. **Sato Y, Asoh T, Kondo I, Satoh K.** Vitamin D deficiency and risk of hip fractures among disabled elderly stroke patients. Stroke 2001;32:1673–1677.

This was a prospective cohort study of patients, aged 65 years and older, with hemiplegia after stroke. Patients with vitamin D deficiency (defined as 25-OHD ≤ 10 ng/mL; deficient group, $n = 88$) were compared to those with vitamin D insufficiency (25-OHD = 10–20 ng/mL; $n = 76$) and those who were vitamin D–sufficient (25-OHD ≥ 21 ng/mL; $n = 72$). Over a 2-year follow-up interval, hip fractures on the paretic side occurred in 7 patients in the deficient group and 1 patient in the insufficient group ($p < 0.05$; hazard ratio = 6.5), whereas no hip fractures occurred in the sufficient group. The 7 hip fracture patients in the deficient group had a 25-OHD level of less than 5 ng/mL. Higher age and severe immobilization were noted in the deficient group, and 25-OHD levels correlated positively with age, Barthel Index, and serum parathyroid hormone.

11. **Diamond T, Smerdely P, Kormas N,** et al. Hip fracture in elderly men: The importance of subclinical vitamin D deficiency and hypogonadism. Med J Aust 1998; 169:138–141.

This study aimed to determine the risk factors for hip fractures for elderly men (>60 years). Forty-one men with hip fractures were compared with 41 hospital inpatient and 41 outpatient control subjects without hip fractures. Osteoporotic risk factors (including age, body weight, comorbid illnesses, alcohol intake, cigarettes smoked, and corticosteroid use) and serum concentrations of creatinine, urea, calcium, albumin, alkaline phosphatase, parathyroid hormone, 25-hydroxyvitamin D, and free testosterone were collected. There were no significant differences between the hip fracture and two control groups on any of the osteoporotic risk factors, but men with hip fractures had significantly lower mean serum 25-OHD (45.6 nmol/L; 95% CI, 36.9–52.3 nmol/L) than both inpatient (61.1 nmol/L; 95% CI, 50.0–72.2 nmol/L) and outpatient (65.9 nmol/L; 95% CI, 59.0–72.8 nmol/L) controls ($p = 0.007$). Subclinical vitamin D deficiency (defined as 25-OHD <50 nmol/L) was seen in 63% of the fracture group, compared with 25% in the control groups combined (odds ratio, 3.9; 95% CI, 1.74–8.78; $p = 0.0007$). In a multiple regression analysis, subclinical vitamin D deficiency was the strongest predictor of hip fracture [beta (regression coefficient), 0.34 ± 0.19; $p = 0.013$].

12. **Lau EM, Woo J, Swaminathan R,** et al. Plasma 25-hydroxyvitamin D concentration in patients with hip fracture in Hong Kong. Gerontology 1989;35:198–204.

Two hundred patients with hip fracture (age range 49–93 years) were compared with 427 elderly subjects living in the community (age range 60–90 years). The mean 25-OHD concentration was significantly lower in the hip fracture group than the controls for all sex and age groups. None of the patients with a low 25-hydroxyvitamin D level had a blood picture suggestive of osteopathy resulting from vitamin D deficiency or frank osteomalacia. Hip fracture patients with a low 25-hydroxyvitamin D level were much less ambulant and went outdoors much less frequently than hip fracture patients with a normal vitamin D level.

13. **Bakhtiyarova S, Lesnyak O, Kyznesova N,** et al. Vitamin D status among patients with hip fracture and elderly control subjects in Yekaterinburg, Russia. Osteoporos Int 2006;17:441–446.

This study investigated the prevalence of vitamin D deficiency in Yekaterinburg, Russia. The study was performed on 63 people with hip fracture (mean age, 68.8 years) and 97 elderly people living independently (mean age, 70.2 years). Serum 25-OHD (mean ± SD) in the hip fracture group was 22.4 ± 11.4 nmol/L, significantly lower than in the control group, which was 28.1 ± 10.1 nmol/L. The percentage of patients with severe hypovitaminosis D (<25 nmol/L) in the hip fracture group was 65%, compared with 47% in the control group ($p < 0.05$). The prevalence of hypovitaminosis D among hip fracture patients, as well as among independently living elderly people in Yekaterinburg, was high.

14. **Seton M, Jackson V, Lasser KE,** et al. Low 25-hydroxyvitamin D and osteopenia are prevalent in persons ≥55 yr with fracture at any site: A prospective, observational study of persons fracturing in the community. J Clin Densitom 2005;8:454–460.

This was a prospective, observational study designed to analyze risk factors for fracture in an ambulatory, ethnically diverse, urban population aged 55 years or older. The goal of the study was to determine the number of fractures associated with hypovitaminosis D (≤15 ng/mL serum 25-hydroxyvitamin D) and osteopenia (T-score <−1.5) by bone mineral density (BMD). From January 1 to July 31, 2001, of 262 persons who fractured in our community, 83 chose to enroll in the study; 88% of the group had evidence of osteopenia or osteoporosis (T-score <1.5) or low 25-OHD.

15. **Gallacher SJ, McQuillian C, Harkness M,** et al. Prevalence of vitamin D inadequacy in Scottish adults with non-vertebral fragility fractures. Curr Med Res Opin 2005;21:1355–1361.

The study investigated the prevalence of vitamin D inadequacy in a population of patients (>50 years old) with nonvertebral fragility fractures. The study had a retrospective arm comprising patients seen over the previous 4 years with hip fracture, and a prospective arm comprising consecutive patients with clinical nonvertebral fragility fracture with osteoporosis, as measured by axial spine or hip dual-energy X-ray absorptiometry (DXA) (T-score < −2.5) after November 2004. In the retrospective arm, (mean age of 80.5 years) the mean 25-OHD was 24.7 nmol/L (9.9 ng/mL) SD = 17; however, it is likely that the true mean is lower, since in approximately 25% of cases vitamin D levels were reported to be less than 15 nmol/L, and these were considered 15 nmol/L in the calculation. In the study, 97.8% had vitamin D levels below 70 nmol/L, and 91.6% had vitamin D levels below 50 nmol/L. There were no significant differences by patient sex, age, or season of presentation. In the prospective arm, (mean age, 65.8 years), the mean vitamin D level was 44.1 nmol/L (18.4 ng/mL), SD = 25.3; 82% had vitamin D levels below 70 nmol/L and 72% had vitamin D levels below 50 nmol/L. The mean vitamin D level in the 13 patients with hip fracture (34.5 nmol/L) was lower than in the 37 with nonhip fractures (48.2 nmol/L).

16. **Sato Y, Inose M, Higuchi I,** et al. Changes in the supporting muscles of the fractured hip in elderly women. Bone 2002;30:325–330.
Gluteal muscle biopsies were performed at surgery in 42 elderly women with hip fracture caused by a fall. On the basis of serum 25-hydroxyvitamin D (25-OHD) concentration, the patients were divided into a sufficient group (25-OHD concentration >39 nmol/L, $n = 20$) and a deficient group (25-OHD concentration <39 nmol/L, $n = 22$). The mean type II fiber diameter in the deficient group (15.4 ± 4.2 μm) was significantly smaller than that in the sufficient group (38.7 ± 8.1 μm) ($p < 0.0001$). In the deficient group, the mean type II fiber diameter correlated with the serum 25-OHD concentration ($r = 0.714$, $p = 0.0011$). This correlation was not observed in the sufficient group. The investigators believe that severe type fiber II atrophy is an independent risk factor for hip fractures and may also have contributed to the poor functional outcome in the deficient group.

17. **Avenell A, Gillespie WJ, Gillespie LD, O'Connell DL.** Vitamin D and vitamin D analogues for preventing fractures associated with involutional and post-menopausal osteoporosis. Cochrane Database Syst Rev 2005:CD000227.
An extensive analysis of literature was done to determine the effects of vitamin D or analogues, with or without calcium, in the prevention of fractures in older people. Two authors independently assessed trial quality, and extracted data. Vitamin D alone showed no statistically significant effect on hip fracture (7 trials, 18,668 participants; RR, 1.17; 95% CI, 0.98–1.41), vertebral fracture [4 trials, 5,698 participants; RR, (random effects) 1.13; 95% CI, 0.50–2.55] or any new fracture (8 trials, 18,903 participants; RR, 0.99; 95% CI, 0.91–1.09). Vitamin D with calcium marginally reduced hip fractures (7 trials, 10,376 participants; RR, 0.81; 95% CI, 0.68–0.96), nonvertebral fractures (7 trials, 10,376 participants; RR, 0.87; 95% CI, 0.78–0.97), but there was no evidence of effect of vitamin D with calcium on vertebral fractures. The effect appeared to be restricted to those living in institutional care. Hypercalcemia was more common when vitamin D or its analogues was given, compared with placebo or calcium (14 trials, 8,035 participants; RR, 2.38; 95% CI, 1.52–3.71). The risk was particularly high with calcitriol (3 trials, 742 participants; RR, 14.94, 95% CI, 2.95–75.61). There was no evidence that vitamin D increased gastrointestinal symptoms [7 trials, 10,188 participants; RR, (random effects) 1.03; 95% CI, 0.79–1.36] or renal disease (9 trials, 10,107 participants; RR, 0.80; 95% CI, 0.34–1.87). Effectiveness of vitamin D alone in fracture prevention is unclear. There is no evidence of advantage of analogues of vitamin D compared with vitamin D. Calcitriol may be associated with an increased incidence of adverse effects.

18. **Papadimitropoulos E, Wells G, Shea B,** et al. Meta-analyses of therapies for postmenopausal osteoporosis. VIII: Meta-analysis of the efficacy of vitamin D treatment in preventing osteoporosis in postmenopausal women. Endocr Rev 2002;23:560–569.
This was a metaanalysis of 25 trials that randomized women to standard or hydroxylated vitamin D with or without calcium supplementation or a control and measured bone density or fracture incidence for at least 1 year. Vitamin D reduced the incidence of vertebral fractures [relative risk (RR), 0.63; 95% confidence interval (CI), 0.45–0.88, $p < 0.01$] and showed a trend toward reduced incidence of nonvertebral fractures (RR, 0.77; 95% CI 0.57–1.04, $p = 0.09$). Hydroxylated vitamin D had a consistently larger impact on bone density than did standard vitamin D. For instance, total body differences in percentage change between hydroxylated vitamin D and control were 2.06 (0.72, 3.40) and 0.40 (−0.25, 1.06) for standard vitamin D. At the lumbar spine and forearm sites, hydroxylated vitamin D doses above 50 μg yield larger effects than lower doses.

19. **Rossini M, Alberti V, Flor L,** et al. Effect of oral vitamin D_2 yearly bolus on hip fracture risk in elderly women: A community primary prevention study. Aging Clin Exp Res 2004;16:432–436.
Oral 400,000 IU vitamin D_2 was offered to all women older than 65 years in the winters of 2000 to 2001 and 2001 to 2002 in a region in Italy. Analysis of hip fracture incidence was carried out for 4 years from 1999 to 2002. In the study, 120 of the women (age 68–90 years) had serum concentrations of 25-OH vitamin D measured from October to June, both before, and 1 and 4 months after, vitamin D administration; 23,325 and 24,747 women received the vitamin D bolus during winters 2000–2001 and 2001–2002, respectively, that is, 45% to 47% of eligible women. The 2-year intervention in the community decreased the incidence

of fracture by 10% ($p = 0.050$) in comparison with the previous 2 years. The age-adjusted risk reduction (RR) of hip fracture during 2001 and 2002 in women who had received vitamin D, with respect to women who had not, decreased by 17% ($p = 0.056$) and 25% ($p = 0.005$), respectively. The RR was considerably greater and statistically significant over both 2001 and 2002 in the cohort aged more than 75 years. 25-OH vitamin D concentrations, in the subset of women in whom it was measured, rose significantly ($p < 0.0001$) by 9 ng/mL over 4 months after administration.

20. **Larsen ER, Mosekilde L, Foldspang A.** Vitamin D and calcium supplementation prevents osteoporotic fractures in elderly community dwelling residents: A pragmatic population-based 3-year intervention study. J Bone Miner Res 2004;19:370–378.

    Community-dwelling residents aged 66 years and older residing in Northern Europe were offered a prevention program of a daily supplement of 1,000 mg of elemental calcium as calcium carbonate and 400 IU (10 μg) of vitamin D_3; 4,957 residents chose to participate in that arm of the study. Another program with evaluation and suggestions for the improvement of the domestic environment was offered to a total of 5,063 participants. Both programs included revision of the resident's current pharmaceutical treatment. Active participation was 50.3% in the Calcium and Vitamin D Program and 46.4% in the Environmental and Health Program. We observed a 16% reduction in fracture incidence rate [relative risk (RR), 0.84; CI, 0.72–0.98; $p < 0.025$] among male and female residents offered the Calcium and Vitamin D Program (intention-to-prevent analysis).

8

Treatment Options

Pauline M. Camacho

Postmenopausal Osteoporosis, 127
Glucocorticoid-induced Osteoporosis, 134
Male Osteoporosis, 135

The National Osteoporosis Foundation has outlined clinical recommendations regarding initiation of therapy for low bone mass and osteoporosis (Table 8.1). According to their guidelines, treatment should be initiated when the T-score is below -1.5 in the presence of at least one risk factor, or if the T-score is below -2.0 in the absence of risk factors. As described in Chapter 3, T-score alone cannot be used to judge when drugs are to be prescribed. The World Health Organization (WHO) is working on a fracture risk assessment scheme that will give the 10-year fracture risk based on the number of risk factors. Low bone mineral density (BMD) is only one of many risk factors in this scheme. Until the results are published, it is important for clinicians to individualize therapy and use their clinical judgments in this decision process. High-risk individuals (e.g., an elderly woman who has suffered from multiple compression fractures) deserve to be treated even if they do not meet densitometric criteria for osteoporosis.

Evaluation and treatment of secondary causes of osteoporosis must be done to ensure success of therapy (see Chapter 6). This chapter will discuss pharmacologic and nonpharmacologic treatment of osteoporosis in various clinical situations; postmenopausal osteoporosis, glucocorticoid-induced osteoporosis (GIO), and male osteoporosis.

POSTMENOPAUSAL OSTEOPOROSIS

Pharmacologic Therapy

Drugs for osteoporosis can be divided into two major classes: antiresorptive and anabolic agents (Table 8.2). Antiresorptive agents inhibit bone resorption, mainly through their action on osteoclasts, whereas anabolic agents stimulate osteoblastic differentiation and activity.

Antiresorptive Therapy

Bisphosphonates

These pyrophosphate analogues bind to hydroxyapatite crystals in the bone, are taken up by osteoclasts in the bone, and exert their action by inhibiting the mevalonate pathway, subsequently leading to inhibition of osteoclast

Table 8.1.   National Osteoporosis Foundation recommendations regarding initiation of pharmacologic therapy

BMD T-scores below −2.0 by central DXA with no risk factors
BMD T-scores below −1.5 by central DXA with one or more risk factors
History of a prior vertebral or hip fracture

BMD, bone mineral density; DXA, dual-energy x-ray absorptiometry.

function and increase in rates of apoptosis. Oral bioavailability is generally low, only 1% to 3%, and is greatly inhibited by food, calcium, iron supplements, and drinks. Patients must be advised to take this medication in the morning, to withhold food and drinks to ensure good absorption, and to remain upright for at least 30 minutes.

Major side effects include erosions and ulcers in the upper gastrointestinal tract. Several studies have attempted to determine which agent is less erosive, but the results were not consistent. With the approval of once-monthly therapy with ibandronate, it remains to be determined whether less frequent exposure of the gut will lead to fewer gastrointestinal adverse events.

The Food and Drug Administration (FDA) has approved three oral bisphosphonates for the prevention and treatment of osteoporosis: alendronate (Fosamax), risedronate (Actonel), and ibandronate (Boniva), as well as an intravenous agent, ibandronate.

Alendronate

This drug is available in 5-, 10-, 35-, and 70-mg tablet forms. The 5-mg once daily or 35 mg once weekly is used for prevention, and 10-mg once daily or 70-mg once weekly for treatment of established osteoporosis. The pivotal study that established the efficacy of alendronate for the treatment of postmenopausal osteoporosis was the Fracture Intervention Trial (FIT) [1,2]. This was conducted on postmenopausal women, who were given alendronate

Table 8.2.   Osteoporosis treatment options

Antiresorptive therapy

Bisphosphonate: alendronate, risedronate, ibandronate
SERM: raloxifene
Calcitonin
Hormone replacement therapy

Anabolic therapy

Teriparatide

Nonpharmacologic therapy

Calcium and vitamin D supplementation
Fall prevention
Weight-bearing exercises

SERM, selective estrogen regulator modulator.

(daily) or placebo for 3 years. The study showed a 47% reduction in new radiographic vertebral fractures, a 55% reduction in clinical vertebral fractures, a 90% reduction in multiple vertebral fractures, and a 51% reduction in hip fractures among women without prior vertebral fractures [1]. Those with prior vertebral fractures experienced a 44% reduction in new radiographic vertebral fractures [2]. Mean increases in BMD were 6% to 8% for the lumbar spine (LS) and 4% to 5% for the hip [1,2]. A metaanalysis of alendronate trials showed similar fracture reduction and BMD benefits for postmenopausal osteoporosis [3,4].

In a follow-up study, postmenopausal osteoporotic women who took 10 mg alendronate daily for 10 years had a total increase of 13.7% in lumbar spine BMD, 10.3% in trochanter, and 5.4% in femoral neck BMD [5]. The BMD gradually declined after a number of years of discontinuation [5]. It appears that if used for only a year, discontinuation of alendronate led to a rate of bone loss that was similar to the group that did not receive the drug; however, at the end of 15 months, there was still a 3% difference in mean LS BMD between the groups, but the femoral neck BMD went back to baseline [6]. Whether fracture protection was indeed lost as bone mass declined is unknown.

The BMD efficacy of weekly alendronate dosing was studied in a 1-year trial that compared 70-mg weekly, 35-mg twice-weekly, and 10-mg daily doses of alendronate. At 1 year, similar increases in LS BMD (range, 5.1%–5.4%) in these three groups were seen, and there were no observed differences in the side effect profiles [7].

A head-to-head study comparing weekly 70 mg alendronate with 35 mg risedronate for 1 year revealed small but significantly greater increases in BMD at 6 and 12 months, and greater degrees of bone suppression in the alendronate group, with similar tolerability [8]. This study was not powered to detect differences in fracture rates.

Risedronate
Risedronate is approved in the 5-mg once-daily or a 35-mg once-weekly dose for prevention and treatment of osteoporosis. Two large randomized placebo-controlled studies of postmenopausal women showed a reduction in radiographic vertebral fractures by 41% to 49% after 3 years of daily risedronate therapy [9,10]. One of these trials was extended to 7 years, and the follow-up revealed persistence of BMD gains and fracture risk reductions through the seventh year of follow-up [11]. In another large study with hip fracture reduction as the primary endpoint [12], risedronate was found to significantly reduce fracture risk by 30%. In the subgroup of patients who entered into the study with BMD criteria for osteoporosis, a significant 40% risk reduction for fracture was seen, but no significant reduction was seen in the subgroup that entered into the study based on age alone. The exact reason why this subgroup did not experience a reduction in fracture risk is not known.

A metaanalysis on the use of risedronate for postmenopausal osteoporosis [13] showed a pooled risk reduction (RR) of 0.64 for vertebral and 0.73 for nonvertebral fractures. The pooled estimate of the differences in percentage of change in BMD between risedronate (5 mg) and placebo was 4.54% at the LS and 2.75% at the femoral neck.

The efficacy of once-weekly risedronate was shown in a randomized placebo-controlled study of 1,456 postmenopausal women with T-scores below −2.5 or below −2.0 with a prevalent vertebral fracture. Risedronate, at 5-mg daily, 35-mg weekly, or 50-mg weekly doses, was given for 1 year. Mean percentage changes in LS BMD after 12 months were similar, as were mean increases in femoral neck BMD in the three groups [14].

Ibandronate

Ibandronate, FDA approved for the treatment and prevention of post-menopausal osteoporosis, is available in two oral forms, 2.5 mg daily and 150 mg monthly, as well as an intravenous form, 3 mg quarterly. The Monthly Oral Pilot Study was a 3-month, Phase 1 randomized, double-blind, multicenter, placebo-controlled study of 144 postmenopausal women who were given 50, 100, or 150 mg of ibandronate or placebo. The main endpoints were changes in serum and urine C-telopeptide (CTX), safety, and AUC. Ibandronate significantly decreased CTX in the 100- or 150-mg groups. No significant differences in adverse events compared with placebo were observed [15]. The MOBILE (Monthly Oral Ibandronate in Ladies) study was a 2-year, randomized, double-blind trial that searched for the appropriate ibandronate dose for the treatment of osteoporosis. The 1,609 women in the study were assigned to four groups: 2.5 mg daily, 50 mg once a month, 100 mg once a month, or 150 mg once a month. Those on monthly ibandronate experienced increases in LS (3.9%, 4.3%, 4.1%, and 4.9%, respectively) and hip (about 2%–3%) BMD. The 150-mg group had a small but significantly greater increase in LS BMD than the daily regimen. In addition, when the groups were evaluated for those who achieved BMD gains above baseline of more than 6% at the LS or 3% at the hip, the 150-mg and 100-mg groups had significantly more patients at these goals than the daily regimen (only 150 mg at the LS with respect to gains above baseline). The frequency of gastrointestinal symptoms with each dose was similar, but there was a small increase in flu-like symptoms with the monthly regimens [16].

In a noninferiority study [DIVA (Dosing Intravenous Administration)], two regimens—2 mg IV every 2 months and 3 mg IV every 3 months—were found to be similar in efficacy to daily ibandronate (2.5 mg) in terms of mean increases in lumbar spine and hip BMD at 1 and 2 years. Safety profiles were similar [17].

Side Effect Profile and Clinical Issues with Bisphosphonates

Oral bisphosphonates are alkaline substances that have the potential to cause esophageal and gastric ulcers. Head-to-head endoscopy studies have shown conflicting results [18,19], perhaps partly because of difference in study design. A metaanalysis of eight trials that included 10,086 patients showed no difference in gastrointestinal adverse events, clinically or endoscopically, in patients treated with risedronate versus placebo [20].

One recent concern raised about bisphosphonate therapy is the possibility of oversuppression of bone turnover, which might lead to increased bone fragility. A case series of nine patients who had taken alendronate for 3 to 8 years described fractures and delayed or no healing. Bone biopsy showed minimal bone formation. More studies need to be done regarding this potential risk and the optimal duration of therapy with bisphosphonates [21].

Osteonecrosis of the jaw has recently received a lot of media attention. To date, hundreds of cases have been reported, but the estimated risk is quite low, at 0.7 cases per 100,000 person-years exposure [22–24]. The vast majority were cancer patients who received intravenous zoledronic acid every month or pamidronate every 3 months. Few patients were on oral bisphosphonates for osteoporosis treatment. The exact etiology is unknown, but an association with recent dental procedure was found.

Raloxifene

Raloxifene is a selective estrogen receptor modulator, with agonistic effects on bone. The major efficacy trial for raloxifene was the Multiple Outcomes of Raloxifene Evaluation (MORE) Trial [25]. The LS BMD increase over the 3-year study period was 2% to 3%, and vertebral fracture reduction rates in women with and without preexisting fractures were 50% and 30%, respectively. No significant difference in nonvertebral and hip fracture reduction was observed, but the study was not powered to detect differences in such fractures. Efficacy of raloxifene was sustained through 4 years of treatment [26].

A metaanalysis of seven trials comparing raloxifene and placebo showed a similar BMD increase at the LS and a 2% increase at the hip [27]. This drug has other potential benefits, including reduction in breast cancer risk and improvement in lipids and markers of cardiovascular disease. In a large study of 10,101 postmenopausal women [Raloxifene Use for The Heart (RUTH) Trial], raloxifene did not show a significant reduction in primary coronary events but showed a reduction in invasive breast cancer [40 vs. 70 events; hazards ratio (HR), 0.56; 95% CI, 0.38–0.83; absolute RR, 1.2 invasive breast cancers per 1,000 women treated for 1 year]; increased risk of fatal stroke (59 vs. 39 events; HR, 1.49; 95% CI, 1.00–2.24; absolute risk increase, 0.7 per 1,000 woman-years) and venous thromboembolism (103 vs. 71 events; HR, 1.44; 95% CI, 1.06–1.95; absolute risk increase, 1.2 per 1,000 woman-years) [28]. Clinical vertebral fractures were reduced (64 vs. 97 events; HR, 0.65; 95% CI, 0.47–0.89) [28].

Calcitonin

Because of its modest effect on BMD, and small fracture risk reduction, calcitonin is rarely used as first-line therapy; rather, owing to its mild analgesic effects, this drug is more commonly used now as an adjunctive therapy after an acute vertebral fracture, usually combined with a stronger antiresorptive. The major efficacy trial was the PROOF (Prevent Recurrence of Osteoporotic Fractures) study, which demonstrated a 1.2% increase in LS BMD and a 33% reduction in vertebral fractures with 200 IU of intranasal calcitonin [29]. No significant reduction was seen in the 100 or 400 international units groups. No significant reduction in nonvertebral and hip fractures was demonstrated in this trial. In a metaanalysis of 30 trials that compared calcitonin with placebo, the smaller studies were found to have more impressive results than the PROOF study [30]. The authors of that metaanalysis alluded to possible publication bias in the smaller studies.

Hormone Replacement Therapy

Hormone replacement therapy (HRT) was the original antiresorptive therapy used for osteoporosis. However, current controversies centered on increased breast cancer, and cardiovascular risks have resulted in a marked decline in use for osteoporosis indications. A metaanalysis of 57 randomized studies, which compared at least 1 year of HRT with controls in postmenopausal women, showed a trend toward reduction of vertebral and nonvertebral fracture incidence. At 2 years, BMD increased by 6.76% in the LS and 4.12% in the femoral neck [31]. Perhaps the best prospective data to date that showed fracture reduction with combined HRT were those established in the Women's Health Initiative study. The incidence of clinical vertebral fractures was reduced by 34%, hip fractures by 34%, and all fractures by 24%. Absolute excess risks per 10,000 person-years attributable to estrogen plus progestin were 8 more coronary heart disease events, 8 more strokes, 8 more pulmonary emboli, and 8 more invasive breast cancers, while absolute RRs per 10,000 person-years were 6 fewer colorectal cancers and 5 fewer hip fractures [32].

Anabolic Therapy

Teriparatide

Synthetic human parathyroid hormone [PTH (1–34)], or teriparatide, is an anabolic agent that has been approved for postmenopausal and male osteoporosis treatment. The landmark trial in postmenopausal women was the Fracture Prevention Trial (FPT). In this study, 1,637 postmenopausal women received 20 or 40 mcg of teriparatide for a mean of 21 months. Vertebral fracture risk was decreased by 65% and 69%, respectively, and nonvertebral fracture risk by 53% and 54%. Mean increases in LS BMD of 9% and 13%, as well as 3% and 6% at the femoral neck, were seen. The most common side effects were nausea and headaches [33].

Teriparatide is approved for only 2 years of use because of a lack of studies that have gone beyond that time frame. Several studies have investigated what happens after the drug is discontinued. Extensions of the FPT have looked at changes in BMD and fracture risk after discontinuation of teriparatide. One study found that 30 months after discontinuation of teriparatide, the hazard ratio for nonvertebral fragility fractures was still significantly lower than placebo but only in the 40-μg group. BMD decreased over this time span in both groups, except in those who received bisphosphonates for at least 2 years during the trial [34]. Another study looked at vertebral BMD changes and fractures 1.5 years after discontinuing teriparatide. There continued to be a statistically significant increase in BMD and a decrease in fractures in those who had been on teriparatide. Those who used bisphosphonates for at least 1 year continued to gain BMD, whereas those who did not lost BMD [35].

The BMD effects of anabolic versus antiresorptive therapy have been compared in a randomized double-blind trial of teriparatide 40 μg versus alendronate 10 mg daily. By 3 months, and through the 14 months of the study, those in the teriparatide group experienced significantly greater increases in LS and hip BMD than those in the alendronate group. Nonvertebral fractures were significantly less in the teriparatide group [36].

What about administration of antiresorptive agents before anabolic therapy? The effects of teriparatide after administration of alendronate or raloxifene have been assessed. The prior raloxifene group had higher gains in BMD at the LS and the hip. The difference in LS BMD was largely due to an increase in the first 6 months [37]. Bone formation markers had a lesser and later peak in the alendronate group.

Combination Therapy

Trials that have studied combination therapy for osteoporosis had BMD and not fracture risk reduction as the primary endpoint. Thus, although the effects appear to be additive, it is unknown whether there is indeed a greater reduction in fracture risk when two agents are combined.

Combined HRT and alendronate have demonstrated superiority in BMD benefit than either agent alone. In a 2-year study of 425 postmenopausal women who were randomly assigned to receive estrogen, alendronate, a combination of the two, or placebo, the mean change in LS BMD was statistically higher with combination therapy than either agent alone [38]. Another trial gave alendronate 10 mg/day or placebo to 428 postmenopausal women on HRT for at least 1 year. After 12 months, alendronate produced significantly greater BMD increases in the LS (3.6% vs. 1.0%) and the hip trochanter (2.7% vs. 0.5%) than did placebo [39].

A study comparing raloxifene 60 mg/day and alendronate 10 mg/day, in combination or alone, in 331 postmenopausal women with femoral neck T-scores below -2 found a significantly greater LS BMD increase in the combination group than with alendronate or raloxifene alone (3.7% vs. 2.7% vs. 1.7%, respectively) [40].

The role of PTH as combination versus monotherapy has been addressed. The results have not been consistent, and similar to previous combination studies, conclusions have mostly been drawn from BMD and bone marker data. A study comparing PTH (1–84) 100 μg daily alone, alendronate alone, and the PTH-alendronate combination found no significant difference in LS BMD between PTH and the combination, but a significantly higher increase in hip BMD was seen in the combination therapy group compared to the PTH group. Rarely hypercalcemia and hypercalciuria were seen in the PTH and combination groups. This study contrasts with the results of the trial conducted by Black et al. [41], which showed that the volumetric increase in trabecular density in the spine of the PTH group was about twice the combination and alendronate-alone group. This, plus the greater increase in formation markers in the PTH-alone group, has led the investigators of this study to conclude that perhaps there was an attenuation of anabolic effect PTH by alendronate [41].

Nonpharmacologic Therapy
Calcium and Vitamin D Supplementation

In a metaanalysis of 15 trials comparing calcium with placebo, the pooled difference in percentage change from baseline was 2.05% for the total body BMD, 1.66% for the LS, and 1.64% for the hip in patients who received calcium. Vertebral fracture risk decreased by 23% and nonvertebral fracture risk by 14% in the calcium group [42].

The recommended intake of elemental calcium is 1,200 to 1,500 mg/day for adults over the age of 50 years. Intake of more than 2,000 to 2,500 mg is not recommended, as this may cause hypercalciuria. Vitamin D supplementation has been found to significantly reduce vertebral fractures by 37% in a metaanalysis of 25 trials. There was a trend toward reduction in nonvertebral fractures, as well (RR, 0.72; $p = 0.09$). Patients who received hydroxylated vitamin D had larger increases in BMD than those who received standard vitamin D [43].

For patients who are not found to be insufficient or deficient in vitamin D, the recommended dose of vitamin D is at least 400 to 800 IU per day (also refer to Chapter 7).

Weight-bearing Exercises

All patients should be counseled on exercises that are appropriate for those with osteoporosis. Benefits of exercise include improved muscle strength, gait, and balance, and better sense of well-being. Exercises should focus on strengthening the back and abdominal muscles, and also on improving overall strength. Motions that expose the spine to extreme forward flexion, should be avoided.

Fall Prevention

The clinician or nurse should spend time explaining ways to avoid falls, particularly to elderly patients who suffer from vision loss and balance problems. Hallways and stairways must be appropriately lit, rugs should be avoided, and stairways kept free of objects.

Hip Protectors

Hip protectors may be useful among nursing home patients and homebound elderly patients who fall frequently. Although the use of hip protectors may reduce hip fractures, adherence is only about 40% [44].

Kyphophasty and Vertebroplasty

These two surgical modalities have been reported to successfully relieve pain from acute compression fractures and decrease kyphosis slightly [45–48]. The procedures entail injection of polymethylmethacralate or bone cement directly into the fractured vertebra in vertebroplasty, and into a balloon within the vertebra, in kyphoplasty. Some of the potential complications include leakage of the cement into the spine, surrounding structures, and vessels, and development of the compression fractures in other vertebrae [49–51].

GLUCOCORTICOID-INDUCED OSTEOPOROSIS

The pathophysiology of glucocorticoid-induced osteoporosis (GIO) has been discussed in Chapter 2. The American College of Rheumatology has recommended the use of pharmacologic agents for the prevention or treatment of GIO when patients' use or anticipated use is more than 5 mg of prednisone (or its equivalent) for longer than 3 months. All patients must be advised to take calcium and vitamin D supplements [52]. If patients are vitamin D–deficient, pharmacologic doses of vitamin D should be prescribed.

Alendronate is approved for the treatment and prevention, and risedronate for the treatment, of GIO. The effect of alendronate on glucocorticoid-induced osteoporosis was studied in a 2-year trial of 477 men and women on glucocorticoids. The study showed significant increases in mean LS BMD by 2.1% and 2.9%, from 5 and 10 mg of alendronate per day. The femoral neck bone density significantly increased by 1.2% and 1.0% in the respective alendronate groups [53]. Risedronate has also been studied among men and women on glucocorticoids and showed significant increases in the LS and hip BMD [54,55]. To our knowledge, no fracture studies have been done in this patient population.

Although teriparatide has not been approved for GIO, increases in lumbar spine BMD and markers of bone formation have been observed among those treated with the drug [56,57].

MALE OSTEOPOROSIS

As mentioned in Chapter 5, the prevalence of secondary causes is much higher among men with osteoporosis. Before an osteoporosis drug is prescribed, a thorough evaluation for these secondary causes must be undertaken. In addition, men who are given androgen deprivation therapy (ADT) for prostate cancer should probably be prescribed bisphosphonates to prevent bone loss associated with testosterone deficiency.

In general, studies on male osteoporosis are smaller than those on postmenopausal women. One 2-year, double-blind, placebo-controlled trial involved 241 men with osteoporosis. The men who received alendronate had a mean increase in BMD of 7.1% at the LS, 2.5% at the femoral neck, and 2.0% for the total body. Vertebral fracture incidence was lower in the treated versus the placebo group (0.8% vs. 7.1%), and height loss was significantly greater in the placebo than alendronate group (2.4 mm vs. 6 mm) [58].

Teriparatide has also been shown to increase bone mass by 13% in the LS and 2.9% in the femoral neck in men with idiopathic osteoporosis [59]. A randomized trial of 83 men, with an LS or femoral neck T-score of less than or equal to -2, compared teriparatide, alendronate, and their combination over 2.5 years (teriparatide was started at month 6). The teriparatide group had significant increases in BMD at the LS and the femoral neck, and these were greater than what was seen in the alendronate and combination groups [60]. In a study that assessed BMD and fractures 30 months after a year of exposure to teriparatide, LS and total hip BMD remained significantly higher in the PTH group than placebo, even though the BMDs decreased after discontinuation [61]. When the subjects were divided according to bisphosphonate use, those who took bisphosphonates had an increase in spine and hip BMD, although significant intergroup differences were lost. Among those who did not take bisphosphonates, the BMD decreased. A significant decrease in moderate-to-severe spine fractures was seen at 18 months of follow-up.

REFERENCES

1. **Black DM, Cummings SR, Karpf DB,** et al. Randomised trial of effect of alendronate on risk of fracture in women with existing vertebral fractures. Fracture Intervention Trial Research Group. Lancet 1996;348:1535–1541.

This is a randomized placebo-controlled trial of 2,027 postmenopausal women aged 55 to 81 years with low femoral neck bone mineral density (BMD) who were assigned to receive placebo (n = 1,005) or daily alendronate (n = 1,022) and were observed during a follow-up for 36 months. Alendronate reduced the risk of new radiographic fractures by 47%. Clinically apparent vertebral fractures were reduced in the alendronate group [2.3 vs. 5.0%; relative hazard (RH), 0.45; CI, 0.27–0.72]. The risk of any clinical fracture was lower in the alendronate group than in the placebo group [139 (13.6%) vs. 183 (18.2%); RH, 0.72 (0.58–0.90)], including a 51% reduction in hip fracture. No significant differences in the number of adverse events in the two groups were seen.

2. **Cummings SR, Black DM, Thompson DE,** et al. Effect of alendronate on risk of fracture in women with low bone density but without vertebral fractures: Results from the Fracture Intervention Trial. JAMA 1998;280:2077–2082.

This was a prospective, double-blind, randomized, placebo-controlled study of 4,432 postmenopausal women aged between 54 and 81 years without preexisting vertebral fractures who were randomly assigned to receive alendronate or placebo and followed up for 4 years. Similar to FIT 1, alendronate was initially given at 5 mg/day for 2 years followed by 10 mg/day. Alendronate increased bone mineral density (BMD) at all sites studied (p < 0.001). Risk of radiographic vertebral fracture was reduced by 44% [RR, 0.56; 95% CI, 0.39–0.80; treatment-control difference, 1.7%; number needed to treat (NNT), 60]. Clinical vertebral fracture reduction was not significantly different; however, in the subset of patients with femoral neck T-scores of −2.5 or lower, alendronate reduced clinical vertebral fractures by 36% (RH, 0.64; 95% CI, 0.50–0.82; treatment-control difference, 6.5%; NNT, 15).

3. **Cranney A, Guyatt G, Griffith L,** et al. Meta-analysis of alendronate for the treatment of postmenopausal women. IX: Summary of meta-analyses of therapies for postmenopausal osteoporosis. Endocr Rev 2002;23:570–578.

This was a metaanalysis of 11 randomized, placebo-controlled trials of alendronate for postmenopausal osteoporosis. The pooled RR for vertebral fracture for the 5-mg dose was 0.52 (95% CI, 0.43–0.65), and for the nonvertebral fracture RR for 10 mg or more was 0.51 (CI, 0.38–0.69). Results for nonvertebral fractures were similar. Two- to 4-year percentage increases in bone mineral density (BMD) between alendronate and placebo were 7.48% (CI, 6.12–8.85) for the LS, 5.6% (CI, 4.8–6.39) for the hip, 2.08% for the forearm (CI, 1.53–2.63), and 2.73% (CI, 2.27–3.2) for the total body. Pooled RR for gastrointestinal side effects was 1.03 (0.81–1.3; p = 0.83).

4. **Papapoulos SE, Quandt SA, Liberman UA,** et al. Meta-analysis of the efficacy of alendronate for the prevention of hip fractures in postmenopausal women. Osteoporos Int 2005;16:468–474.

This was a metaanalysis of 6 randomized trials of alendronate that lasted from 1 to 4.5 years. At least 95% received 5 to 10 mg of alendronate daily. The subjects with a vertebral fracture or T-scores less than or equal to 2.0 who were on alendronate had a hip fracture risk reduction of 45% (CI, 16%–64%; p = 0.007); those with osteoporosis by T-score had a 55% reduced risk (CI, 29%–72%; p = 0.0008).

5. **Bone H, Hosking D, Devogelaer JP,** et al. Ten years' experience with alendronate for osteoporosis in postmenopausal women. N Engl J Med 2004;350:1189–1190.

This extension of a multicenter, randomized, double-blind study, originally of 994 postmenopausal women, assessed the bone mineral density (BMD) changes in 804 of them over 10 years. The original cohort was divided into four dosage groups: 20 mg for 2 years and then 5 mg for the third year; 5 mg, 10 mg, or placebo for 3 years. In the extension period, those in the 5-mg and 10-mg groups remained on their respective doses. The group originally on 20 mg, then 5 mg, remained on 5 mg for 2 more years, and then they were placed on placebo. The placebo group received 10 mg for the first 2 years of the extension, after which they did not take any further study medication. The most significant BMD changes were seen in those on 10 mg for 10 years. This group's BMD at the lumbar spine increased by a mean of 13.7% (CI, 12%–15.5%), at the trochanter by a mean of 10.3% (CI, 8.1%–12.4%), at the femoral neck by a mean of 5.4% (CI, 3.5%–7.4%), and by a mean of 6.7% at the proximal femur (CI, 4.4%–9.1%).

6. **Uusi-Rasi K, Sievanen H, Heinonen A,** et al. Effect of discontinuation of alendronate treatment and exercise on bone mass and physical fitness: 15-month follow-up of a randomized, controlled trial. Bone 2004;35:799–805.

These investigators conducted a 15-month extension of a 1-year trial examining the effect of alendronate and exercise on bone mineral density (BMD) and physical fitness parameters. Of the 152 original postmenopausal female subjects, 102 of them participated in the follow-up trial. After 1 year, alendronate was discontinued. Over the next 15 months, those in the prior alendronate group lost bone mass at a rate similar to that in the placebo group. Although a difference in mean BMD of 3.2% (CI, 1%–5.4%) persisted at the lumbar spine between the treatment and placebo groups, there was no difference at the femoral neck at the end of the follow-up phase.

7. **Schnitzer T, Bone HT, Cripaldi G,** et al. Therapeutic equivalence of alendronate 70 mg once-weekly and alendronate 10 mg daily in the treatment of osteoporosis. Alendronate Once-Weekly Study Group. Aging (Milano) 2000;12:1–12.

The efficacy and safety of treatment with oral once-weekly alendronate 70 mg, twice-weekly alendronate 35 mg, and daily alendronate 10 mg were compared in a 1-year, double-blind, multicenter study of postmenopausal women with osteoporosis by T-score or previous vertebral or hip fracture. Mean increases in lumbar spine (LS) bone mineral density (BMD) at 12 months were 5.1% (CI, 4.8–5.4) in the 70-mg once-weekly group, 5.2% (CI, 4.9–5.6) in the 35-mg twice-weekly group, and 5.4% (CI, 5.0–5.8) in the 10-mg daily treatment group. Increases in BMD at the total hip, femoral neck, trochanter, and total body were similar for the three groups. Reduction in markers of bone resorption [urinary N-telopeptide (NTX)] and bone formation [serum bone-specific alkaline phosphatase (BSAP)] was similar across three groups into the middle of the premenopausal reference range. Upper gastrointestinal adverse experiences were similar, with a trend toward a lower incidence of esophageal events in the once-weekly dosing group.

8. **Rosen CJ, Hochberg MC, Bonnick SL,** et al. Treatment with once-weekly alendronate 70 mg compared with once-weekly risedronate 35 mg in women with post-menopausal osteoporosis: a randomized double-blind study. J Bone Miner Res 2005; 20:141–151.

This randomized, double-blind, active-controlled, multicenter trial assessed bone mineral density (BMD) and bone turnover marker changes, as well as side effects, in 1,053 post-menopausal osteoporotic women who were randomized to alendronate 70 mg weekly or risedronate 35 mg weekly for 12 months. At 1 year, those on alendronate had small but significant increases in BMD over the subjects on risedronate, with treatment differences of 1.4% at the trochanter (CI, 0.8%–1.9%; $p < 0.001$), 1.1% at the hip (CI, 0.7%–1.4%; $p < 0.001$), 0.7% at the femoral neck (0.1%–1.2%; $p = 0.005$), and 1.2% at the lumbar spine (CI, 0.7%–1.6%; $p < 0.001$). Significant differences at all sites in BMD were seen at 6 months, as well. In the study, 10.3% more patients in the alendronate group demonstrated at least a 3% increase in trochanter BMD at 1 year (CI, 4%–16.7%; $p = 0.002$), and 16.7% more patients on alendronate rather than risedronate exhibited a maintenance or gain in trochanter BMD at 12 months ($p < 0.001$). CTX, N-telopeptide (NTX), bone-specific alkaline phosphatase (BSAP), and aminoterminal propeptide of type I collagen (PINP) were all depressed more with alendronate ($p < 0.001$). No significant differences in adverse events were noted between the two groups.

9. **Harris ST, Watts MB, Gennant HK,** et al. Effects of risedronate treatment on vertebral and nonvertebral fractures in women with postmenopausal osteoporosis: A randomized controlled trial. Vertebral Efficacy With Risedronate Therapy (VERT) Study Group. JAMA 1999;282:1344–1352.

In this randomized, double-blind, placebo-controlled trial, 2,458 postmenopausal women younger than 85 years of age and with at least one vertebral fracture were randomly assigned to receive 3 years of risedronate (2.5 or 5 mg/day) or placebo. All subjects received calcium (1,000 mg/day), and cholecalciferol (up to 500 IU/day) was provided if baseline levels of 25-OHD were low. The 2.5 mg/day of risedronate arm was discontinued after 1 year. Treatment with 5 mg/day of risedronate decreased incidence of new vertebral fracture risk by 41% (CI, 18%–58%) over 3 years (11.3% vs. 16.3%; $p = 0.003$). Vertebral fracture reduction of 65% (CI, 38%–81%) was seen after the first year (2.4% vs. 6.4%; $p < 0.001$). Nonvertebral fracture incidence over 3 years was reduced by 39% (CI, 6%–61%) (5.2% vs. 8.4%; $p = 0.02$). Bone mineral density (BMD) increased significantly compared with placebo at the lumbar spine (5.4% vs. 1.1%), femoral neck (1.6% vs. 21.2%), femoral trochanter (3.3% vs. 20.7%), and midshaft of the radius (0.2% vs. 21.4%). Bone biopsies obtained showed histologically normal bone.

10. *(1A)* **Reginster J, Minne HW, Sorensen OH,** et al. Randomized trial of the effects of risedronate on vertebral fractures in women with established postmenopausal osteoporosis. Vertebral Efficacy with Risedronate Therapy (VERT) Study Group. Osteoporos Int 2000;11:83–91.

The design of this European arm of the VERT study was similar to that of the U.S. arm. The study included 1,226 postmenopausal women. Risedronate reduced the risk of new vertebral fractures by 49% over 3 years compared with placebo ($p < 0.001$). A significant reduction of 61% was seen within the first year ($p = 0.001$). The risk of nonvertebral fractures was reduced by 33% compared with placebo over 3 years ($p = 0.06$). Risedronate significantly increased bone mineral density (BMD) at the spine and hip within 6 months. The adverse event profile of risedronate was not significantly different from that of placebo.

11. **Mellstrom DD, Sorensen OH, Goemaere S,** et al. Seven years of treatment with risedronate in women with postmenopausal osteoporosis. Calcif Tissue Int 2004;75:462–468.

This was the second 2-year extension of an originally 3-year randomized placebo-controlled trial that assessed the effect of risedronate on bone mineral density (BMD) and fractures. In this portion of the trial, 164 subjects enrolled and 83% of them (136 subjects) completed the 2-year phase. All patients received 5 mg/day of risedronate. In those who had been on treatment prior to this extension, their BMD gains persisted or improved. The incidence of vertebral fractures remained similar in years 4 through 7. Those who were in the placebo group prior to this extension experienced significant BMD gains; they also noted decreases in fracture rates to those similar to the treatment group.

12. **McClung MR, Geusens P, Miller PD,** et al. Effect of risedronate on the risk of hip fracture in elderly women. Hip Intervention Program Study Group. N Engl J Med 2001;344:333–340.

In this study, 5,445 postmenopausal women, 70 to 79 years old with osteoporosis (femoral neck T-score −4 or less or below −3 with a nonskeletal risk factor for hip fracture, such as poor gait or a propensity to fall; group 1) and 3,886 women at least 80 years old who had at least one nonskeletal risk factor for hip fracture or low bone mineral density (BMD) at the femoral neck (T-score below −4 or below −3 with a hip axis length ≥ 11.1 cm; group 2) were randomly assigned to receive oral risedronate (2.5 or 5.0 mg/day) or placebo for 3 years. The incidence of hip fracture among all the women in the risedronate group was reduced significantly (RR, 0.7; CI, 0.6–0.9; $p = 0.02$). In group 1, there was a significant reduction in hip fractures compared with placebo (RR, 0.6; CI, 0.4–0.9; $p = 0.009$). In group 2, incidence of hip fracture was not significantly different between the two groups ($p = 0.35$).

13. **Cranney A, Tugwell P, Adachi J,** et al. Meta-analyses of therapies for postmenopausal osteoporosis. III. Meta-analysis of risedronate for the treatment of postmenopausal osteoporosis. Endocr Rev 2002;23:517–523.

This was a metaanalysis of eight randomized trials that compared risedronate with placebo. The pooled RR of vertebral fractures in postmenopausal women given 2.5 mg or more of risedronate was 0.64 (CI, 0.54–0.77). The pooled RR of nonvertebral fractures was 0.73 (CI, 0.61–0.87). Mean percentage change difference between risedronate and placebo was 4.54% (CI, 4.12–4.97) in the lumbar spine and 2.75% (CI, 2.32–3.17) in the femoral neck.

14. **Brown JP, Kendler DL, McClung MR,** et al. The efficacy and tolerability of risedronate once a week for the treatment of postmenopausal osteoporosis. Calcif Tissue Int 2002;71:103–111.

This study's design included a randomized double-blind active controlled group of 1,456 postmenopausal women 50 years and older with T-score of less than −2.5 or less than −2.0 with at least one prevalent fracture. Risedronate, 35 mg once weekly, 50 mg once weekly, and 5 mg once daily, had similar efficacy and safety profiles. The mean percentage change in LS bone mineral density (BMD) after 12 months was 4.0% (0.2%) in the 5-mg daily group, 3.9% (0.2%) in the 35-mg group, and 4.2% (0.2%) in the 50-mg group.

15. **Reginster J, Wilson K, Dumont E,** et al. Monthly oral ibandronate is well tolerated and efficacious in postmenopausal women: Results from the Monthly Oral Pilot Study. J Clin Endocrinol Metab 2005;90:5018–5024.

In this randomized, double-blind, multicenter, placebo-controlled study, 144 postmenopausal women were given 50 mg, 100 mg, or 150 mg of ibandronate or placebo monthly. They were followed for 3 months for tolerability and changes in the bone turnover marker C-telopeptide (CTX). No significant differences in adverse events compared with placebo were discovered. CTX significantly decreased over these 3 months in those on 100- and 150-mg dosages (serum −40.7% and −56.7%, respectively, $p < 0.001$; urinary −34.6% and −54.1%, respectively, $p < 0.001$).

16. **Miller PD, McClung MR, Macovei L,** et al. Monthly oral ibandronate therapy in postmenopausal osteoporosis: 1-year results from the MOBILE study. J Bone Miner Res 2005;20:1315–1322.

This was a randomized, double-blind trial that searched for the appropriate ibandronate dose for the treatment of osteoporosis. The 1,609 postmenopausal osteoporotic women in the study were assigned to four groups: 2.5 mg daily, 50 mg/50 mg once a month, 100 mg once a month, or 150 mg once a month, and they were followed up for 2 years. Those on monthly ibandronate experienced increases in lumbar spine (3.9%, 4.3%, 4.1%, and 4.9%, respectively) and similar increases in hip bone mineral density (BMD) (about 2%–3%). The 150-mg group had small but significantly greater increases in lumbar spine BMD than the daily regimen ($p < 0.0001$). When the groups were evaluated for those who achieved BMD gains above baseline as well as over 6% at the LS or 3% at the hip, the 150-mg and 100-mg groups had significantly more patients at these goals than the daily regimen at the LS and at the hip (only 150 mg at the LS with respect to gains above baseline). Regarding side effects, the frequency of gastrointestinal symptoms with each dose was similar, but there was a small increase in flu-like symptoms with the monthly regimens (6.6% in the 50/50-mg group, 6.8% in the 100-mg group, 8.3% in the 150-mg group, and 2.8% in the daily group).

17. **Delmas PD, Adami S, Strugala C,** et al. Intravenous ibandronate injections in postmenopausal women with osteoporosis: One-year results from the dosing intravenous administration study. Arthritis Rheum 2006;54:1838–1846.

This was a noninferiority study of two regimens of intermittent intravenous injections of ibandronate (2 mg every 2 months and 3 mg every 3 months) and 2.5 mg of oral ibandronate daily. The study enrolled 1,395 postmenopausal women (ages 55–80 years) with osteoporosis [lumbar spine (L2–L4) bone mineral density (BMD) T-score less than −2.5]. Participants also received daily calcium (500 mg) and vitamin D (400 IU). At 1 year, mean lumbar spine BMD increases were as follows: 5.1% among 353 patients receiving 2 mg of ibandronate every 2 months, 4.8% among 365 patients receiving 3 mg of ibandronate every 3 months, and 3.8% among 377 patients receiving 2.5 mg of oral ibandronate daily. The intravenous (IV) regimens were superior to the oral regimen ($p < 0.001$). Hip BMD increases (at all sites) were also greater in the IV groups than in the oral group. Robust decreases in the serum CTX level were observed in all arms of the study. Both of the intravenous regimens were well tolerated and no adverse effects on renal function were noted.

18. **Lanza F, Schwartz H, Sahba B,** et al. An endoscopic comparison of the effects of alendronate and risedronate on upper gastrointestinal mucosae. Am J Gastroenterol 2000;95:3112–3117.

This was a multicenter, randomized, parallel-group, double-blind, placebo-controlled trial of 235 patients (men or postmenopausal women, aged 45–80 years) with normal upper gastrointestinal endoscopies at baseline. They received 28 days of the following therapy: alendronate 40 mg/day, risedronate 30 mg/day, placebo, or placebo with aspirin 650 mg four times a day for the last 7 days. Endoscopy was repeated on day 29. After 28 days of treatment, the alendronate and risedronate groups had comparable mean gastric and duodenal erosion scores, which were significantly lower than those in the aspirin group. Esophageal scores were comparable in all groups. Gastric ulcers alone, or combined with large numbers of gastric erosions, occurred in about 3% of alendronate and risedronate patients versus 60% in those treated with aspirin and placebo.

19. **Lanza FL, Hunt RH, Thomson AB,** et al. Endoscopic comparison of esophageal and gastroduodenal effects of risedronate and alendronate in postmenopausal women. Gastroenterology 2000;119:631–638.

Healthy postmenopausal women were randomly assigned to receive 5 mg risedronate or 10 mg alendronate for 2 weeks. Endoscopies were performed at baseline and on days 8 and 15. Gastric ulcers were observed during the treatment period in 9 of 221 (4.1%) evaluable subjects on risedronate compared with 30 of 227 (13.2%) on alendronate ($p < 0.001$). Mean gastric endoscopy scores for the risedronate group were lower than those for the alendronate group at days 8 and 15 ($p \leq 0.001$). Mean esophageal and duodenal endoscopy scores were similar in the two groups at days 8 and 15. Esophageal ulcers were noted in three evaluable subjects in the alendronate group, compared with none in the risedronate group, and duodenal ulcers were noted in one evaluable subject in the alendronate group and two in the risedronate group.

20. **Taggart H, Bolognese MA, Lindsay R,** et al. Upper gastrointestinal tract safety of risedronate: A pooled analysis of 9 clinical trials. Mayo Clin Proc 2002;77:262–270.

    The nine included studies enrolled 10,068 men and women who received placebo or 5 mg of risedronate sodium for up to 3 years (intent-to-treat population). The treatment groups were similar with respect to baseline gastrointestinal tract disease and use of concomitant treatments during the studies. There was no significant difference in upper gastrointestinal tract adverse events in the risedronate and placebo groups (29.8% and 29.6%, respectively). Risedronate-treated patients with preexisting active upper gastrointestinal disease did not experience worsening of their underlying conditions or an increased frequency of upper gastrointestinal adverse events. Concomitant use of nonsteroidal anti-inflammatory drugs (NSAIDs), requirement for gastric antisecretory drugs, or the presence of active gastrointestinal tract disease did not result in a higher frequency of upper gastrointestinal tract adverse events in the risedronate-treated patients compared with findings in controls. Endoscopy, performed in 349 patients, demonstrated no statistically significant differences across treatment groups.

21. **Odvina C, Zerwekh JE, Rao DS,** et al. Severely suppressed bone turnover: A potential complication of alendronate therapy. J Clin Endocrinol Metab 2005;90:1294–1301.

    This is a case report of nine osteoporotic patients on calcium and alendronate 10 mg daily or 70 mg weekly for 3 to 8 years. They each suffered a nonvertebral fragility fracture on this bisphosphonate, and two-thirds either did not heal this fracture or healed it slowly. Bone biopsies in these patients revealed decreased bone volume and minimal bone formation. Seven of the nine patients demonstrated few, if any, osteoblasts. Of note, osteocalcin was low-normal to low in these patients.

22. **Bagan JV, Jimenez Y, Murillo J,** et al. Jaw osteonecrosis associated with bisphosphonates: Multiple exposed areas and its relationship to teeth extractions. Study of 20 cases. Oral Oncol 2006;42:327–329.

    This is a case report of 20 cases of osteonecrosis of the jaw.

23. **Ruggiero SL, Mehrotra B, Rosenberg TJ, Engroff SL.** Osteonecrosis of the jaws associated with the use of bisphosphonates: A review of 63 cases. J Oral Maxillofac Surg 2004;62:527–534.

    Sixty-three patients were identified to have osteonecrosis of the jaw, presenting as nonhealing extraction sockets or exposed jaw bone. Fifty-six patients had received intravenous bisphosphonates for at least 1 year, and seven patients were on chronic oral bisphosphonate therapy. Biopsy of these lesions showed no evidence of metastatic disease.

24. **Camacho P, Girgis M, Sapountzi P, Sinacore J.** Correlations between vitamin D, parathyroid hormone, urinary calcium excretion, markers of bone turnover and bone density of patients referred to an osteoporosis center. J Bone Miner Res 2005;20(Suppl 1):S389.

    The primary aim of the study was to characterize the relationships between 25-OHD,1-25 OHD, intact parathyroid hormone (PTH), ionized calcium, phosphorus, 24-hour urine calcium excretion (UrCa), bone-specific alkaline phosphatase, urinary N-telopeptide (NTX)/creatinine, and bone density. In this study, 163 patients (143 female, 20 male; mean age, 62.5 years) evaluated for low bone mass at Loyola University Osteoporosis and Metabolic Bone Disease Center were studied. The strongest indirect relationship seen was between PTH and UrCa ($r = -0.496$; $p < 0.001$). 25-OHD showed a significant correlation with UrCa ($r = 0.420$; $p < 0.001$), PTH ($r = -0.215$; $p = 0.014$), BSAP ($r = -0.288$; $p = 0.010$), and a trend with spine bone mineral density (BMD) ($r = -0.156$; $p = 0.071$). Analysis of the subgroup with 25-OHD less than or equal to 20 ng/mL (26% of the group) showed that 25-OHD correlated significantly with PTH ($r = -0.354$; $p = 0.027$). The strong indirect correlation between PTH and UrCa ($r = -0.540$; $p = 0.021$) remained in this group. 1,25-OHD showed a trend associated with UrCa ($r = 0.459$; $p = 0.064$) and spine BMD ($r = -0.356$; $p = 0.069$). Ionized calcium, phosphorus, or NTX/creatinine did not show significant correlations with PTH or vitamin D levels. The difference between the means of PTH above and below a 25-OHD level of 30 ng/mL was significant. At 35 ng/mL, the significance was lost. The same 25-OHD level of 30 ng/mL showed significant differences in the UrCa of patients with 25-OHD above and below this threshold. This relationship was also significant at 35 ng/mL and was lost at 40 ng/mL. A level of 30 ng/mL was concluded as the cut-off of vitamin D deficiency. This was seen in 48% of the population.

25. **Ettinger B, Black DM, Mitlak BH,** et al. Reduction of vertebral fracture risk in postmenopausal women with osteoporosis treated with raloxifene: Results from a 3-year randomized clinical trial. Multiple Outcomes of Raloxifene Evaluation (MORE) Investigators. JAMA 1999;282:637–645.

This is a multicenter, randomized, blinded, placebo-controlled trial of 7,705 postmenopausal women with osteoporosis. They were randomly assigned to receive 60 or 120 mg/day of raloxifene or placebo. At 36 months, the risk of vertebral fracture was reduced in both study groups receiving raloxifene (60 mg/day group: RR, 0.7; and CI, 0.5–0.8; 120 mg/day group: RR, 0.5; and CI, 0.4–0.7). Frequency of vertebral fracture was reduced both in women with (50% reduction) and in women without prevalent fractures (30% reduction). Nonvertebral fracture reduction was not significant. Raloxifene increased BMD in the femoral neck by 2.1% (60 mg) and 2.4% (120 mg) and in the spine by 2.6% (60 mg) and 2.7% (120 mg) ($p < 0.001$ for all comparisons). Women receiving raloxifene had increased risk of venous thromboembolus compared with placebo (RR, 3.1; CI, 1.5–6.2).

26. **Delmas PD, Ensrud KE, Adachi JD,** et al. Efficacy of raloxifene on vertebral fracture risk reduction in postmenopausal women with osteoporosis: Four-year results from a randomized clinical trial. J Clin Endocrinol Metab 2002;87:3609–3617.

This was a 4-year extension of the Multiple Outcomes of Raloxifene Evaluation (MORE) trial. The 4-year cumulative RRs for one or more new vertebral fractures were 0.64 (CI, 0.53–0.76) with raloxifene 60 mg/day and 0.57 (CI, 0.48–0.69) with raloxifene 120 mg/day. The nonvertebral fracture risk was not significantly reduced (RR, 0.93; CI, 0.81–1.06). The safety profile after 4 years was similar to that observed after 3 years.

27. **Cranney A, Tugwell P, Zytaruk N,** et al. IV. Meta-analysis of raloxifene for the prevention and treatment of postmenopausal osteoporosis. Endocr Rev 2002;23:524–528.

This was a metaanalysis of seven trials comparing raloxifene with placebo. Pooled mean percentage increase in lumbar spine (LS) bone mineral density (BMD) was 2.51% (CI, 2.21–2.82), hip was 2.11 (CI, 1.68–2.53), total body was 1.33% (CI, 0.37–2.30), and forearm was 2.05% (CI, 0.71–3.39). Vertebral fracture reduction was 40% (CI, 0.5–0.7). Nonvertebral fracture reduction was not significant.

28. **Barrett-Connor E, Mosca L, Collins P,** et al. Effects of raloxifene on cardiovascular events and breast cancer in postmenopausal women. N Engl J Med 2006;355:125–137.

In this study, 10,101 postmenopausal women (mean age, 67.5 years) with coronary heart disease (CHD) or multiple risk factors for CHD were given 60 mg of raloxifene daily or placebo and followed for a median of 5.6 years. As compared with placebo, raloxifene had no significant effect on the risk of primary coronary events, and reduced the risk of invasive breast cancer. There was no significant difference in the rates of death from any cause or total stroke but raloxifene was associated with an increased risk of fatal stroke and venous thromboembolism. Raloxifene did reduce the risk of clinical vertebral fractures (64 vs. 97 events; HR, 0.65; 95% CI, 0.47–0.89; absolute RR, 1.3 per 1,000).

29. **Chestnut CH, Silverman S, Andriano K,** et al. A randomized trial of nasal spray calcitonin in postmenopausal women with established osteoporosis. The Prevent Recurrence of Osteoporotic Fractures Study. Am J Med 2000;109:267–276.

This was a 5-year, prospective, randomized placebo-controlled study of 1,255 postmenopausal women with one or more vertebral compression fractures and with a lumbar spine (LS) T-score of −2 or lower. The incidence of new vertebral fractures decreased significantly by 33% ($p = 0.05$) only in the calcitonin 200-IU group but not the 100-IU or 400-IU dose. There was no significant difference in nonvertebral fracture risk reduction between placebo and calcitonin.

30. **Cranney A, Tugwell P, Zytaruk N,** et al. VI. Meta-analysis of calcitonin for the treatment of postmenopausal osteoporosis. Endocr Rev 2002; 23:540–551.

In this metaanalysis of 30 studies, calcitonin reduced the incidence of vertebral fractures by 54% (CI, 0.25–0.87) over placebo. In a large randomized trial, the RR was 0.79 (CI, 0.62–1.0). The pooled RR for nonvertebral fractures was 0.52 (CI, 0.22–1.23). In the largest trial, this was not significant. Pooled increases in weighted mean difference were 3.74 (CI, 2.04–5.43) for the lumbar spine, 3.02 (CI, 0.98–5.07) at the combined mean forearm, and 3.80 ($p = 0.07$) at the femoral neck.

31. **Wells G, Tugwell P, Shea B,** et al. Meta-analysis of the efficacy of hormone replacement therapy in treating and preventing osteoporosis in postmenopausal women. Endocr Rev 2002;23: 529–539.

    This metaanalysis of 57 randomized studies showed a trend toward reduction of incidence of vertebral fractures (RR, 0.66; CI, 0.41–1.07; 5 trials) and nonvertebral fractures (RR, 0.87; CI, 0.71–1.08; 6 trials) with HRT. Bone mineral density (BMD) increase was 6.76% at 2 years in the lumbar spine (LS) (21 trials), 4.12% (9 trials) in the femoral neck, and 4.53% (14 trials) in the forearm.

32. **Writing Group for the Women's Health Initiative Investigators**. Risks and benefits of estrogen plus progestin in healthy postmenopausal women: Principal results from the Women's Health Initiative (WHI) randomized controlled trial. JAMA 2002;288:321–333.

    In this randomized control study of more than 16,000 postmenopausal women, Prempro [a proprietary named for conjugated equine estrogens (CEE) 0.625 mg and medroxyprogesterone 2.5 mg] significantly reduced the risk of clinical vertebral fractures by 34%, hip fractures by 34%, and all fractures by 24% over placebo over 5 years. Increased breast cancer and cardiovascular risk led to discontinuation of this treatment arm. Estimated hazard ratios were as follows: congestive heart disease 1.29 (CI, 1.02–1.63); breast cancer 1.26 (CI, 1.00–1.59); stroke 1.41 (CI, 1.07–1.85); pulmonary embolism 2.13 (CI, 1.39–3.25); colorectal cancer 0.63 (CI, 0.43–0.92); endometrial cancer 0.83 (CI, 0.47–1.47); hip fracture 0.66 (CI, 0.45–0.98); death due to other causes 0.92 (CI, 0.74–1.14).

33. **Neer RM, Arnaud CD, Zanchetta JR,** et al. Effect of parathyroid hormone (1–34) on fractures and bone mineral density in postmenopausal women with osteoporosis. N Engl J Med 2001;344: 1434–1441.

    In this study, 1,637 postmenopausal women with prior vertebral fractures were randomly assigned to once-daily 20 or 40 µg SC of parathyroid hormone [PTH (1–34)] or placebo for a median of 21 months. RRs of fracture in the 20- and 40-µg groups, compared with placebo, were 0.35 (CI, 0.22–0.55) and 0.3 (CI, 0.19–0.50). Nonvertebral fracture RRs were 0.47 (CI, 0.25–0.88) and 0.46 (CI, 0.25–0.861). Compared with placebo, the 20- and 40-µg doses of PTH increased LS bone mineral density (BMD) by 9% and 13%, and by 3% and 6% in the femoral neck; the 40-µg dose decreased BMD at the shaft of the radius by 2%, but total body BMD was increased by 2% to 4%. Most common side effects included nausea and headache.

34. **Prince R, Sipos A, Hossain A,** et al. Sustained nonvertebral fragility fracture risk reduction after discontinuation of teriparatide treatment. J Bone Miner Res 2005;20: 1507–1513.

    This observational study assessed nonvertebral changes in 1,262 of the Fracture Prevention Trial (FPT) subjects for 30 months after discontinuation of teriparatide. Although the hazard ratios for nonvertebral fragility fractures remained significantly less in the treatment groups when the entire 50 weeks were analyzed, if the period of time after teriparatide discontinuation was solely assessed, only the 40-mg group had a significant decrease. Bone mineral density (BMD) decreased after teriparatide discontinuation in both groups, except in those on bisphosphonates for at least 2 years during the trial.

35. **Lindsay R, Scheele WH, Neer R,** et al. Sustained vertebral fracture risk reduction after withdrawal of teriparatide in postmenopausal women with osteoporosis. Arch Intern Med 2004;164: 2024–2030.

    This is an observational study of 1,262 Fracture Prevention Trial (FPT) subjects who were followed up for 18 months after teriparatide discontinuation. The treatment groups continued to have a significantly decreased risk of vertebral fractures (41% for 20-µg, $p = 0.004$, and 45% for 40-µg, $p = 0.001$). The absolute vertebral fracture risk reduction was about 13% for both treatment groups. In addition, although lumbar spine (LS) bone mineral density (BMD) was still significantly greater in the treatment groups at the end of the follow-up study, those who used bisphosphonates for at least 1 year continued to gain BMD, whereas those not on bisphosphonates lost BMD.

36. **Body J, Gaich GA, Scheele WH,** et al. A randomized double-blind trial to compare the efficacy of teriparatide [recombinant human parathyroid hormone (1–34)

with alendronate in postmenopausal women with osteoporosis. J Clin Endocrinol Metab 2002;87:4528–4545.

In this randomized trial, 146 postmenopausal women with osteoporosis were studied for a median of 14 months. They received either 40 µg of teriparatide and a placebo tablet or 10 mg of alendronate and a placebo injection. A significantly greater increase in lumbar spine (LS) bone mineral density (BMD) was seen in the teriparatide group by the third month (p < 0.001). At the study's end, significantly greater increases in LS, femoral neck, and total body BMD were noted in the teriparatide group. However, a significant decrease in one-third distal radius BMD occurred in the teriparatide group ($p \leq 0.05$). The teriparatide group also experienced a significant decrease in nonvertebral fracture incidence (4.1% vs. 13.7%; $p < 0.05$).

37. **Ettinger B, San Martin J, Crans G, Pavo I**. Differential effects of teriparatide on BMD after treatment with raloxifene or alendronate. J Bone Miner Res 2004; 19:745–751.

This is an 18-month observational study of 59 postmenopausal women, with a T-score of at least −2, on 20 µg of teriparatide after 1.5 to 3 years of either alendronate or raloxifene. Those in the alendronate group started with lower bone turnover markers. The markers in the raloxifene group tended to be higher, but the difference was not statistically significant except for bone-specific alkaline phosphatase (BSAP), osteocalcin, and PINP at 1 month. At 3 and 6 months, those in the prior raloxifene group had significant lumbar spine (LS) bone mineral density (BMD) increases (2.1% at 3 months and 5.2% at 6 months), whereas the prior alendronate group did not. After the first 6 months, the rates of increase in both groups were similar. At 18 months, the raloxifene group had gained 10.2% in LS BMD, compared with 4.1% in the alendronate group ($p < 0.001$). At the hip during the first 6 months, BMD in the raloxifene group changed little, whereas that in the alendronate group decreased by 1.8%. After 6 months, both groups had about an 1.5% increase in hip BMD.

38. **Bone HG, Greenspan SL, McKeever C,** et al. Alendronate and estrogen effects in postmenopausal women with low bone mineral density. Alendronate/Estrogen Study Group. J Clin Endocrinol Metab 2000;85:720–726.

This was a prospective, double-blind, placebo-controlled, randomized clinical trial in which 425 postmenopausal women who had previously undergone hysterectomy with low bone mass were randomly assigned to receive placebo, oral alendronate, 10 mg/day; conjugated estrogen, 0.625 mg/day; or a combination of the two drugs. At 2 years, mean percentage changes in lumbar spine (LS) bone mineral density (BMD) were 0.6% for placebo, 6% for alendronate ($p < 0.001$ vs. placebo), 6% for conjugated equine estrogens (CEE) ($p < 0.001$ vs. placebo), and 8.3% for combination therapy ($p < 0.001$ vs. placebo and CEE; $p = 0.022$ vs. alendronate). The corresponding changes in total proximal femur BMD were 4.0%, 3.4%, 4.7%, and 0.3% for the alendronate, estrogen, alendronate plus estrogen, and placebo groups, respectively. Greater reductions in urinary N-telopeptide (NTX) and bone-specific alkaline phosphatase (BSAP) were seen in the combination therapy than either one alone.

39. **Lindsay R, Cosman F, Lobo RA,** et al. Addition of alendronate to ongoing hormone replacement therapy in the treatment of osteoporosis: A randomized, controlled clinical trial. J Clin Endocrinol Metab 1999;84:3076–3081.

In this randomized, placebo-controlled trial of 428 postmenopausal women with osteoporosis who had been receiving hormone replacement therapy (HRT) for at least 1 year, alendronate 10 mg/day plus HRT produced significantly greater increases in bone mineral density (BMD) of the LS (3.6% vs. 1.0%; $p < 0.001$) and hip trochanter (2.7% vs. 0.5%; $p < 0.001$) compared with HRT alone; the intergroup difference in BMD at the femoral neck was not significant (1.7% vs. 0.8%; $p = 0.072$). Serum bone-specific alkaline phosphatase (BSAP) and urine N-telopeptide (NTX) decreased significantly at 6 and 12 months with alendronate plus HRT, after which they remained within premenopausal levels. No differences in upper gastrointestinal adverse events or fractures were seen.

40. **Johnell O, Scheele WA, Lu Y,** et al. Additive effects of raloxifene and alendronate on bone density and biochemical markers of bone remodeling in postmenopausal women with osteoporosis. J Clin Endocrinol Metab 2002;87:985–992.

This study was a phase 3, randomized, double-blind, 1-year trial that evaluated the effects of combined raloxifene and alendronate in 331 postmenopausal women with osteoporosis. Patients received placebo, raloxifene 60 mg/day, alendronate 10 mg/day, or a combination of the latter two. Mean lumbar spine (LS) bone mineral density (BMD) increases over baseline were 2.1%, 4.3%, and 5.3% in the raloxifene, alendronate, and combination groups, respectively ($p < 0.05$). The mean increase in femoral neck BMD in the combination group was 3.7% compared with the 2.7% and 1.7% increases in the alendronate ($p = 0.02$) and raloxifene ($p < 0.001$) groups, respectively. The changes from baseline to 12 months in bone markers ranged from -7.1% to -16.0% with placebo, -23.8% to -46.5% with raloxifene, -42.3% to -74.2% with alendronate, and -54.1% to -81.0% in the raloxifene–alendronate combination group. Although the alendronate group had changes in BMD and bone markers that were approximately twice the magnitude as found in the raloxifene group, clinical correlation to fractures is not known. Combined therapy reduced markers of bone turnover to a greater degree than either drug alone.

41. **Black DM, Greenspan SL, Ensrud KE,** et al. The effects of parathyroid hormone and alendronate alone or in combination in postmenopausal osteoporosis. N Engl J Med 2003;349:1207–1215.

This was a 1-year study of 238 postmenopausal women with T-scores of less than -2.5, or a T-score of less than -2.0 with an additional risk factor for osteoporosis who were randomly assigned to daily treatment with parathyroid hormone [PTH (1–84)] (100 µg; 119 women), alendronate (10 mg; 60 women), or both (59 women). Lumbar spine bone mineral density (BMD) increased in all the treatment groups, and there was no significant difference in the increase between the PTH group and the combination-therapy group. However, in terms of the volumetric density of the trabecular bone at the spine, the increase in the PTH group was about twice that found in either of the other groups. Bone formation increased markedly in this group but not in the combination-therapy group. Bone resorption decreased in the combination-therapy group and the alendronate group.

42. **Shea B, Wells G, Cranney A,** et al. Meta-analysis of calcium supplementation for the prevention of postmenopausal osteoporosis. Endocr Rev 2002;23:552–559.

This is a metaanalysis of 15 trials comparing calcium with placebo. The pooled difference in percentage change from baseline was 2.05% for the total body bone mineral density (BMD), 1.66% for the lumbar spine (LS), 1.64% for the hip in patients who received calcium. Vertebral fracture RR was 23% and nonverterbral fracture reduction was 14%.

43. **Papadimitropoulos E, Wells G, Shea B,** et al. Meta-analysis of the efficacy of vitamin D treatment in preventing osteoporosis in postmenopausal women. Endocr Rev 2002;23:560–569.

This was a metaanalysis of 25 randomized trials of vitamin D with or without calcium versus control. The incidence of vertebral fractures was reduced (RR, 0.63; CI, 0.45–0.88; $p < 0.01$) and nonvertebral fracture incidence showed a trend toward reduction (RR, 0.77; CI, 0.57–1.04; $p = 0.09$). Hydroxylated vitamin D had a more profound effect on bone mineral density (BMD) than standard vitamin D. Total body BMD was increased by 2.06% in patients who received hydroxylated vitamin D compared with 0.4% in those who received standard vitamin D.

44. **Cameron ID, Venman J, Kurrle ST,** et al. Hip protectors in aged-care facilities: A randomized trial of use by individual higher-risk residents. Age Ageing 2001;30: 477–481.

This was a randomized controlled trial of 174 women who lived in nursing homes or aged-care facilities and who had two or more falls or at least one fall that required hospital admission in the previous 3 months. During follow-up, a mean of 4.6 falls per person occurred. There was no difference in mortality. Eight hip fractures occurred in the intervention group and seven in the control group (HR, 1.46; CI, 0.53–4.51). No hip fractures occurred when hip protectors were being worn as directed. Adherence was about 57% over the duration of the study, and hip protectors were worn at the time of 54% of falls in the intervention group.

45. **Berlemann U, Franz T, Orler R, Heini PF.** Kyphoplasty for treatment of osteoporotic vertebral fractures: A prospective non-randomized study. Eur Spine J 2004; 13:496–501.

This study presented 1-year results of 27 kyphoplasty procedures for osteoporotic compression fractures. All but one patient experienced pain relief following the procedure, and all 25 patients exhibited a lasting effect over the follow-up period. An average vertebral kyphosis reduction of 47.7% was achieved with no loss of reduction after 1 year. During follow-up, one fracture adjacent to a treated level was observed.

46. **Machinis TG, Fountas KN, Feltes CH,** et al. Pain outcome and vertebral body height restoration in patients undergoing kyphoplasty. South Med J 2006;99: 457–460.

Twenty-four patients underwent kyphoplasty for a total of 37 compression fractures. Mean VAS score improved and all patients returned to their daily activities within 24 hours. There was no observed significance in restoration of vertebral body height.

47. **Pradhan BB, Bae HW, Kropf MA,** et al. Kyphoplasty reduction of osteoporotic vertebral compression fractures: Correction of local kyphosis versus overall sagittal alignment. Spine 2006;31:435–441.

In 65 consecutive patients who underwent kyphoplasty, local kyphotic deformity at the fractured vertebra was reduced by an average of 7.3 degrees (63% of preoperative kyphosis); however, this did not translate to similar correction in overall sagittal alignment.

48. **McGraw JK, Lippert JA, Minkus KD,** et al. Prospective evaluation of pain relief in 100 patients undergoing percutaneous vertebroplasty: results and follow-up. J Vasc Interv Radiol 2002;13(9 Pt 1):883–886.

One hundred patients (156 fractures) who underwent vertebroplasty were asked to quantify their pain on a visual analog scale (VAS) and complete a follow-up questionnaire. One patient sustained a sternal fracture and one experienced a transient radiculopathy. In this study, 97% of the patients reported significant pain relief 24 hours after treatment; 93% reported significant improvement in back pain and noted improved ambulation.

49. **Baumann A, Tauss J, Baumann G,** et al. Cement embolization into the vena cava and pulmonal arteries after vertebroplasty: interdisciplinary management. Eur J Vasc Endovasc Surg 2006;31:558–561.

A case report of cement embolization into the IVC and pulmonary arteries. The large embolus from the IVC was extracted and the patient was given anticoagulant therapy for 3 months. One year later the patient was asymptomatic.

50. **Syed MI, Jan S, Patel NA,** et al. Fatal fat embolism after vertebroplasty: Identification of the high-risk patient. AJNR Am J Neuroradiol 2006;27:343–345.

A case report of fat embolism after vertebroplasty in 3 levels. Cement was not found to have leaked or embolized.

51. **Trout AT, Kallmes DF, Kaufmann TJ.** New fractures after vertebroplasty: adjacent fractures occur significantly sooner. AJNR Am J Neuroradiol 2006;27:217–223.

This was a report of 186 new vertebral fractures that occurred in 86 (19.9%) of 432 patients. Seventy-seven (41.4%) fractures were of vertebrae adjacent to the level treated with vertebroplasty. Median times until diagnosis of new adjacent and nonadjacent level fractures were 55 days and 127 days, respectively. Distance of the new fracture from the treated level was also significantly associated with time to new fracture ($p < 0.0001$). Relative risk of adjacent level fracture was 4.62 times that for nonadjacent level fracture.

52. **American College of Rheumatology Ad Hoc Committee on Glucocorticoid-Induced Osteoporosis.** Recommendations for the prevention and treatment of glucocorticoid-induced osteoporosis: 2001 update. Arthritis Rheum 2001;44:1496–1503.

The main recommendation was that all patients be advised to take calcium and vitamin D supplements. Bisphosphonates should be prescribed to those who are anticipated to use prednisone at greater than or equal to 5 mg/day for more than 3 months, or those on long-term glucocorticoids in whom the bone mineral density (BMD) T-score at either the lumbar spine or the hip is below normal.

53. **Saag K, Emkey R, Schnitzer TJ,** et al. Alendronate for the prevention and treatment of glucocorticoid-induced osteoporosis. Glucocorticoid-Induced Osteoporosis Intervention Study Group. N Engl J Med 1998;339:292–299.

Two 48-week, randomized, placebo-controlled studies of two doses of alendronate were conducted on 477 men and women on glucocorticoids. The mean bone mineral density (BMD) of the lumbar spine (LS) increased by 2.1% ± 0.3% and 2.9% ± 0.3% in the groups that received 5 mg and 10 mg of alendronate per day, respectively ($p < 0.001$), and decreased by 0.4% ± 0.3% in the placebo group. The femoral neck bone density increased by 1.2% ± 0.4% and 1.0% ± 0.4% in the respective alendronate groups ($p < 0.01$) and decreased by 1.2% ± 0.4% in the placebo group ($p < 0.01$). The BMD of the trochanter and total body also increased significantly in the patients on alendronate. There were proportionally fewer new vertebral fractures in the alendronate groups (overall incidence, 2.3%) than in the placebo group (3.7%; RR, 0.6; CI, 0.1–4.4). Markers of bone turnover decreased significantly in the alendronate groups ($p < 0.001$). There were no differences in serious adverse effects among the three groups, but there was a small increase in minor upper gastrointestinal effects in the 10-mg group.

54. **Eastell R, Devogelaer JP, Peel NF,** et al. Prevention of bone loss with risedronate in glucocorticoid-treated rheumatoid arthritis patients. Osteoporos Int 2000;11:331–337.

    This was a 2-year, double-masked, placebo-controlled trial with a third year of nontreatment follow-up in which 120 women on long-term glucocorticoid therapy (>2.5 mg/day prednisolone) were randomly assigned to receive daily placebo, risedronate 2.5 mg/day, or cyclic risedronate (15 mg/day for 2 of 12 weeks). At the end of 97 weeks, bone mineral density (BMD) was maintained at the lumbar spine (LS) (1.4%) and trochanter (0.4%) in the daily 2.5-mg risedronate group, whereas significant bone loss occurred in spine and hip of the placebo group (-1.6%; $p = 0.03$; and -4.0%; $p < 0.005$, respectively). At the femoral neck, there was an insignificant bone loss in the daily 2.5-mg risedronate group (-1.0%), whereas in the placebo group, bone density decreased significantly (-3.6%; $p < 0.001$). The difference between placebo and daily 2.5-mg risedronate groups was significant at the LS ($p = 0.009$) and trochanter ($p = 0.02$) but was not significant at the femoral neck. Although not significantly different from placebo at the LS, the overall effect of the cyclic regimen was similar to that of the daily 2.5-mg risedronate regimen. After treatment was withdrawn, there was significant bone loss at the LS. Adverse events (including upper gastrointestinal events) were similar across treatment groups.

55. **Reid DM, Hughes RA, Laan RF,** et al. Efficacy and safety of daily risedronate in the treatment of corticosteroid-induced osteoporosis in men and women: A randomized trial. European Corticosteroid-Induced Osteoporosis Treatment Study. J Bone Miner Res 2000;15:1006–1013.

    This was a multicenter, double-blind, placebo-controlled study of 290 men and women on high-dose oral corticosteroid therapy (prednisone at least 7.5 mg/day or higher or equivalent) for 6 or more months. Risedronate 2.5 or 5 mg/day or placebo was administered for 12 months. All patients received 1 g calcium and 400 IU vitamin D daily. The primary endpoint was LS bone mineral density (BMD) at month 12. Overall, there were statistically significant treatment effects on BMD at 12 months at the lumbar spine (LS) ($p < 0.001$), femoral neck ($p = 0.004$), and trochanter ($p = 0.010$). Risedronate 5 mg increased BMD at 12 months by an SEM of 2.9% (0.49%) at the LS, 1.8% (0.46%) at the femoral neck, and 2.4% (0.54%) at the trochanter, whereas BMD was maintained only in the control group. The incidence of vertebral fractures was reduced by 70% in the combined risedronate treatment groups, relative to placebo ($p = 0.042$). No difference in gastrointestinal adverse events was noted between the risedronate and placebo groups.

56. **Lane NE, Sanchez S, Modin GW,** et al. Parathyroid hormone treatment can reverse corticosteroid-induced osteoporosis. Results of a randomized controlled clinical trial. J Clin Invest 1998;102:1627–1633.

    One-year randomized clinical trial of human parathyroid hormone [PTH (1–34)] in postmenopausal women (mean age, 63 years) with osteoporosis who were taking corticosteroids and hormone replacement therapy. The mean ($\pm$ SE) changes in bone mineral density (BMD) of the lumbar spine by quantitative computed tomography (QCT) and dual-energy x-ray absorptiometry (DXA) in the PTH group were 35 $\pm$ 5.5% and 11 $\pm$ 1.4%, respectively, significantly greater than the small change of 1.7 $\pm$ 1.8% and 0 $\pm$ 0.9% observed in the estrogen-only group. The differences in mean percentage between the groups at 1 year were 33.5% for the lumbar spine by QCT ($p < 0.001$) and 9.8% for the lumbar spine by DXA ($p < 0.001$). The changes in the hip and forearm were not significantly different between or within the groups. Markers of bone formation increased to nearly 150% in the first 3 months of therapy, whereas markers of bone resorption increased only 100%

57. **Lane NE, Sanchez S, Modin GW,** et al. Bone mass continues to increase at the hip after parathyroid hormone treatment is discontinued in glucocorticoid-induced osteoporosis: Results of a randomized controlled clinical trial. J Bone Miner Res 2000;15:944–951.

    Patients in this study continued to have an increase in bone mineral density (BMD); the total change in lumbar spine BMD by quantitative CT and dual-energy x-ray absorptiometry

(DXA) at 24 months was 45.9 ± 6.4% and 12.6 ± 2.2% ($p < 0.001$). The change in total hip and femoral neck BMD was not significant at 12 months but increased to 4.7 ± 0.9% ($p < 0.01$) and 5.2 ± 1.3% at 24 months, respectively. The estrogen group had a small change of 1.3 ± 0.9% and 2.6 ± 1.7%. Biochemical markers remained elevated throughout 12 months, and returned to baseline within 6 months of discontinuing the parathyroid hormone (PTH).

58. **Orwoll E, Ettinger M, Weiss S,** et al. Alendronate for the treatment of osteoporosis in men. N Engl J Med 2000;343:604–610.

This is a 2-year, double-blind, placebo-controlled trial. The effect of daily alendronate (10 mg) or placebo on bone mineral density (BMD) in 241 men with osteoporosis was evaluated. About one-third had low serum-free testosterone concentrations at baseline; the rest had normal concentrations and no other secondary causes of osteoporosis. The men who received alendronate had a mean (±SE) increase in BMD of 7.1% ± 0.3% at the lumbar spine (LS), 2.5% ± 0.4% at the femoral neck, and 2.0% ± 0.2% for the total body ($p < 0.001$ for all comparisons with baseline). In contrast, men who received placebo had an increase in LS BMD of 1.8% ± 0.5% ($p < 0.001$ for the comparison with baseline) and no significant changes in femoral-neck or total-body BMD. Vertebral fracture incidence was lower in the alendronate group than in the placebo group (0.8% vs. 7.1%; $p = 0.02$), and height loss was significantly greater in the placebo than in the alendronate group (2.4 vs. 0.6 mm; $p = 0.02$).

59. **Bilezikian JP, Kurland ES**. Therapy of male osteoporosis with parathyroid hormone. Calcif Tissue Int 2001;69:248–251.

This was the first controlled, randomized, double-blind study of parathyroid hormone (PTH) in men with idiopathic osteoporosis. Twenty-three men, aged 30 to 64 years, with Z-scores below −2.0, were assigned to placebo or treatment. After 18 months, there were significant increases in lumbar spine (LS) bone mineral density (BMD) (13.5% ± 3%) and femoral neck BMD (2.9% ± 1.5%). The distal radius site did not change. There was no further increase in BMD in the LS, but the femoral neck continued to show gains during the 12-month extension. Markers of bone formation and resorption increased in the PTH arm, reaching a peak between 9 and 12 months of therapy and declining thereafter.

60. **Finkelstein J, Hayes A, Hunzelman JL,** et al. The effects of parathyroid hormone, alendronate, or both in men with osteoporosis. N Engl J Med 2003;349:1216–1226.

This is a randomized trial of 83 men, with a lumbar spine (LS) or femoral neck T-score of at least −2, that compared daily teriparatide 40 µg, alendronate 10 mg, and their combination over 2.5 years (teriparatide was started at month 6). Significant increases in bone mineral density (BMD) at the lumbar spine (LS) (posterior-anterior view 7.9% vs. 18.1% vs. 14.8%;, respectively; $p < 0.001$) and the femoral neck [3.2% vs. 9.7% ($p < 0.001$) vs. 6.2% ($p = 0.01$)] in the teriparatide group were seen over those on either alendronate or the combination. The differences between the alendronate and the combination groups were not significantly different, except at the spine. Significant increases in alkaline phosphatase were noted in the teriparatide group ($p < 0.001$).

61. **Kaufman J, Orwoll E, Goemaere S,** et al. Teriparatide effects on vertebral fractures and bone mineral density in men with osteoporosis: Treatment and discontinuation of therapy. Osteoporos Int 2005;16:510–516.

This observational study of bone mineral density (BMD) and fractures over 30 months, in 355 men who were exposed to 1 year of teriparatide, showed that lumbar spine (LS) and hip BMD remained significantly higher in the teriparatide group than placebo ($p \leq 0.001$), even though BMD decreased overall. Those on bisphosphonates had an increase in spine and hip BMD, although the significant intergroup difference was lost. In those not on bisphosphonates, the BMD decreased. Also, a significant decrease in moderate-to-severe spine fractures was seen (83%; $p = 0.01$) at 18 months.

9

Tailoring Therapy to Individual Patients

Paul D. Miller

Patients with Prior Fragility Fractures, 151
Postmenopausal Patients with Low Bone Mineral Density without
  Prior Fracture, 152
Fall Prevention Strategies, 157
Treatment to Reduce Risk of Specific Types of Fractures or in
  Patients with Specific Needs, 158

The pharmacological agents for the prevention and treatment of post-menopausal osteoporosis (PMO) registered with the Food and Drug Administration (FDA) are listed in Table 9.1.

The FDA has distinguished between prevention and treatment registrations for PMO. In order to gain a prevention indication, an agent needs to show that bone mineral density (BMD) loss can be prevented in early post-menopausal women as compared with placebo. For a treatment indication, an agent must show evidence of significant vertebral fracture risk reduction over a 3-year period as compared with placebo. Hence, there are agents that have FDA labels for both indications, and agents that have evidence for only a prevention indication [e.g., hormonal replacement therapy (HT)].

It is also important to put the HT registration in historical perspective: When HT was FDA approved for PMO, the "prevention vs. treatment" registration distinction did not exist. The treatment (e.g., fracture) distinction was created by the FDA when the evidence became available that sodium fluoride increased BMD in a linear manner yet was not associated with any reduction in vertebral fracture risk [1]. In fact, in the U.S. fluoride study just cited, nonvertebral fracture events were greater in the treated (fluoride) group than placebo. Due to this disconnect between improvements in BMD and lack of risk reduction, the FDA changed the registration requirements for a "treatment" indication to fracture risk reduction as opposed to maintenance of BMD. However, the doses of fluoride used in the pivotal U.S. fluoride study induced a very abnormal bone histology, which explained the poor bone quality and strength despite improvements in BMD. Nevertheless, requirements for registration for osteoporosis agents now had two categories: prevention and treatment. Notwithstanding, data from the large, prospective Women's Health Initiative (WHI) study [2] were the

Table 9.1.   FDA-approved medications for use in osteoporosis

Generic Name	Trade Name	Prevention	Treatment
Hormone therapy		X	
Calcitonin	Miacalcin		X
Raloxifene	Evista	X	X
Alendronate	Fosamax	X	X
Risedronate	Actonel	X	X
Ibandronate	Boniva		X
Teriparatide	Forteo		X

Adapted from Miller PD, personal communication.

first to show evidence for significant reduction in both vertebral as well as nonvertebral fracture risk. However, to gain a "new" label, the end point must be the primary end point, and in the WHI dataset, fracture risk assessment was a secondary end point. Hence, there is still no FDA label for HT for "treatment." In a similar manner, cyclical administration of the first-generation nonamino bisphosphonate etidronate did not gain FDA registration for "treatment," since the FDA treatment requirement is evidence over 3 years of significant vertebral fracture risk reduction. In the pivotal clinical trials, etidronate did achieve significant fracture risk reduction over 2 but not through 3 years, as compared with placebo [3]. Etidronate registration got "caught" in the FDA registration requirement change (BMD to fracture) as a result of the fluoride studies, since when the etidronate clinical trials were planned, the FDA requirement for registration was a BMD, not fracture, end point. The etidronate clinical trials were statistically powered for a BMD, not a fracture, end point (e.g., smaller sample sizes). Etidronate thus never gained FDA registration for the treatment of PMO, due in larger part to a change in the registration data requirement. Nevertheless, cyclical etidronate is registered in more than 30 other countries for the treatment of PMO and still is used for the treatment of PMO in the United States in specific circumstances (e.g., intolerability to newer amino bisphosphonates).

Table 9.1 shows the FDA-registered therapies for PMO at the current time. Nasal or injectable calcitonin, raloxifene, alendronate, risedronate, ibandronate, and teriparatide are registered for the treatment of PMO [4–13]. This chapter will focus on these registered products, recognizing that physicians also utilize in an "off-label" fashion intravenous pamidronate, zolendronic acid, and HT for treatment (now defined as risk reduction) in individual patients for particular clinical reasons. In that vein, strontium ranelate (Protelos), registered in Europe for treatment of PMO, may also become available for off-label use in the United States, by patients obtaining access via other nations' pharmacy availability [14]. In addition, the 1–84 parathyroid hormone (PTH; PREOS) formulation was recently also approved for the treatment of PMO in Europe and is under consideration for registration in the United States [15].

Individual treatment decisions for selecting therapy for PMO are complex. Although there are "guidelines" published for whom to treat and when to treat to prevent BMD loss or to reduce the risk of fracture by specific highly acknowledged organizations [National Osteoporosis Foundation (NOF), American Association for Clinical Endocrinologists (AACE)], treatment decisions are often individualized by clinicians based on case-by-case individual circumstances [16,17]. Although important health-economic considerations for treatment "thresholds" based on public-policy considerations are critical to putting the costs of osteoporosis treatment in the proper perspective of global health-economics and competition for public expenditures for many other chronic diseases, the physician and patient embark on decisions often based on what an individual patient needs. So, although the important considerations for health-economic-based decisions are very necessary, this chapter will try to incorporate the issues of evidence of efficacy of therapies with opinion-based decisions based on broad clinical experience.

PATIENTS WITH PRIOR FRAGILITY FRACTURES

Postmenopausal women with prior fragility fracture are at high risk for future fracture [18–22]. These patients are at high risk for future fractures within a short period of time after a fracture—even at skeletal sites that are distant from where the original fracture occurred (Table 9.2) [22]. These fragility fractures are predictive of future fracture risk, independent of the prevailing BMD (or T-score) [23]. Exactly why a prior fragility fracture at one skeletal site conveys a high risk for a future fracture at a distant skeletal site is unclear. Perhaps, in the untreated postmenopausal population, a fragility fracture is symbolic of systemic skeletal fragility. In those patients with hip fractures, evidence indicates that the older the patient, the less important low BMD becomes as a contributor for the hip fracture, and that falls are a larger component of the risk [24]. In the National Osteoporosis Risk Assessment (NORA) dataset, even in those women who have reported a prior wrist fracture after the age of 45 years, there is a greater risk for all (global) fractures at nonwrist skeletal sites [25]. Even though a solid reason for why there is a greater risk for a second fracture following the first fracture is not definitive, the reality is that it is—and these are patients who need the strongest considerations for treatment interventions.

One of the limitations of the pharmacological clinical trials that have shown evidence for fracture risk reduction in postmenopausal women is

Table 9.2. Prior fractures as a predictor

Prior fracture	Relative Risk of Future Fractures		
	Wrist	Vertebra	Hip
Wrist	3.3	1.7	1.9
Vertebra	1.4	4.4	2.3
Hip	NA	2.5	2.3

From **Klotzbuecher CM, Ross PD, Landsman PB,** et al. Patients with prior fractures have an increased risk of future fractures: A summary of the literature and statistical synthesis. J Bone Miner Res 2000;15:721–739, with permission.

that the patients randomized between treatment and placebo groups have been randomized based on a prior vertebral fracture and/or a low BMD (e.g., T-score of −2.0 or below) and are 60 years of age or older. Though a prior fragility fracture of the forearm, hip, or shoulder conveys a high risk for future fracture, it is unknown if treatment with the FDA-approved osteoporosis-specific pharmacological agents reduces the risk in the other postmenopausal populations who have higher BMD levels or who are under the age of 60 years. Nevertheless, clinicians should seriously consider treatment intervention beyond adequate vitamin D and calcium in postmenopausal women who sustain a fragility fracture after the age of 45 to 50 years. The exception is the data from the Women's Health Initiative (WHI), which did show a benefit of HT in reducing fractures in a population generally considered not to have had osteoporosis by World Health Organization (WHO) criteria and in subgroups of the WHI under the age of 60 years [26].

POSTMENOPAUSAL PATIENTS WITH LOW BONE MINERAL DENSITY WITHOUT PRIOR FRACTURE

Patients who have "osteoporosis" or "osteopenia" by WHO criteria are at increased risk for fragility fractures—based simply on their low BMD alone. In fact, whether the technique for measuring BMD uses central or peripheral bone mass measuring devices, there are a greater number of post-

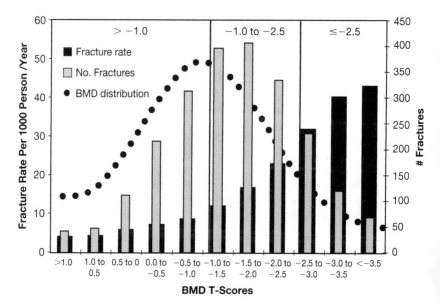

Figure 9.1. Fracture rate and total fracture number as a function of the bone mineral density (BMD) T-score from the National Osteoporosis Risk Assessment (NORA) study. As BMD declines, fracture rate increases. The total number of fractures is more in the osteopenic as compared to the osteoporotic population because there are more osteopenic than osteoporotic women. (From Siris E, Miller P, Barrett-Connor E, et al. Identification and fracture outcomes of undiagnosed low bone mineral density in postmenopausal women: Results from the National Osteoporosis Risk Assessment (NORA). JAMA 2001;286:2815–2822, with permission.)

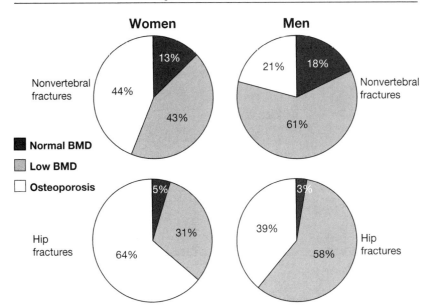

Figure 9.2. The distribution of nonvertebral and hip fractures in postmenopausal women and elderly men as a function of the femoral neck T-score classification of the World Health Organization (WHO). A large proportion of fractures are not osteoporotic by WHO criteria. BMD, bone mineral density. (From Wainwright SA, Marshall LM, Ensrud KE, et al. Study of Osteoporotic Fractures Research Group. Hip fracture in women without osteoporosis. J Clin Endocrinol Metab 2005;90:2787–2793, with permission.)

menopausal women who sustain fractures that have WHO "osteopenia" rather than osteoporosis—because there are simply more people with osteopenia than osteoporosis [27–29] (Figs. 9.1 and 9.2). The latter observations present a conundrum—how to stratify risk to select those patients who are at greater risk for fracture who do not have WHO osteoporosis without overtreating those with osteopenia that have a lower fracture risk.

A number of papers have been published that look at the interaction of risk factors and fracture risk prediction [30–32]. All of these studies show that as the number of risk factors increases, the risk for hip or all fractures also increases. In addition, above a certain number of risk factors [4,5] the risk for fracture begins to plateau, and it is clear that certain risk factors have more power to predict risk than others: prior fracture, increased age, low BMD, and family history of osteoporosis are easily captured in clinical practice. The risk factor assessment also shows that a "T-score is not a T-score is not a T-score." For example, in the 5-year fracture risk score by Black et al. [31] (Fig. 9.3), Mrs. L, with a T-score of −2.8, has a lower 5-year fracture risk than Mrs. R, with a T-score of −1.7. This is related to the fact that the fracture risk of Mrs. L is based on the risk calculated from low BMD and age alone, whereas the presence of a prior fracture and smoking in Mrs. R puts her at greater risk for fracture, even though her T-score is better. Thus, just basing risk and intervention decisions on a BMD (or T-score) level alone for the osteopenic population becomes problematic. What level of BMD or T-score should be a cutoff

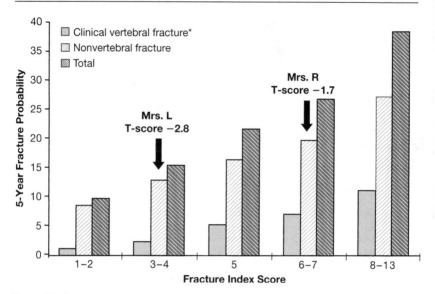

Figure 9.3. Five-year fracture risk as a function of the number of specific risk factors. Mrs. R has a higher fracture risk than Mrs. L, despite a better T-score, due to a greater number of risk factors in Mrs. R. (From Black DM, Steinbuch M, Palermo L, et al. An assessment tool for predicting fracture risk in postmenopausal women. Osteoporos Int 2001;12:519–528, with permission.)

for intervention? There is no clear answer, but progress in this arena has been made.

It appears that the WHO diagnostic threshold for osteoporosis of a T-score of −2.5 is close to an intervention threshold of −2.5 for treating a postmenopausal woman at age 50 years with the intent of reducing the 10-year absolute fracture risk for all (global) fractures to less than 10% [33] (Fig. 9.4). The WHO absolute fracture risk validation data have spear-headed the establishment of intervention thresholds based on 10-year longitudinal population studies representing data collection from more than 90,000 untreated postmenopausal women. The individual risk factors that have been validated as consistently predicting fracture risk are shown in Table 9.3. The 10-year risk for all fractures at age 50 years and a T-score of −2.5 is 10%. What level of risk is an unacceptable risk? This question may be answered from both a health-economic and a clinical point of view. From the WHO perspective, the treatment threshold is a health-economic one and may be decided from country to country based on the gross domestic product (GDP) of each nation and the disutility costs of the fracture(s). The treatment threshold will also vary according to the cost of the specific pharmacological therapy. For example, for the United States, the intervention threshold may be set at 10% fracture risk or greater. Hence, from the health-economic perspective, physicians and payors may provide treatment based on a risk for all fractures over 10 years of 10% or greater. This would mean at age 50 years, a postmenopausal woman with a T-score of −2.5 or lower [at the femoral neck, based on calculation from the National Health

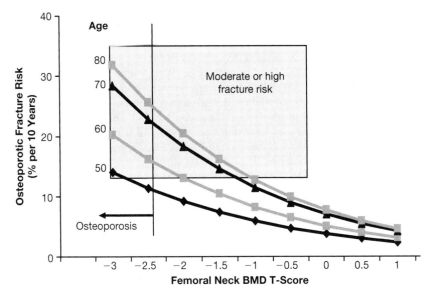

Figure 9.4. Relationship between age and femoral neck T-score and the 10-year risk for all (global) fracture risk. At the same bone mineral density (BMD), risk increases with age. (From Kanis JA, Johnell O, Oden A, et al. Ten year probabilities of osteoporotic fractures according to BMD and diagnostic thresholds. J Bone Miner Res 2001;16:S19–S24, with permission.)

and Nutrition Examination Survey III (NHANES III) database] would receive treatment for osteoporosis.

The treatment threshold would be different (e.g., T-score of −1.5) if the patient had additional risk factors that, when added to low BMD and age alone, would also yield a fracture risk over 10 years of 10% or more. Hence, a postmenopausal woman at age 50 years with a family history of osteoporosis and who is also a smoker would be treated at a T-score of −1.5. Thus, the WHO absolute fracture risk validated data will allow the tailoring of treatment based on decisions that incorporate more than just the T-score level and help move the field forward to a risk-based treatment decision process.

Table 9.3. World Health Organization population-based validated risk factors for global fracture risk over a 10-year period

Low bone mineral density
Older age
Prior fragility fracture
Any history of steroid use
Rheumatoid arthritis
Smoking
Excess alcohol
Family history

From a clinical point of view, the WHO absolute fracture risk model has limitations. The WHO model does not include morphometric vertebral fractures or bone turnover markers, both of which are known to independently predict fracture risk as well [34,35]. The WHO risk project did not include morphometric vertebral fractures or bone turnover markers in the risk model because these two risk factors were not captured in the 12 population studies that were used to validate the other risk factors.

In all clinical trial datasets that have led to FDA approval of all of the pharmacological therapies for PMO, the presence of a morphometric vertebral fracture is consistently associated with an increased risk for future fracture in the placebo arms. Had the WHO been able to add morphometric vertebral fractures into the risk predictive model, the 10-year risk would be greater than the risk based on T-score and age without a morphometric fracture. Since more morphometric vertebral fractures than clinical (painful) vertebral fractures occur in women and men after the age of 50 years, risk could be underestimated if morphometric vertebral fractures are missed.

How do clinicians resolve this important issue—to use the WHO absolute fracture risk model that, it is hoped, will be added to the dual-energy x-ray absorptiometry (DXA) computer printouts, yet also judge treatment if a morphometric vertebral fracture is identified?

The International Society for Clinical Densitometry (ISCD) has spearheaded the application of vertebral fracture assessment (VFA) by DXA as a respected means of identifying vertebral fractures and has developed indications for VFA performance and Medicare reimbursement [36]. The National Osteoporosis Foundation (NOF) is charged with leading the implementation of the use of the WHO absolute fracture risk model in the United States. It is probable that the NOF clinical report on the WHO risk model will also state that the identification of a morphometric vertebral fracture means that treatment should be considered, even if the WHO absolute calculated risk is not 10% or more. This is because of the high risk of future fracture (for all fractures) that is seen from the placebo arms of the clinical trials once a morphometric vertebral fracture is identified. In addition, from specific population data as well, the presence of a morphometric vertebral fracture is also associated with a greater risk for future fracture [37,38]. Hence, individual physicians will be able to tailor treatment decisions based on risk beyond just the WHO absolute model alone. This individual decision is clear if a prior morphometric vertebral fracture is identified.

Other risk factors that clinicians often use to individualize treatment are bone turnover markers (BTMs), especially markers of bone resorption. In several studies, a high rate of bone turnover is associated with a greater risk for fracture, independent of the prevailing BMD [34,35,39]. In addition, published studies indicate that the rate of postmenopausal bone loss has some correlation to the baseline level of bone turnover—for example, the higher the BTM, the greater the rate of bone loss [36]. Hence, a clinical decision may be made if the BTM is high as opposed to normal. For example, one might consider treatment in a postmenopausal woman with a T-score of -1.4 if her resorption marker is high as opposed to normal or low. Although there is no evidence that response to osteoporosis pharmacological therapy is greater (e.g., fracture risk reduction) if the BTM is high or normal, the decision to treat may be triggered if one believes that a woman who is concerned about osteoporosis prevention has a greater rate of loss and fracture risk based on a high BTM. Much of this type of decision based on BMD and bone turnover marker levels has to do with individual patient concerns about maintaining BMD at the current level. In theory, this approach is based on maintenance of BMD, such that the BMD will not be lower 10 years later when the fracture risk could be higher due to older age. Other considerations include preserving BMD at the current level to reduce the lifetime risk of fracture, an untested consideration. Here, the concept is that if BMD continues to decline over a patient's lifetime, the risk for fracture is greater as the patient gets older. Though the lifetime fracture risk as a function of the menopausal BMD (or T-score) is not validated, the concept is valid—based on the continual rate of bone loss seen after the menopause in untreated women, the lower the BMD will become as age increases. Accompanying a lower BMD and an older age will be a greater fracture risk. Thus, earlier intervention in younger postmenopausal women without osteoporosis by WHO criteria is often tailored to mitigating lifetime fracture risk.

A few other non-WHO-validated independent risk factors for fracture include a long hip axis length (HAL), hip structural analysis (HSA), and the Femur Strength Index (FSI). These parameters, which are capable of being measured by DXA and are available in specific DXA softwares, have been shown in small studies to predict hip fracture risk, independent of the hip BMD level [40–42]. The most recent report of these DXA-derived strength parameters is the Hip Strength Analysis Program, which incorporates the HAL, cross-sectional moment of inertia (CSMI), and the Femur Strength Index. The FSI is the ratio of the estimated compressive yield strength of the femoral neck to the expected compressive stress of a fall on the greater trochanter [43]. The FSI was significantly lower in hip-fractured patients as compared with controls, as the HAL was significantly higher than in controls, and these two strength parameters predicted hip fracture independent of the prevailing T-score. Hence, once these interesting preliminary findings are validated in larger sample sizes and we develop means of modifying these parameters, these DXA software applications will take on greater clinical meaning both for risk prediction and for additional therapeutic interventions.

The considerations for tailoring therapy to individual patients should include strategies to modify frailty. Abundant literature shows that frailty can be quantitated in the elderly population, and that certain "frailty scores" are associated with a greater risk for falling and hip fractures [44]. In addition, certain frailty parameters can be modified to reduce frailty and reduce the risk for falls [45]. For example, lower-extremity muscle tone and balance can be improved with specific interventions and are associated with a lower hip fracture risk [46].

FALL PREVENTION STRATEGIES

Falls are a greater contribution to hip fracture than low BMD in the more elderly population [24]. In addition, specific pharmacological therapy that reduces hip fracture risk in specific populations may not be as effective in the more elderly population [11]. In this latter cited clinical trial, falls were not captured in the dataset in this population, 80 years of age and older, randomized on the basis of risk factors for falling, so it remains unknown if more falls were the reason that pharmacological treatment was ineffective. Notwithstanding, it seems logical to target fall prevention strategies in frail individuals that may have a greater impact on reducing hip fractures than pharmacological therapies.

TREATMENT TO REDUCE RISK OF SPECIFIC TYPES OF FRACTURES OR IN PATIENTS WITH SPECIFIC NEEDS

Early Postmenopausal Women

HT is useful in preventing postmenopausal bone loss; in women who also have menopausal symptoms, it is the intervention of choice that can accomplish two end points. Whereas menopausal symptoms are the first indication for HT, the physician can also feel confident that for the majority of women who receive proper formulations of HT, their skeleton can also be protected [2]. The WHI data are very clear on this outcome. The dose of conjugated equine estrogen (0.625 mg/day) reduced both clinical vertebral as well as hip fractures. While not FDA labeled for the treatment of PMO, the lack of an FDA registration does not mean that there is a lack of evidence for a fracture reduction benefit.

The same statement can be said of many agents FDA registered for the treatment of PMO. Although the pivotal clinical trial that led to the FDA registration of raloxifene—MORE (multiple outcomes raloxifene evaluation)—had powerful vertebral fracture reduction data, no effect was demonstrated on a risk reduction for nonvertebral or hip fractures [5]. Although this lack of efficacy does not necessarily mean that raloxifene could not reduce the risk of nonvertebral or hip fractures in the context of a different clinical trial design, it does suggest that the target population for raloxifene should be postmenopausal women with a low spine BMD and normal hip BMD, or younger (50–65 years) postmenopausal women with a vertebral fracture and low risk for hip fracture.

One of the hypotheses for why bisphosphonates show evidence for reduction in vertebral, nonvertebral, and hip fracture risk (especially nonvertebral fracture risk) is that they induce a greater reduction in BTMs and a greater increase in hip BMD (in metaanalysis) than other antiresorptive agents [47]. Hence, in targeting specific therapy for the reduction of nonvertebral or hip fractures in patients with prior nonvertebral fractures or a low hip BMD, bisphosphonates have become the mainstay of therapy. Although different bisphosphonates have different evidence for risk reduction or FDA "labels," and the marketing of bisphosphonates involves claims of one specific benefit over another (e.g., alendronate has a FDA label for hip fracture reduction, and risedronate does not have this FDA endorsement), the evidence from clinical trial data is that bisphosphonates have a global effect of risk reduction. The exception is the oral ibandronate data that did not show evidence in any prospective manner for reduction in nonvertebral or hip fracture risk [12]. Ibandronate did show evidence for reduction in nonvertebral fracture risk in a post hoc analysis in those postmenopausal women with lower hip BMD. To the extent that ibandronate reduces BTMs and increases BMD in a similar fashion to the other bisphosphonates, there is no reason to believe its skeletal distribution or effect on nonvertebral bone strength would differ from that of the other available bisphosphonates.

It is also important to emphasize that the FDA approval of all of the intermittent bisphosphonate formulations (weekly, monthly, quarterly) was not based on any fracture-reduction data, but rather on noninferiority statistical end points: The intermittent formulations increased BMD to the equal degree as the fracture-proven daily formulations [48–50]. Hence, the use of intermittent formulations is based on the trust that within the same class of compounds, risk reduction is the same as for the fracture-proven daily formulations. For the patient with a higher risk for nonvertebral or hip fracture, bisphosphonates have become strongly considered as one of the treatments of choice.

What Specific Populations Should Be Targeted for the Use of Teriparatide?

Teriparatide, the first registered anabolic agent for the treatment of PMO, is also the first agent that affects bone by a totally different mechanism of action than that of the antiresorptive agents. Teriparatide adds new bone to the periosteal surface, increases trabecular bone volume and connectivity, and offers a means of affecting bone strength not offered by antiresorptive agents.

What patients should be targeted to receive teriparatide? Two separate reviews have suggested which patients should be considered for teriparatide intervention [51,52]. There seems to be agreement that teriparatide should be targeted toward high-risk populations. What constitutes high risk? Patients with prior fragility fractures and older (>65 years) patients who have T-scores of −3.0 or lower are generally considered at high risk for future fractures. Even though the teriparatide clinical trial that led to the FDA registration of teriparatide did not show evidence for hip fracture reduction, there is strong indirect evidence that hip strength is increased with teriparatide use [53]. Hence, clincians should not be reluctant to initiate teriparatide as first-line therapy in elderly patients with low hip BMD.

An additional group of patients for whom teriparatide might be used as initial treatment are those who cannot tolerate an oral bisphosphonate or in whom an oral bisphosphonate is unsafe (e.g., patients with esophageal stricture). For these, teriparatide offers a safe alternate [nongastrointestinal (non-GI)] route of administration. Even though intravenous bisphosphonates may also be considered in patients with gastrointestinal diseases for which oral bisphosphonates may be unsafe or not absorbed (celiac disease, bowel resections, etc.), there is plausible reason to still use this anabolic agent as first-line therapy for 18 to 24 months. Opinions that teriparatide should be initiated before bisphosphonates—for example, the treatment sequence should be teriparatide followed by an antiresorptive agent—have been expressed. This opinion is based on several observations: that prior exposure to bisphosphonates might mitigate or delay the anabolic effect of teriparatide [54,55] and that after teriparatide is discontinued, axial BMD declines, unless an antiresorptive agent is applied [56,57]. In addition, data show that when a bisphosphonate is applied after discontinuation of PTH therapy, the BMD may even increase more [56,58]. Hence, the concept of using an anabolic agent first and then an antiresorptive agent has wide appeal.

What about the use of PTH as first-line therapy in a lower-risk postmenopausal population? The clinical trial that examined the 1–84 PTH effect on fracture risk in postmenopausal women (Treatment of Osteoporosis with PTH, or TOP) randomized greater than 80% of the population without a prevalent vertebral fracture [15]. There was a significant reduction in the first incident vertebral compression fracture in this population. Thus, evidence exists that PTH reduced risk in a lower-risk population. Certainly for the bone biological reasons previously cited, treating treatment-naive patients first with an anabolic agent to "make new bone" unencumbered by any prior antiresorptive effect on bone turnover could also lead to treating a lower-risk postmenopausal population first with PTH.

Treating Populations with Parathyroid Hormone and Raloxifene

The selective estrogen receptor modulator (SERM) raloxifene is FDA approved to prevent as well as treat postmenopausal osteoporosis. There is also evidence that raloxifene reduces the risk of specific forms of breast cancer in postmenopausal women both at low risk and at high risk for breast cancer [59]. Hence, it is plausible that in specific populations, raloxifene might be considered (still off-label) for breast cancer prevention, and PTH in the same population at risk for nonvertebral or hip fracture.

What are the bone biological implications of PTH-raloxifene combinations? Data suggest that prior or concomitant administration of raloxifene may not mitigate the anabolic effect of PTH as assessed by improvements in BMD or the rise in bone formation markers [60,61]. It could be that this possible lower degree of the inhibition of the PTH anabolic effect is due to the lower degree of bone turnover that is induced by raloxifene as compared with bisphosphonates.

Tailoring Therapy to Premenopausal Women or Younger Men

There are specific clinical circumstances in which pharmacological intervention might be considered in premenopausal women or younger men. These are highly specialized situations that are clearly off-label use of bisphosphonates or teriparatide and that are best handled by specialists in metabolic bone disease.

The use of bisphosphonates or teriparatide in glucocorticoid-induced or post–solid-organ-transplantation bone loss, or osteogenesis imperfecta (OI), is the subject of separate chapters in this book. Occasionally, however, the younger patient with fragility fractures of the appendicular or axial skeleton comes to the specialist. It is important to emphasize that neither bisphosphonates nor teriparatide should be used in these patients solely on the basis of low BMD or T-scores. Young women and men with low BMD (or T-scores) alone usually are healthy and have low peak adult bone mass, are not losing BMD, and are not at any increased risk for fracture. Specifically, women on DeproProvera for birth control or endometriosis may lose BMD on this agent, but there is no evidence that they are at any increased risk for fracture or respond to bisphosphonates or PTH. In addition, once the DeproProvera is discontinued, they recover most, if not all, of the BMD that might have been lost during the DeproProvera use [62].

Nevertheless, when a younger woman or man presents with unusual fragility fractures, careful assessment is needed for secondary conditions that might lead to fracture. It most cases, a secondary condition can be identified (celiac disease, Cushing disease, mastocytosis, prolactinoma, renal tubular acidosis, and so on). Double tetracycline–labeled bone biopsy might be useful in this situation, not only to exclude mastocytosis (which may be missed by only a bone marrow aspiration), but also to possibly discover occult osteomalacia and low bone turnover. The latter might be related to inadequate production of insulin-like growth factor 1 (IGF-1) or IGF-2 and could lead to a consideration of teriparatide as opposed to bisphosphonate use. If no etiology for recurrent fragility fractures can be discovered (including forms of OI), then a bisphosphonate or teriparatide may be offered for a brief period of time because idiopathic juvenile osteoporosis (IJO) may respond to these therapies and patients with unexplained fragility may increase their bone strength with therapy. Fragility (stress) fractures of metatarsals or metacarpals should not be considered in the same category as other nonvertebral fractures, and this author would not consider pharmacological therapy in such cases.

Obviously, bisphosphonate use in special circumstances must be applied with the clear informed consent that there are no scientific data on their efficacy in conditions beyond OI and IJO in younger populations and that bisphosphonates do cross the placenta. Although there are no reported teratogenic cases in women on bisphosphonates who have had successful pregnancies (e.g., post–solid-organ-transplant patients or those on chronic glucocorticoids), there also has never been a systematic review of this population. Hence, any bisphosphonate in premenopausal women must be used with caution and only in very specific circumstances. In addition, use should be limited to as brief a period as clinically necessary.

Hypogonadism is also a cause of fragility fractures in the younger population but represents a specific etiology. The cause of the hypogonadism should be defined and gonadal steroid replacement for bone effects considered.

Two special circumstances in which fragility fractures may occur and be related, in part, to hypogonadism are anorexia nervosa and fractures in athletes [63–65]. Although both may be associated with either amenorrhea or hypomenorrhea, there are patients in either subset who may have fragility fractures (even hip) and may not be hypogonadal. Low body mass index (BMI) and disorders of nutrition also contribute to impaired bone strength in these populations. In the case of elite athletes, fractures are seen in those patients who also apply impact to their skeleton—runners, ballet dancers, and gymnasts. It is very rare to see fragility fractures in swimmers or bikers. Treatment in these specific populations should be directed at the complex issues that underlie the anorexia or low BMI, and, if possible, gonadal steroid replacement should be given when indicated. The use of bisphosphonates or teriparatide in these groups has not been studied, though there might be specific circumstances in which their use might be justified on a clinical basis.

Finally, there is wide use of teriparatide for nonunion of fractures, and there is also an ongoing FDA registration study examining the effect of teriparatide versus placebo in promoting union of forearm fractures. The consideration of this off-label use of teriparatide for recalcitrant nonunion of fractures should be fully discussed with the patient as well as the other physicians responsible for the care of the patient.

The tailoring of therapy to specific indications or to specific populations is an important application of the available treatments that can improve bone strength and reduce risk for fragility fractures. Although evidence may not exist from clinical trial data to support the use of osteoporosis-specific pharmacological agents in many clinical circumstances that the clinician may face, there are specific populations for which which use of agents that alter bone remodeling and may improve bone strength should be considered.

REFERENCES
Annotations by Alexandra Reiher

1. **Riggs BL, Hodgsan SF, O'Fallon WM,** et al. Effect of fluoride treatment on the fracture rate in postmenopausal women with osteoporosis. N Engl J Med 1990;322: 802–809.

   This was a 4-year randomized, prospective trial in 202 postmenopausal women with osteoporosis and vertebral fractures assigned to receive 75 mg/day sodium fluoride or placebo. All subjects received a daily calcium supplement of 1,500 mg. Increases in median bone mineral density (BMD) were seen in the treatment group of 35% ($p < 0.0001$) in the lumbar spine, 10% ($p < 0.0001$) in the femoral trochanter, and 12% ($p < 0.0001$) in the femoral neck, as compared with the placebo group. However, a 4% ($p < 0.02$) decrease in BMD was observed in the radial shaft. The treatment and placebo group had similar amounts of new vertebral fractures (p not significant), but there were more nonvertebral fractures in the treatment group (72 vs. 24; $p < 0.01$). Major side effects included lower extremity pain and gastrointestinal symptoms, and were significant enough to necessitate decreased dosage in 54 fluoride-treated subjects and 24 from the placebo group.

2. **Writing Group for The Women's Health Initiative Investigators.** Risks and benefits of estrogen plus progestin in healthy postmenopausal women: principal results from the women's health initiative randomized control trial. JAMA 2002;288:321–323.

   The Women's Health Initiative, a randomized controlled primary prevention trial, included 16,608 postmenopausal osteoporotic women, ages 50 to 79 years old and with an intact uterus, and evaluated the risks and benefits of treatment with estrogen plus progestin. Coronary heart disease was the primary outcome, and invasive breast cancer was the primary adverse outcome. Subjects received conjugated estrogens, 0.625 mg/day, plus medroxyprogesterone acetate, 2.5 mg/day, or placebo. After a mean of 5.2 years of follow-up (planned length was 8.5 years), the trial was stopped early because the test statistic for invasive breast cancer exceeded the predetermined stopping boundary, and the global index statistics were consistent with risks exceeding benefits. Estimated hazard ratios (HRs; nominal 95% CIs) were CHD, 1.29 (1.02–1.63); breast cancer, 1.26 (1.00–1.59); stroke, 1.41 (1.07–1.85); pulmonary embolism (PE), 2.13 (1.39–3.25); colorectal cancer, 0.63 (0.43–0.92); endometrial cancer, 0.83 (0.47–1.47); hip fracture, 0.66 (0.45–0.98); and death due to other causes, 0.92 (0.74–1.14). Corresponding HRs (nominal 95% CIs) for composite outcomes were 1.22 (1.09–1.36) for total cardiovascular disease (arterial and venous disease), 1.03 (0.90–1.17) for total cancer, 0.76 (0.69–0.85) for combined fractures, 0.98 (0.82–1.18) for total mortality, and 1.15 (1.03–1.28) for the global index. Absolute risk reductions per 10,000 person-years were 6 fewer colorectal cancers and 5 fewer hip fractures. Absolute excess risks per 10,000 person-years attributable to estrogen plus progestin were 8 more strokes, 8 more PEs, 7 more coronary heart disease (CHD) events, and 8 more invasive breast cancers. The absolute excess risk of events included in the global index was 19 per 10,000 person-years.

3. **Watts NB, Harris ST, Genant HK,** et al. Intermittent cyclical etidronate treatment of postmenopausal osteoporosis. N Engl J Med 1990;323:73–79.

This multicenter, prospective, randomized, double-blind, placebo-controlled study evaluated the effects of etidronate in 429 women with one to four vertebral compression fractures and radiographic evidence of osteopenia. Over 2 years, patients received treatment with phosphate (1.0 g) or placebo twice daily on days 1–3, etidronate (400 mg) or placebo daily on days 4 through 17, and supplemental calcium (500 mg) daily on days 18 through 91 (group 1: placebo and placebo; group 2: phosphate and placebo; group 3: placebo and etidronate; and group 4: phosphate and etidronate). Treatment cycles were repeated eight times. The etidronate groups (groups 3 and 4) had significant increases in their mean ($\pm$SE) spinal bone mineral density (BMD) after 2 years (4.2 $\pm$ 0.8% and 5.2 $\pm$ 0.7%, respectively; $p < 0.017$). Among the etidronate groups (groups 3 and 4 combined), the rate of new vertebral fractures was cut in half compared with the patients not receiving etidronate (groups 1 + 2 combined; 29.5% vs. 62.9% fractures per 1,000 patient-years; $p = 0.043$). The most impressive treatment effects were among patients in the subgroup with the lowest spinal BMD at baseline, as their fracture rates decreased by two-thirds (42.3 vs. 132.7 fractures per 1,000 patient-years; $p = 0.004$). Phosphate provided no added benefit. No significant adverse effects of treatment were observed.

4. **Chesnut CH III, Silverman S, Andriano K,** et al. A randomized trial of nasal spray salmon calcitonin in postmenopausal women with established osteoporosis: The prevent recurrence of osteoporotic fractures study. PROOF Study Group. Am J Med 2000;109:267–276.

The effects of salmon calcitonin nasal spray were analyzed in this 5-year, randomized, double-blind, placebo-controlled study in 1,255 osteoporotic postmenopausal women. Patients received calcitonin nasal spray (100, 200, or 400 IU) or placebo daily, and all patients received elemental calcium (1,000 mg) and vitamin D (400 IU) daily. The primary efficacy end point was the risk of new vertebral fractures in the 200-IU calcitonin group compared with placebo. The risk of new vertebral fractures was significantly decreased by 33% in the 200 IU calcitonin group compared with placebo [200 IU: 51/287, placebo: 70/270, relative risk (RR) = 0.67; 95%CI, 0.47–0.97; $p = 0.03$]. Of the 817 women with one to five known vertebral fractures at enrollment, the risk was reduced by 36% (RR = 0.64; 95% CI, 0.43–0.96; $p = 0.03$). All active treatment groups had significant increases in lumbar bone mineral density (BMD) from baseline (1% to 1.5%; $p < 0.01$). No significant differences were observed for the reductions in vertebral fractures in the 100-IU group (RR = 0.85; 95% CI, 0.60–1.21) and the 400-IU group (RR = 0.84; 95% CI, 0.59–1.18) when compared with placebo. Suppression of serum type-I collagen cross-linked telopeptide (C-telopeptide) by 12% in the 200-IU group ($p < 0.01$) and by 14% in the 400-IU group ($p < 0.01$) as compared with placebo provided evidence of bone turnover inhibition.

5. **Ettinger B, Black DM, Mitlak BH,** et al. Reduction of vertebral fracture risk in postmenopausal women with osteoporosis treated with raloxifene: Results from a 3-year randomized clinical trial. JAMA 1999;282:637–645.

The effects of raloxifene in postmenopausal women (of at least 2 years) with osteoporosis were evaluated in this multicenter, randomized, blinded, placebo-controlled trial. A total of 7,705 women ages 31 to 80 years old received 60 mg/day or 120 mg/day of raloxifene or placebo for up to 40 months of follow-up. All subjects received supplemental calcium and cholecalciferol. At 36 months, 7.4% of women had at least one new vertebral fracture found radiographically, which included 10.1% of women receiving placebo, 6.6% of women receiving 60 mg/day of raloxifene, and 5.4% of the 120 mg/day raloxifene group. Both groups receiving raloxifene had a decreased risk of vertebral fractures. (For 60 mg/day group: RR = 0.7; 95% CI, 0.5–0.8. For 120 mg/day group: RR = 0.5; 95% CI, 0.4–0.7.) Also, the occurrence of vertebral fractures was reduced in women whether or not they had previous fractures. No significant difference was observed for the risk of nonvertebral fracture in raloxifene versus placebo groups (RR, 0.9; 95% CI, 0.8–1.1, for both raloxifene groups combined). Raloxifene increased bone mineral density (BMD) in the femoral neck by 2.1% (60 mg) and 2.4% (120 mg) and in the spine by 2.6% (60 mg) and 2.7% (120 mg) ($p < 0.001$ for all comparisons) when compared with placebo. An increased risk of venous thromboembolism was found in the raloxifene group versus placebo groups (RR, 3.1; 95% CI, 1.5–6.2). Raloxifene was associated with a lower incidence of breast cancer and did not cause breast pain or vaginal bleeding.

6. **Black DM, Cummings SR, Karpf DB,** et al. Randomized trial of the effect of alendronate on risk of fracture in women with existing vertebral fractures. Fracture Intervention Trial Research Group. Lancet 1996;348:1535–1541.

This randomized, double-blind, placebo-controlled trial examined the effects of alendronate on the risk of radiographic and clinically evident fractures in postmenopausal women with low bone mass and the presence of existing vertebral fractures. Based on the presence or absence of existing vertebral fractures, 2,077 women ages 55 to 81 with low femoral-neck bone mineral density (BMD) were randomly assigned to receive alendronate or placebo for 36 months. The initial dose of alendronate, 5 mg daily, was increased to 10 mg daily at 24 months. The primary end point was vertebral fractures, defined as a 20% decrease and 4-mm decrease in at least one vertebral height as compared with baseline radiographs. Eight percent of women receiving alendronate had at least one new vertebral fracture on lateral spine radiographs, compared with 15% of the placebo group (RR, 0.53; 95% CI, 0.41–0.68); 2.3% of the alendronate group and 5.0% of the placebo group developed clinically apparent fractures [RH, 0.45 (0.27–0.72)]. The main secondary end point was the risk of any clinical fracture, and was found to be lower in the alendronate group (13.6%) than in the placebo group [18.2%; RH, 0.72 (0.58–0.90)]. Relative hazards for hip and wrist fracture for alendronate versus placebo were 0.49 (0.23–0.99) and 0.52 (0.31–0.87). Adverse experiences, including upper gastrointestinal disorders, were not significantly different between the groups.

7. **Cummings SR, Black DM, Thompson DE,** et al. Effect of alendronate on risk of fracture in women with low bone density but without vertebral fractures: Results from the Fracture Intervention Trial. JAMA 1998;280:2077–2082.

This randomized, double-blind, placebo-controlled trial examined the effects of alendronate on the risk of radiographic and clinically evident fractures in postmenopausal women with low bone mass but without existing vertebral fractures. Over 4 years, women ages 54 to 81 with a femoral bone mineral density (BMD) of 0.68 g/cm^2 or less but no vertebral fracture received alendronate or placebo. All subjects with reported low calcium intake received supplemental calcium and cholecaliferol. Subjects received 5 mg daily or placebo for the first 2 years, and then all subjects received 10 mg daily for the second 2 years. Alendronate increased BMD at all examined sites ($p < 0.001$) and decreased clinical fractures from 312 in the placebo group to 272 in the intervention group, but not to a significant degree (14% reduction; RH, 0.86; 95% CI, 0.73–1.0). Alendronate decreased the occurrence of clinical fractures by 36% in women with baseline osteoporosis at the femoral neck (>2.5 SDs below the normal young adult mean; RH, 0.64; 95% CI, 0.50–0.82; treatment-control difference, 6.5%; NNT: 15), but did not significantly reduce clinical fractures among women with higher BMD (RH, 1.08; 95% CI, 0.87–1.35). Radiographic evidence of vertebral fractures was decreased by 44% overall with alendronate treatment (RR, 0.56; 95% CI, 0.39–0.80; treatment-control differences, 1.7%; NNT, 60). Adverse events were not increased by treatment with alendronate.

8. **Harris ST, Watts NB, Genant H. K.,** et al. Effects of risedronate treatment on vertebral and nonvertebral fractures in women with postmenopausal osteoporosis: A randomized controlled trial. JAMA 1999;282:1344–1352.

Over 3 years, postmenopausal women with osteoporosis and younger than 85 years old were assigned to receive oral risedronate (2.5 or 5 mg daily) or placebo in this randomized, double-blind, placebo-controlled study. All participants ($n = 458$) had evidence of at least one vertebral fracture at baseline. All women received calcium, and vitamin D if baseline levels were low. After 1 year, the 2.5-mg risedronate group was discontinued, while the other 2 groups were enrolled for a total of 3 years. The cumulative incidence of new vertebral fractures was decreased by 41% in the 5 mg/day risedronate group, as compared with placebo (95% CI, 18%–58%) over 3 years (11.3 vs. 16.3%; $p = 0.003$). A 65% fracture reduction (95% CI, 38%–81%) was observed after the first year (2.4% vs 6.4%; $p < 0.001$). Nonvertebral fracture cumulative incidence was decreased by 39% (95% CI, 6%–61%) (5.2% vs. 8.4%; $p = 0.02$). The lumbar spine bone mineral density (BMD) increased significantly compared with placebo (5.4% vs. 1.1%); significant increases were also seen at the femoral trochanter (3.3% vs. −0.7%), femoral neck (1.6% vs. −1.2%), and at the radial midshaft (0.2% vs. −1.4%). Bone formation during treatment with risedronate was histologically normal. The safety profile of risedronate was similar to that of the placebo group.

9. **Reginster J-Y, Minne HW, Sorensen OH,** et al. Randomized trial of the effects of risedronate on vertebral fractures in women with established postmenopausal osteoporosis. Osteoporos Int 2000;11:83–91.

This randomized, double-blind, placebo-controlled study evaluated the efficacy of risedronate in postmenopausal women with at least two vertebral fractures. All subjects received supplemental calcium, and also vitamin D if baseline levels were low. Patients received risedronate 2.5 mg or 5 mg daily or placebo. The 2.5 mg/day risedronate group was stopped after 2 years, but the 5 mg/day risedronate group and placebo group continued for 3 years' duration. The risk of new vertebral fractures was decreased by 49% over 3 years in the 5 mg/day risedronate group compared with control ($p < 0.001$). A significant reduction of 61% in the treatment group versus control was observed within the first year ($p = 0.001$). Between the 2.5 mg/day and 5 mg/day risedronate groups, fracture reduction was similar over 2 years. Over 3 years, the treatment group experienced a 33% reduction in risk of nonvertebral fractures compared with placebo ($p = 0.06$). Bone mineral density (BMD) was increased significantly within 6 months at the spine and hip in the risedronate group. The adverse events observed were similar between the control and risedronate groups.

10. **Sorensen OH, Crawford GM, Mulder H,** et al. Long-term efficacy of risedronate: A 5-year placebo-controlled clinical experience. Bone 2003;32:120–126.

To examine the long-term effects of risedronate, this study extended a 3-year, placebo-controlled vertebral fracture study in osteoporotic women by 2 years. The subjects in the extension study continued to receive 5 mg risedronate or placebo based on original randomization, with maintenance of blinding. Similar results to the original study were observed for fracture reduction in the study extension. New vertebral fracture risk was significantly decreased with risedronate in years 4 and 5 by 59% (95% CI, 19–79%; $p = 0.01$), compared with a 49% reduction in the first 3 years. The observed increases in spine and hip bone mineral density (BMD) during the first 3 years were preserved or increased during the additional 2 years. Mean increase from baseline in lumbar BMD over the 5 years was 9.3% ($p < 0.001$). The rapid and significant decreases in bone turnover markers that occurred during the first 3 years were similarly sustained with the additional 2 years of treatment.

11. **McClung MR, Geusens P, Miller PD,** et al. Effect of risedronate on the risk of hip fracture in elderly women. N Engl J Med 2001;344:333–340.

This multicenter, randomized, placebo-controlled trial investigated whether risedronate prevents hip fracture in elderly women with and without osteoporosis. Women ages 70 to 79 years old with osteoporosis and women of at least 80 years with at least one nonskeletal risk factor for hip fracture or low bone mineral density (BMD) at the femoral neck were enrolled. Treatment assigned was either oral risedronate (2.5 or 5.0 mg daily) or placebo for 3 years. The incidence of hip fracture for the risedronate group was 2.8% overall, compared with 3.9% for the placebo group (RR, 0.7; 95% CI, 0.6–0.9; $p = 0.02$). Osteoporotic women (those ages 70–79) taking risedronate had a significantly lower incidence of hip fracture (1.9%) as compared with the control group (3.2%) (RR, 0.6; 95% CI, 0.4–0.9; $p = 0.009$). Among women with nonskeletal risk factors (those age 80 or above), the hip fracture incidence was 4.2% for the risedronate group versus 5.1 percent for the placebo group, lacking significant differences ($p = 0.35$).

12. **Delmas PD, Recker RR, Chesnut CH III,** et al. Daily and intermittent oral ibandronate normalize bone turnover and provide significant reduction in vertebral fracture risk: Results from the BONE study. Osteoporos Int 2004;15:792–798.

Oral ibandronate taken daily (2.5 mg/day) or intermittently (20 mg every other day for 12 doses every 3 months) and its effects on bone mineral density (BMD), new fractures, and bone turnover markers were studied in this multinational, randomized, double-blind, placebo-controlled trial. Both daily and intermittent doses of ibandronate significantly decreased the risk of vertebral fractures by 62% and 50%, respectively, and produced significant and maintained reductions in all measured biochemical bone turnover markers. The bone turnover rate at 3 months was decreased by close to 50 to 60%, with maintenance of this level of suppression for the rest of the study.

13. **Neer RM, Arnaud CD, Zanchetta JR,** et al. Effect of parathyroid hormone (1–34) on fractures and bone mineral density in postmenopausal women with osteoporosis. N Engl J Med 2001;344:1434–1441.

This randomized, placebo-controlled trial evaluated the effects of parathyroid hormone [PTH (1–34)] at doses of 20 or 40 μg daily (administered subcutaneously) in postmenopausal women with prior vertebral fractures. Among women in the PTH group, 5% from the 20-μg and 4% from the 40-μg groups experienced new fractures, as compared with 14% in the placebo group. Relative risks of fracture in the 20-μg and 40-μg PTH groups, compared with the placebo group, were 0.35 and 0.31 (95% CI, 0.22–0.55 and 0.19–0.50). Six percent of women receiving placebo had new nonvertebral fragility, as compared with 3% in each PTH group [RR, 0.47 and 0.46, respectively (95% CI, 0.25–0.88 and

0.25–0.86)]. The lumbar spine bone mineral density (BMD) was increased by 9 and 13 more percentage points in the 20- and 40-μg groups compared with placebo, respectively, and by 3 and 6 more percentage points in the femoral neck. BMD was decreased at the shaft of the radius by 2 more percentage points in the 40-μg dose group. Total BMD was increased by 2% to 4% more for both PTH doses compared with placebo. Side effects from PTH were minor and included occasional headache and nausea.

14. **Meunier PJ, Roux C, Seeman E,** et al. The effects of strontium ranelate on the risk of vertebral fracture in women with postmenopausal osteoporosis. N Engl J Med 2004;350:459–468.

   This phase 3 trial examined the efficacy of strontium ranelate in preventing vertebral fractures. Postmenopausal women with osteoporosis and at least one vertebral fracture were randomly assigned to receive 2 g oral strontium ranelate per day or placebo for 3 years, along with calcium and vitamin D. Fewer patients in the strontium group had new vertebral fractures compared with placebo, and the risk reduction was 49% for the first year of treatment and 41% over the 3-year period (RR, 0.59; 95% CI, 0.48–0.73). Bone mineral density (BMD) was increased at 36 months by 14.4% at the lumbar spine and 8.3% at the femoral neck in the treatment group ($p < 0.001$ for both comparisons). Adverse events were not significantly different between groups.

15. **Greenspan SL, Ettinger MP, Bone HG,** et al. PTH (1–84) prevents first vertebral fracture in postmenopausal women with osteoporosis: Results from the TOP study. Ann Intern Med (in press).

16. **National Osteoporosis Foundation.** Osteoporosis: Review of the evidence for prevention, diagnosis, and treatment and cost-effectiveness analysis. Osteoporos Int 1998;8(Suppl 4):S1–S88.

17. **Hodgson S, Watts NB, Bilezikian JP,** et al, for the AACE Osteoporosis Taskforce. American Association of Clinical Endocrinologists medical guidelines for clinical practice for the prevention and treatment of postmenopausal osteoporosis: 2001 edition, with selected updates for 2003. Endocr Pract 2003;9:544–564.

18. **Holmberg AH, Johnell O, Nilsson PM,** et al. Risk factors for fragility fracture in middle age. A prospective population-based study of 33,000 men and women. Osteoporos Int 2006;17:1065–1077.

   This prospective study investigated risk factors for low-energy fractures in men ($n = $ 22,444) and women ($n = $ 10,902), with mean ages of 44 and 50 years, respectively. Follow-up for incident fractures lasted close to 19 years for men and 15 years for women. Diabetes (RR, 2.38; CI 95%, 1.65–3.42) and mental health hospitalizations (RR, 1.91; CI 95%, 1.47–2.51) were the risk factors with the greatest association with low-energy fractures among the men. Mental health and lifestyle factors significantly increased fracture risk in most of the specific fracture groups: Hospitalizations for mental health (RR, 2.28–3.38), poor self-rated health (RR, 1.80–1.83), sleep disturbances (RR, 1.72–2.95), smoking (RR, 1.70–2.72), and poor appetite (RR, 3.05–3.43). For women, diabetes was associated with the highest risk of developing fractures (RR, 1.87; CI 95%, 1.26–2.79), and previous fracture was also strongly associated with an increased risk of fracture (RR, 2.00; CI 95%, 0.81–0.96). Middle-aged men and women had similar risk factors for fracture, but gender differences existed for forearm, vertebral, proximal humerus, and hip fracture.

19. **Lindsay R, Silverman SL, Cooper C,** et al. Risk of new vertebral fracture in the year following a fracture. JAMA 2001;285:320–323.

   To evaluate the risk of having a vertebral fracture within a year of having a vertebral fracture, this study examined data from four large multinational, 3-year, randomized, placebo-controlled osteoporosis treatment trials. The women enrolled in all trials had a mean age of 74 years and had a mean of 28 years since menopause. In the first year, there was a cumulative incidence of 6.6% for new vertebral fractures. The risk of having a vertebral fracture in the first year was increased by fivefold in patients who had the presence of one or more vertebral fractures at baseline, as compared with subjects without vertebral fractures at baseline (RR, 5.1; 95% CI, 3.1–8.4; $p < 0.001$). Among those who developed an incidental vertebral fracture, the incidence of a new vertebral fracture in the following year was 19.2% (95% CI, 13.6%–24.8%). Among those with prevalent vertebral fractures, this risk was also increased (RR, 9.3; 95% CI, 1.2–71.6; $p < 0.03$).

20. **Gallagher JC, Genant HK, Crans GG,** et al. Teriparatide reduces fracture risk associated with increasing number and severity of osteoporotic fractures. J Clin Endocrinol Metab 2005;90:1583–1587.

21. **Miller P, Siris E, Barrett-Connor E,** et al. Prediction of fracture risk in postmenopausal white women with peripheral bone densitometry: Evidence from the National Osteoporosis Risk Assessment (NORA) program. J Bone Miner Res 2002; 17:2222–2230.

    This study measured bone mineral density (BMD) at peripheral sites in 149,524 postmenopausal white women who did not carry a diagnosis of osteoporosis, to compare results at these locations with the "gold" standard test of dual-energy x-ray absorptiometry (DXA) measurements at the hip and spine. BMD was measured at the hip, wrist, forearm, spine, and ribs. New fractures were reported at 1 year in 2,259 women. Multivariable adjusted analyses and equipment manufacturers' normative data were used to determine that women with T-scores less than or equal to −2.5 SD were 2.15 (finger) to 3.94 (heel ultrasound) times more likely to develop a fracture than women with normal BMD. Risk prediction was comparable whether calculated from the manufacturers' young normal T-values (T-scores) or using SDs from the mean age of the NORA population. All measured sites and devices predicted fracture equally well. The area under receiving operating characteristic (ROC) curves for hip fracture was similar to those published using measurements at hip sites. The authors predict that a low BMD found by peripheral measurements is associated with at least a twofold increased fracture risk within 1 year, regardless of the site measured.

22. **Klotzbuecher CM, Ross PD, Landsman PB,** et al. Patients with prior fractures have an increased risk of future fractures: A summary of the literature and statistical synthesis. J Bone Miner Res 2000;15:721–739.

    This study summarized trials that reported increased risk of fracture among individuals with a history of a previously clinically diagnosed fracture or with radiographic evidence of a prior fracture. The strongest associations were found between prior and future vertebral fractures; women with pre-existing fractures had a four times greater risk of future vertebral fracture than those without prior fractures. As the number of prior fractures increased, so did the risk. Relative risks of about 2 for other combinations of prior and future fracture sites were reported in most studies. Using the confidence profile method, a single pooled estimate from the studies with enough data for other combinations of prior and future fracture sites was determined. Peri- and postmenopausal women with previous fractures had 2.0 (95% CI, 1.8, 2.1) times the risk of future fracture compared with women without prior fractures. Other studies including men and women of all ages had risks increased by 2.2 (1.9, 2.6) times.

23. **Siris E, Miller P, Barrett-Connor E,** et al. Identification and fracture outcomes of undiagnosed low bone mineral density in postmenopausal women: Results from the National Osteoporosis Risk Assessment (NORA). JAMA 2001;286:2815–2822.

    This longitudinal observational study described the occurrence of low bone mineral density (BMD) in postmenopausal women, its risk factors, and fracture incidence during a follow-up of 12 months. Using the WHO criteria, 39.6% had osteopenia (T-score of −1 to −2.49) and 7.2% had osteoporosis (T-score ≤ −2.5). Factors associated with increased likelihood of osteoporosis included age, personal or family history of fracture, Asian or Hispanic heritage, smoking, and cortisone use. Factors associated with a significant decrease in likelihood of osteoporosis included higher body mass index, African American heritage, estrogen or diuretic use, exercise, and alcohol consumption. Of the 167 patients who had follow-up, osteoporosis was associated with a fracture rate approximately 4 times that of normal bone mineral density (BMD) (rate ratio, 4.03; 95% CI, 3.59–4.53) and osteopenia was associated with a 1.8-fold higher rate (95% CI, 1.49–2.18).

24. **Dargent-Molina P, Favier F, Grandjean H,** et al. Fall-related factors and risk of hip fracture: The EPIDOS prospective study. Lancet 1996;348:145–149.

    Women age 75 or older were evaluated in this study of the role of fall-related factors in relation to bone mineral density (BMD) in predicting risk of hip fractures. Age-adjusted multivariate analyses were used to determine four independent fall-related predictors of hip fracture: difficulty in doing a tandem walk [1.2 for 1 point on the difficulty score (1.0–1.5)], slower gait speed (RR = 1.4 for 1 SD decrease; 95% CI, 1.1–1.6), small calf circumference [1.5 (1.0–2.2)], and reduced visual acuity [2.0 for acuity ≤2/10 (1.3–1.7)]. Neuromuscular impairment—gait speed, tandem walk and poor vision were significantly associated with an increased risk of future hip fracture after adjusting for femoral-neck BMD. The rate of hip fracture among women with a high risk classification, based on both a high fall-risk status and low BMD, was 29 per 1,000 woman-years, compared with 11 per 1,000 for women classified as high risk by either a high fall-risk status or low BMD; women with a low risk classification based on both criteria had a rate of 5 per 1,000.

25. **Kanis JA, Johnell O, De Laet C,** et al. A meta-analysis of previous fracture and subsequent fracture risk. Bone 2004;375–382.

    This metaanalysis investigated prior fractures as a risk factor for subsequent fractures on an international basis and if this risk is related to age, sex, and bone mineral density (BMD). A Poisson model was used for each sex from each cohort, and covariates were age, sex, and BMD. Prior fracture history resulted in a significantly increased risk for any fracture when compared with individuals without a previous fracture (RR = 1.86; 95% CI, 1.75–1.98). Similar risk ratios were observed for the outcomes of osteoporotic fractures or hip fractures. No significant difference in risk ratio was observed between men and women. A small portion of the risk for any fracture (8%) and for hip fracture (22%) was related to low BMD. The risk ratio was stable with age except for hip fracture outcomes, in which the risk ratio significantly decreased with age.

26. **Cauley JA, Robbins J, Chen Z,** et al., for the Women's Health Initiative Investigators. Effects of estrogen plus progestin on risk of fracture and bone mineral density: The Women's Health Initiative randomized trial. JAMA 2003;290:1729–1738.

    As part of the Women's Health Initiative (WHI), a randomized, placebo-controlled trial evaluating estrogen-plus-progestin treatment, the study examined whether the relative risk reduction of estrogen plus progestin for fractures would change based on risk factors for fractures. In the study, 8.6% of women in the treatment arm and 11.1% of women receiving placebo suffered a fracture (HR, 0.76; 95% CI, 0.69–0.83). The results did not differ in women stratified by age, body mass index (BMI), smoking status, history of falls, personal and family history of fracture, calcium intake, previous hormone therapy, bone mineral density (BMD), or summary fracture risk score. Total hip BMD increased 3.7% after treatment for 3 years, compared with 0.14% in the placebo group ($p < 0.001$). HR for the global index was comparable across all tertiles of the fracture risk scale (lowest fracture risk tertile, HR, 1.20; 95% CI, 0.93–1.58; middle tertile, HR, 1.23; 95% CI, 1.04–1.46; highest tertile, HR, 1.03; 95% CI, 0.88–1.24) (p for interaction = 0.54). Although estrogen plus progestin increases BMD and decreases fracture risk in postmenopausal women, there is no global net benefit for this treatment in other disease outcomes.

27. **Siris E, Chen Y-T, Abbott TA,** et al. Bone mineral density thresholds for pharmacological intervention to prevent fractures. Arch Intern Med 2004;164:1108–1112.

    This study evaluated the WHO diagnostic criteria for osteoporosis and the National Osteoporosis Foundation treatment criteria to evaluate how efficient the thresholds are for identifying postmenopausal women at risk of fractures. Of the women who reported new fractures in the first year, only 6.4% had baseline T-scores of −2.5 or less (WHO criteria for osteoporosis). These women had the highest fracture rates, but they suffered only 26% of the hip fractures and 18% of the osteoporotic fractures. By National Osteoporosis Foundation criteria, 22.6% of women had T-scores of 2.0 or less, or −1.5 or less with at least one clinical risk factor. Although lower fracture rates were observed for these women, 53% of hip fractures and 45% of osteoporotic fractures occurred in these women. Eighty-two percent of postmenopausal women with fractures had T-scores better than −2.5 using peripheral measurement devices.

28. **Wainwright SA, Marshall LM, Ensrud KE,** et al. Study of Osteoporotic Fractures Research Group. Hip fracture in women without osteoporosis. J Clin Endocrinol Metab 2005;90:2787–2793.

29. **Schuit SC, van der Klift M, Weel AE,** et al. Fracture incidence and association with bone mineral density in elderly men and women: The Rotterdam Study. Bone 2004;34:195–202.

    This prospective, population-based cohort study of men and women ages 55 and older (n = 7,806) examined the incidence of all nonvertebral fractures and the relation to bone mineral density (BMD). The study also evaluated the sensitivity of using a T-score at or below −2.5 for identifying individuals at risk for fracture. Hip, wrist, and upper humerus fractures were the most frequent fractures in both sexes. Femoral neck BMD was an equally important risk factor in both sexes and is particularly related to hip fracture. For all nonvertebral fractures, the age-adjusted hazard ratio (95% CI) per standard deviation decrease in femoral neck BMD was 1.5 (1.4–1.6) for women and 1.4 (1.2–1.6) for men. For hip fractures, the hazard ratios were 2.1 (1.7–2.5) for women and 2.3 (1.6–3.3) for men. Forty-four percent of all nonvertebral fractures occurred in women with a T-score below −2.5; in men, this percentage was just 21%.

30. **Cummings SR, Nevitt MC, Browner WS,** et al. Risk factors for hip fracture in white women: Study of osteoporotic fractures. N Engl J Med 1995;332:767–773.

31. **Black DM, Steinbuch M, Palermo L,** et al. An assessment tool for predicting fracture risk in postmenopausal women. Osteoporos Int 2001;12:519–528.

The authors developed a FRACTURE Index to help identify variables that could be readily determined by clinicians or postmenopausal individuals. The seven variables include age, bone mineral density (BMD) T-score, fracture after age 50 years, maternal hip fracture after age 50, weight less than or equal to 125 lb (57 kg), smoking status, and use of arms to stand up from a chair. The index was validated using the EPIDOS fracture study. The FRACTURE Index can be used by postmenopausal women or clinicians to estimate the 5-year risk of hip and other osteoporotic fractures, with or without BMD testing.

32. **Miller PD, Barlas S, Brenneman SK,** et al. An approach to identifying osteopenic women at increased short-term risk of fracture. Arch Intern Med 2004;164: 1113–1120.

A classification algorithm was developed in this study to identify women with osteopenia (T-scores of −2.5 to −1.0) who have an increased risk of fracture within 1 year of peripheral bone mineral density (BMD) testing. The most important determinants of short-term fracture risk were found to be previous fracture, self-rated poor health status, poor mobility, and a T-score at a peripheral site of −1.8 or less. Increased fracture risk was identified in 55% of women. Regardless of T-score, women with prior fracture had a risk of 4.1%, women with a T-score of −1.8 or less and poor health status had a risk of 2.2%, and women with poor mobility had a risk of 1.9%. Seventy-four percent of women who experienced a fracture were correctly identified by the algorithm.

33. **Kanis JA, Johnell O, Oden A,** et al. Ten year probabilities of osteoporotic fractures according to BMD and diagnostic thresholds. J Bone Miner Res 2001;16:S19–S24.

This study estimated 10-year probabilities of osteoporotic fractures in women and men based on age and bone mineral density (BMD) at the femoral neck. The 10-year probability of any fracture increased with age and T-score, except for forearm fractures in men. Fracture probabilities for any age with low BMD were comparable between men and women for hip and spine fractures. Age affects risk independently of BMD, suggesting that intervention thresholds should vary based on absolute probabilities instead of at fixed T-scores. Intervention thresholds based on hip BMD T-scores were similar between sexes.

34. **Garnero P, Hausherr E, Chapuy M-C,** et al. Markers of bone resorption predict hip fracture in elderly women: The EPIDOS prospective study. J Bone Miner Res 1996;11:1531–1538.

Increased bone turnover as a risk factor for osteoporotic hip fracture was examined in this prospective, cohort study evaluating healthy women older than 75 years of age. Increased bone resorption and formation occurred in elderly women compared with healthy premenopausal women. Patients with hip fracture had greater urinary excretion of C-telopeptide (CTX) and free deoxypyridinoline (D-Pyr), but not other markers, than age-matched controls ($p = 0.02$ and 0.005, respectively). An increased fracture risk was found to be associated with urinary excretion of CTX and free D-Pyr above the upper limit of the premenopausal range with an odds ratio (95% CI) of 2.2 (1.3–3.6) and 1.9 (1.1–3.2), respectively, but formation markers were not associated with an increased fracture risk. Increased bone resorption was found to predict hip fracture independent of bone mass. The women at greatest risk of hip fracture had both a femoral bone mineral density (BMD) of at least 2.5 SD below the mean of young adults and either high CTX or high free D-Pyr levels, with an odds ratio of 4.8 and 4.1, respectively, compared to individuals with only high bone resorption or low BMD.

35. **Watts NB, Miller PD.** Changing perceptions in osteoporosis. Markers should be used as adjunct to bone densitometry. BMJ 1999;319:1371–1372.

This letter to the editor argues against an article by Wilkins, who wrote in regard to a study published by Marshall, which stated that bone mineral density (BMD) "cannot identify individuals who will have a fracture." The authors contend that BMD is a means to identify who is at high risk, much like a lipid panel cannot predict who will have a heart attack, but can identify high risk individuals who could benefit from treatment. The authors also point out how effective bisphosphonates have been for long-term treatment of osteoporosis.

36. **Vokes T, Bachman D, Baim S,** et al. Vertebral fracture assessment: The 2005 ISCD Official Position. J Clin Densitom 2006;9:37–46.

    This article presents the International Society for Clinical Densitometry (ISCD) Official Positions on Vertebral Fracture Assessment (VFA), including the indications for using VFA, methodology for diagnosis of vertebral fractures using VFA, and indications for using additional imaging after VFA.

37. **Jackson SA, Tenenhouse A, Robertson L.** Vertebral fracture definition from population-based data: Preliminary results from the Canadian Multicenter Osteoporosis Study (CAMOS). Osteoporos Int 2000;11:680–687.

    This population-based prospective study enrolled both male and female participants to study osteoporosis in the Canadian population. Using 3 SD as a limit of normality, the male prevalence (21.5%) was comparable to the female prevalence of 23.5%. Using 4 SD, the prevalence was decreased to 7.3% and 9.3%, respectively. Younger men (ages 50–59) had a higher prevalence of fractures than women and had a smaller increase of prevalence with age. Among older participants (over 80 years), the female prevalence was 45% and male prevalence was 36% using 3 SD (grade 1) to define normal limits. On average, females presented with more severe fractures than males.

38. **Black DM, Arden NK, Palmero L, Cummings SR.** Study of osteoporotic fractures research group. Prevalent vertebral deformities predict hip and new vertebral deformities but not wrist fractures. J Bone Miner Res 1999;14:821–828.

    This prospective study evaluated the ability of vertebral fractures to predict other nonvertebral fractures. Prevalent vertebral fractures were associated with a fivefold increased risk (RR, 5.4; 95% CI, 4.4, 4.6) of developing another vertebral fracture, and the risk increased substantially with both the severity and number of fractures. The risks of hip and any nonvertebral fractures were increased with baseline vertebral fractures, with relative risks of 2.8 (95% CI, 2.3, 3.4) and 1.9 (95% CI, 1.7, 2.1), respectively. Risk increased with severity and number of fractures, and associations remained significant after adjusting for age and calcaneal bone mineral density (BMD). There was a small increased risk of wrist fracture, but it was not significant after adjusting for age and BMD.

39. **Melton LJ III, Khosla S, Atkinson EJ,** et al. Relationship of bone turnover to bone density and fractures. J Bone Miner Res 1997;12:1083–1089.

    Serum and urine biochemical markers of bone turnover were measured from an age-stratified random sample of women. All biochemical markers (OC, BAP, PICP, urine NTx, urine Pyd and Dpd) were positively associated with age among the postmenopausal women, and the elevated turnover prevalence (>1 SD above the premenopausal mean) varied from 9% (PICP) to 42% (Pyd). Among the premenopausal women, PICP, NTx, and Dpd were negatively associated with age. Most markers were negatively correlated with bone mineral density (BMD) after adjusting for age, and osteoporotic women were more likely to have elevated bone turnover. A decreased hip BMD and elevated Pyd was found to be associated with a history of osteoporotic fractures of the hip, spine, or distal forearm. Reduced bone formation, determined by OC, was associated with previous osteoporotic fractures after adjusting for lower BMD and increased bone resorption.

40. **Faulkner KG.** Improving femoral bone density measurements. J Clin Densitom 2003;6:353–358.

    This article examines the use of femoral bone mineral density (BMD) and its ability to assess the risk of developing hip fractures. Upper femoral neck BMD and hip axis length have reportedly been associated with hip fractures. Bilateral femur BMD decreases precision error compared with a single measurement and could be a new location for monitoring changes in BMD compared with the standard spinal BMD.

41. **Khoo BC, Beck TJ, Qiao QH,** et al. *In vivo* short-term precision of hip structure analysis variables in comparison with bone mineral density using paired dual-energy X-ray absorptiometry scans from multi-center clinical trials. Bone 2005;37:112–121.

This study analyzed the precision of hip structural analysis (HSA) variables in determining bone mineral density (BMD) using dual-energy x-ray absorptiometry (DXA) scans. Section modulus (Z), a key HSA variable that is biomechanically indicative of bone strength during bending, had a short-term precision percentage coefficient of variation (CV%) in the femoral neck of 3.4 to 10.1%, depending on the manufacturer or DXA equipment model. Cross-sectional area, closely aligned with conventional DXA bone mineral content, had a range of CV% from 2.8% to 7.9%. Decreased precision was associated with inadequate inclusion of the femoral head or femoral shaft in the DXA-scanned hip region. HSA-derived BMD precision varied between 2.4% and 6.4%, whereas DXA BMD precision varied from 1.9% and 3.4%. The precision of HSA variables was overall not dependent on magnitude, subject height or weight, or conventional femoral neck densitometric variables.

42. **Faulkner KG, Wacker WK, Barden HS,** et al. Femur strength index predicts hip fracture independent of bone density and hip axis length. Osteoporos Int 2006;17: 593–599.
This study used dual-energy x-ray absorptiometry (DXA) measurements in a group of women (50 years or older) with and without fracture, and compared femoral bone density, structure, and the femur strength index (FSI) to evaluate their relationship with the risk of developing hip fractures. The fracture group had significantly lower femoral neck bone mineral density (BMD) and significantly higher HAL (hip axis length) compared with the control group. Mean cross-sectional moment of inertia (CSMI) was not significantly different between fracture patients and controls after adjusting for HAL and BMD. After adjusting for T score and HAL, FSI was significantly lower in the fracture group.

43. **Yoshikawa T, Turner CH, Peacock M,** et al. Femur Strength Index. J Bone Miner Res 1994;9:1053–1064.
Proximal femurs from cadavers of white adults and an aluminum step wedge were scanned to confirm the cross-sectional moment of inertia (CSMI) calculation from dual-energy x-ray absorptiometry (DXA) scans. Scanning three healthy young women evaluated the reproducibility of geometric measurements using DXA. A strong linear association was observed between directly measuring CSMI (by sectioning the cadaver femurs at the narrowest point) and using DXA in both cadaver bones (r^2 = 0.96) and the aluminum step wedge (r^2 = 0.99). Repeated measurements using DXA produced a coefficient of variation for CSMI less than 3%. No strong correlation was found between CSMI and age in normal subjects of either sex; however, safety factor (an index of strength of the femoral neck during walking) and fall index (an index of the strength of the femoral neck during a fall) did decrease with age in both sexes.

44. **Faulkner KG, Cauley J, Zmuda JM,** et al. Ethnic differences in the frequency and circumstances of falling in older community-dwelling women. J Am Geriatr Soc 2005; 53:1774–1779.
Caucasian and African American women (mean age 76 ± 5 years) were evaluated for frequency of falls and fall circumstances. There was a 0.48 falls per woman annual rate (95% CI = 0.43–0.53). Age-adjusted falls were not significantly higher in Caucasians than African Americans; for women less than 75 years of age, fall rates were similar between the two groups. Among women older than 75 years, Caucasians had 50% higher fall rates than African Americans, but this difference was not significant. Caucasian women were more likely to fall outdoors versus indoors compared with African Americans [odds ratio (OR) = 1.6, 95% CI = 1.0–2.7] and laterally versus forward (OR = 2.0, 95% CI = 1.1–3.4). Caucasian women were less likely to fall on their hands or wrists [OR = 0.6; 95% CI = 0.3–1.0], and 98% of individuals who did fall on their hands or wrists stated they were trying to break their fall.

45. **Wehren LE, Magaziner J.** Hip fracture: Risk factors and outcomes. Curr Osteoporos Rep 2003;1:78–85. Review.
This article evaluated the burden of hip fractures on public and personal health, and estimates close to $9 billion was spent in 1995 in the United States for hip fracture management. After hip fracture, mortality is significantly increased, and less than 50% of individuals with a hip fracture will have functional recovery. Also, almost 25% of patients with a hip fracture will live in a long-term-care facility for at least a year after the fracture.

46. **Resnick B, Orwig D, Wehren LE,** et al. The Exercise Plus Program for older women post hip fracture: Participant perspectives. Gerontologist 2005;45:539–544.
Themes that improved participation in exercise were determined through interviewing older women who had a hip fracture 12 months earlier. These themes included real and

expected benefits, visual cues and knowing what to do, simplicity, individualized care, verbal encouragement to exercise, regular schedule, confidence (i.e., self-efficacy), determination, social support, reciprocity, and goal identification. Unpleasant sensations, constraints to exercise, and getting back to baseline were identified as reasons why individuals were not willing to exercise.

47. **Hochberg MC, Greenspan SL, Wasnich RD,** et al. Changes in bone density and turnover explain the reductions in incidence of nonvertebral fractures that occur during treatment with antiresorptive agents. J Clin Endocrinol Metab 2002;87: 1586–1592.

A metaanalysis of all randomized, placebo-controlled trials of the effects of antiresorptive agents in postmenopausal women with osteoporosis was studied. Greater increases in bone mineral density (BMD) and greater reductions in biochemical markers (BCMs) of bone turnover were significantly associated with larger reductions in risk of nonvertebral fractures. Each 1% increase in spine BMD at 1 year was associated with an 8% reduction in nonvertebral fracture risk ($p = 0.02$). Mean BMD changes at the hip were less than at the spine, but the predicted net effect on fracture risk was similar. From the results, it was predicted that a 70% decrease in resorption BCM would reduce risk by 40%, and a 50% reduction in formation BCM would reduce risk by 44%. A separate variable for treatment was not independently significant in any models, suggesting that either BMD or BCM changes are able to explain the effect of treatment.

48. **Schnitzer T, Bone HG, Crepaldi G,** et al. Therapeutic equivalence of alendronate 70 mg once-weekly and alendronate 10 mg daily in the treatment of osteoporosis. Aging Clin Exp Res 2000;12:1–12.

This double-blind study investigated whether changing the dosing regimen of alendronate would affect its safety or efficacy as compared with the standard daily dose regimen. Postmenopausal women were assigned to receive either oral once-weekly alendronate 70 mg, twice-weekly alendronate 35 mg, or daily alendronate 10 mg for 1 year. Mean increases in lumbar spine bone mineral density (BMD) at 12 months were 5.1% (95% CI, 4.8, 5.4) in the 70-mg once-weekly group, 5.2% (4.9, 5.6) in the 35-mg twice-weekly group, and 5.4% (5.0, 5.8) in the 10-mg daily alendronate group. Bone resorption biochemical markers and bone formation markers were similarly decreased in all three treatment groups into the middle premenopausal reference range. Bone mineral density (BMD) at the total hip, trochanter, femoral neck, and total body was comparably increased for all groups. Adverse events were minimal, and the incidence of upper gastrointestinal (GI) events was similar for all treatment regimens. However, the once-weekly dosing group experienced fewer serious upper GI adverse events and had fewer esophageal incidents than the daily dosing group, supporting preclinical data that found once-weekly dosing may have better GI tolerability.

49. **Brown JP, Kendler DL, McClung MR,** et al. The efficacy and tolerability of risedronate once a week for the treatment of postmenopausal osteoporosis. Calcif Tissue Int 2002;71:103–11.

Once-weekly risedronate (35 mg and 50 mg) was compared with 5-mg-daily risedronate in this randomized, double-blind, active-controlled study in postmenopausal osteoporotic women over 2 years. The primary endpoint was mean percent change (SE) in lumbar spine bone mineral density (BMD) after 1 year, and was 4.0% (0.2%) in the 5-mg-daily group, 3.9% (0.2%) in the 35-mg group, and 4.2% (0.2%) in the 50-mg group. From these data, it was determined that each once-a-week treatment was as effective as daily treatment. All regimens had comparable safety profiles. Also, since the 35-mg and 50-mg doses had the same efficacy and safety, it was concluded that the lower weekly dose (35 mg) would be an optimal regimen for women who wish to have a once-a-week treatment.

50. **Miller PD, McClung M, Macovei L,** et al. Monthly oral ibandronate therapy in postmenopausal osteoporosis: One year results from the MOBILE study. J Bone Miner Res 2005;20:1315–1322.

This was a randomized, double-blind, phase III, noninferiority trial examining whether monthly treatment with oral ibandronate has similar efficacy and safety as daily treatment with oral ibandronate. Postmenopausal women were assigned to receive 2.5 mg daily, 50 mg/50 mg monthly (single doses, consecutive days), 100 mg monthly, or 150 mg monthly of oral ibandronate. Lumbar spine bone mineral density (BMD) increased by 3.9%, 4.3%, 4.1%, and 4.9% in the 2.5, 50-mg/50-mg, 100-mg, and 150-mg arms, respectively, after 1 year. Of all the monthly regimens, only the 150-mg regimen was proven superior to the daily regimen. Serum levels of C-telopeptide (a biochemical marker of bone resorption) were comparably reduced in all treatment groups. Similar increases in BMD were observed for all monthly regimens, and were greater than the increases seen in the daily regimens. There was a significantly larger proportion of women from the 100-mg and 150-mg monthly treatment groups that achieved the predefined threshold levels for percent change from baseline in lumbar spine (6%) or total hip BMD (3%) when compared with the daily regimen groups. Safety efficacy was similar for all groups.

51. **Miller PD, Bilezikian JP, Deal C,** et al. Clinical use of teriparatide in the real world: Initial insights. Endocr Pract 2004;10:139–148.
    This is a summary of treatment with teriparatide and practical issues related to its use since being approved by the FDA in 2002.

52. **Hodsman AB, Bauer DC, Dempster D,** et al. Parathyroid hormone and teriparatide for the treatment of osteoporosis: A review of the evidence and suggested guidelines for it use. Endocr Rev 2005;10:2004–2006.
    Parathyroid hormone (PTH) and its analog, teriparatide, are a new class of anabolic treatment for severe osteoporosis, and have potential to improve skeletal architecture. Phase III trials of teriparatide showed significant reductions in vertebral and appendicular skeletal fracture rates. Teriparatide is significantly more expensive than bisphosphonates and has not been proven superior to bisphosphonates for antifracture efficacy. Also, therapy with teriparatide is not recommended for more than 24 months, which is partly based on the induction of osteosarcoma in a rat model of carcinogenicity. Serum calcium levels should be monitored closely with teriparatide. Presently, it is not recommended to combine teriparatide therapy with bisphosphonates.

53. **Sato M, Westmore M, Ma YL,** et al. Teriparatide [PTH(1–34)] strengthens the proximal femur of ovariectomized nonhuman primates despite increasing porosity. J Bone Miner Res. 2004 Apr;19:623–629.

54. **Black DM, Greenspan SL, Ensrud KE,** et al. The effects of parathyroid hormone and alendronate alone or in combination in postmenopausal osteoporosis. N Engl J Med 2003;349:1207–1215.
    Synergy between parathyroid hormone (PTH) and alendronate was investigated in this randomized, double-blind, clinical study comparing PTH or alendronate treatment alone with combination therapy. Postmenopausal women were randomly assigned to receive daily treatment with PTH (100 μg), alendronate (10 mg), or both, and were followed for 12 months. Spinal bone mineral density (BMD) increased in all treatment groups, with no significant difference in the increase between the combination group and the PTH group. Bone formation increased substantially in the PTH group, but not in the combination-therapy group. Bone resorption decreased in the alendronate group and in the combination-therapy group. A considerable increase in volumetric density of trabecular bone at the spine occurred in all groups, but the PTH increase was almost twice that found in the combination-therapy or alendronate group.

55. **Finkelstein JS, Hayes A, Hunzelman JL,** et al: The effects of parathyroid hormone, alendronate, or both in men with osteoporosis. N Engl J Med 2003;349: 1216–1226.
    Combination therapy with alendronate and PTH versus treatment with only PTH or alendronate was investigated in this randomized study. Men with low bone mineral density (BMD) were randomly assigned to receive alendronate (10 mg daily), PTH (40 μg subcutaneously), or both. Alendronate was given for 30 months; PTH was begun at month 6. BMD at the lumbar spine increased significantly more in men treated with PTH alone than in those in the other groups ($p < 0.001$ for both comparisons). The BMD at the femoral neck increased significantly more in the PTH group than in the alendronate group ($p < 0.001$) or the combination-therapy group ($p = 0.01$). BMD of the lumbar spine increased significantly more in the combination-therapy group than in the alendronate group ($p < 0.001$). Serum alkaline phosphatase levels were significantly higher in the PTH group at 12 months than in the alendronate group or in the combination-therapy group ($p < 0.001$ for both comparisons). These results suggest that alendronate negatively affects the ability of PTH to increase BMD at the femoral neck and lumbar spine in men.

56. **Black DM, Bilezikian JP, Ensrud KE,** et al. One year of alendronate after one year of parathyroid hormone (1–84) for osteoporosis. N Engl J Med 2005;353: 555–565.

This randomized study investigated whether antiresorptive therapy is necessary to maintain the increases in bone mineral density (BMD) that occur after 1 year of treatment with parathyroid hormone (PTH). This was a continuation of a trial that examined combination therapy with PTH and alendronate versus either treatment alone. Women who had received PTH for 1 year were randomly reassigned to receive an additional year with either placebo or alendronate. Those who had received alendronate monotherapy for 1 year continued with this treatment for year 2. Subjects who received combination therapy in year 1 received alendronate in year 2. Alendronate therapy after PTH therapy led to significant increases in BMD compared with the results for placebo after PTH therapy over 2 years. This difference was especially evident for BMD in trabecular bone at the spine on quantitative computed tomography (CT) (an increase of 31% in the PTH-alendronate group as compared with 14% in the PTH-placebo group). A large decrease in BMD was observed in the placebo group during year 2. These results suggest the BMD gained during treatment with PTH is lost if treatment is not followed by treatment with an antiresportive agent.

57. **Kurland ES, Heller SL, Diamond B,** et al. The importance of bisphosphonate therapy in maintaining bone mass in men after therapy with teriparatide [human parathyroid hormone (1–34)]. Osteoporos Int 2004;15:992–997.

   After 18 to 24 months of treatment with teriparatide, 21 men were followed to examine changes in bone mineral density (BMD) after discontinuing PTH and either starting bisphosphonate treatment (immediately or delayed) or opting out of treatment. After 1 year, lumbar spine BMD increased an additional 5.1 ± 1.0% in the bisphosphonate group, while it decreased by 3.7 ± 1.7% in those receiving no medication ($p < 0.002$). Delaying bisphosphonate treatment until 1 year after teriparatide withdrawal showed subsequent gains in the second year of 2.6 ± 1.7%, but this still placed them below the peak gains they achieved on teriparatide. Their cumulative gains over 4 years at the lumbar spine were 11.1 ±3.4%. The 12 men who began bisphosphonates immediately and continued treatment for the entire 2-year, post-PTH period had continued gains at the lumbar spine, 8.9 ±1.5% above their post-PTH values ($p = 0.002$). For the 4-year period, including 2 years of teriparatide and 2 years of bisphosphonate, their total gains at the lumbar spine were 23.6 ± 2.9%. The three men who received no bisphosphonate treatment after teriparatide treatment had cumulative gains of only 5.5 ± 3.7%.

58. **Rittmaster RS, Bolognese M, Ettinger MP,** et al. Enhancement of bone mass in osteoporotic women with parathyroid hormone followed by alendronate. J Clin Endocrinol Metab 2000;85:2129–2134.

   Postmenopausal osteoporotic women were treated for 1 year with parathyroid hormone (PTH) (50 μg, 75 μg, or 100 μg) or placebo, followed by 10 mg alendronate daily for an additional year, to examine whether alendronate could maintain or increase bone mineral density (BMD) in individuals previously treated with PTH. For women receiving PTH (all doses), changes in BMD (mean ± BMD) during the first year were 7.1 ± 5.6% (spine), 0.3 ± 6.2% (femoral neck), and −2.3 ± 3.3% (total body). Treatment with alendronate for 1 year after previously receiving PTH for 1 year resulted in mean changes in BMD of 13.4 ± 6.4% (spine), 4.4 ± 7.2% (femoral neck), and 2.6 ± 3.1% (whole body). Among patients who had received the highest dose of PTH, the mean increase in vertebral BMD was 14.6 ± 7.9%. Treatment with PTH resulted in increases in all markers of bone turnover; these levels decreased to below baseline after 1 year of alendronate.

59. **Lippman, ME, Cummings SR, Disch DP,** et al. Effect of raloxifene on the incidence of invasive breast cancer in postmenopausal women with osteoporosis categorized by breast cancer risk. Clin Cancer Res 2006;12:5242–5247.

60. **Ettinger B, San Martin J, Crans G, Imre P.** Response of markers of bone turnover and bone density to teriparatide in postmenopausal women previously treated with an antiresorptive drug. J Bone Miner Res 2004;19:745–751.

61. **Deal C, Omizo M, Schwartz EN,** et al. Combination teriparatide and raloxifene therapy for postmenopausal osteoporosis: Results from a 6-month, double-blind, placebo-controlled trial. J Bone Miner Res 2005;20:905–911.

   This double-blind, placebo-controlled trial compared combination treatment with teriparatide plus raloxifene with teriparatide alone in postmenopausal osteoporotic women over a 6-month period. Bone formation (aminoterminal propeptide of type I collagen,

PINP) increased similarly in both groups, but there was a significantly smaller increase in bone resorption (C-telopeptide, CTX) in the combination group than in the teriparatide-alone group ($p = 0.015$). A significant increase in lumbar spine bone mineral density (BMD) ($5.19 \pm 0.67\%$ from baseline) was observed in the teriparatide-alone group. In the combination group, lumbar spine ($6.19 \pm 0.65\%$), femoral neck ($2.23 \pm 0.64\%$), and total hip ($2.31 \pm 0.56\%$) BMD significantly increased from baseline to study end point, and the increase in total hip BMD was significantly larger than in the teriparatide-alone group ($p = 0.04$). In the teriparatide-alone group, mean serum calcium levels increased (0.30 ± 0.06 mg/dL; $p < 0.001$), but mean serum phosphate remained unchanged. In the combination group, mean serum calcium was unchanged, and mean serum phosphate decreased (-0.20 ± 0.06 mg/dL; $p < 0.001$). Changes in serum calcium ($p < 0.001$) and phosphate ($p < 0.004$) were significantly different between treatment groups. Safety profiles were similar between groups.

62. **Kaunitz A, Miller PD, McClung M,** et al. Bone mineral density in women aged 25 to 35 years receiving depo medroxyprogesterone acetate: Recovery following discontinuation. Contraception 2006;74:90–99.

63. **Keene AD, Drinkwater B.** Irreversible bone loss in former amenorrheic athletes. Osteoporos Int 1997;7:311–315.

This study evaluated whether bone mineral density (BMD) would normalize in former oligomenorrheic or amenorrheic athletes after several years of oral contraceptive therapy or normal menses. Vertebral BMD was significantly lower in women who had never menstruated regularly compared with women who always regularly menstruated at both the initial time and after normal menses or treatment with oral contraceptives ($p < 0.05$). These findings support the need for early intervention to prevent irreversible bone loss in oligo/amenorrheic athletes.

64. **Drinkwater B.** Exercise and bones. Lessons learned from female athletes. Am J Sports Med 1996;24(6 Suppl):S33–35. Review

65. **Otis CL, Drinkwater B, Johnson M,** et al. American College of Sports Medicine position stand. The Female Athlete Triad. Med Sci Sports Exerc 1997;29:1–10.

This article defines the Female Athlete Triad, who is at risk, and the need to identify individuals at risk quickly to avoid associated morbidities and mortality. The Female Athlete Triad is defined as a syndrome that occurs in physically active girls and women with interrelated components of disordered eating, amenorrhea, and osteoporosis.

10

Determining Success of Therapy and What to Do When Therapy Fails

Paul D. Miller

Osteoporosis therapies are designed to improve bone strength and reduce the risk for fracture. When the capacity to reduce fracture is assessed, these therapies reduce risk either expressed as relative risk (RR) or absolute risk (AR) within the context of clinical trials [1,2]. Whether or not risk reduction is expressed as either RR reduction (the ratio of absolute risk reduction in the treated group to absolute risk reduction in the placebo group) or absolute risk reduction (absolute number of fractures over a specified period of time), no osteoporosis treatment abolishes risk. People may still develop fragility fractures even when the osteoporosis-specific pharmacological therapy is altering bone strength in the best biological manner that the agent can induce. In biology, no pharmacological therapy abolishes risk for any specific event. In that regard, for example, patients with high cholesterol still have heart attacks, even though their cholesterol has been normalized by a cholesterol-lowering drug. In the same way, clinicians caring for individual patients will have patients who will suffer fractures while on osteoporosis-specific pharmacological agents; the clinician must then decide if the therapy is "working or not." Measuring optimal bone biological effect (efficacy) of a bone antiresorptive or anabolic agent is not easy to define—and in that regard, clinicians also use surrogate markers [changes in bone mineral density (BMD) or bone turnover markers (BTMs)] in addition to fracture events as measures of the effectiveness of an agent, since we have no clinical tool that is office-based to measure bone strength [3–6]. Hence, the efficacy of intervention is measured in four ways:

1. Fracture event(s)
2. Changes in BMD
3. Changes in biochemical BTM
4. Change in height as assessed by serial stadiometer measurements

Waiting for a fracture to occur or not occur is not a highly appealing efficacy end point for either physicians or patients, and, when a fracture does occur during therapy, both physician and patient feel that the specific treatment has failed, even though both parties may know that no treatment abolishes risk. Nevertheless, when a fracture occurs during treatment, the clinician should first review a checklist with the patient to ensure that everything is being done to guarantee treatment success. This checklist includes queries about adherence and persistence, and queries about following the proper adherence to the dosing instructions.

Specific laboratory tests should also be examined or reexamined that, when found to be abnormal, might contribute to "treatment failure." A few of these laboratory tests, if abnormal, may contribute to inadequate pharmacological response. These include a low 25-hydroxyvitamin D level; an elevated serum parathyroid hormone level; a low or high 24-hour urine calcium excretion; and a positive serum transglutaminase IgA antibody, the latter test a good screen for asymptomatic celiac disease.

Vitamin D insufficiency is prevalent in all populations, even in the United States, at all latitudes [7,8]. Low vitamin D levels may contribute to inadequate pharmacological response to osteoporosis therapies due, in part, to inadequate calcium absorption or the secondary hyperparathyroidism that often accompanies poor calcium absorption [9]. Celiac disease is also very prevalent; it exists in 1 of every 250 Caucasian Americans and, in certain other ethnic populations, as high as 1 in 50 persons [10,11]. Celiac disease is often completely asymptomatic and yet may lead to the specific malabsorption of calcium or iron, and is one of the most common secondary causes of osteoporosis [12,13]. Serum vitamin D levels are often normal in patients with celiac disease because vitamin D is absorbed in the terminal ileum and celiac disease begins in the proximal duodenum. It may take many years for celiac disease to migrate down the small bowel. As celiac disease advances down the small bowel, patients then may develop clinical symptoms such as bloatedness, diarrhea, and frank malabsorption, and in these more advanced subsets, 25-hydroxyvitamin D levels may finally become low. Most of the fractures or losses of BMD in patients being treated with bisphosphonates who have celiac disease are treatment failures because bisphosphonates are not absorbed in the presence of celiac disease. The transglutaminase IgA antibody is the best screening test for celiac disease, but its sensitivity is not nearly as good in asymptomatic as opposed to symptomatic celiac disease (~70% vs. ~90) [14]. Hence, a small bowel biopsy, the gold standard for the diagnosis of celiac disease (histological diagnosis), should still be done for patients with osteoporosis treatment failure who have a negative transglutaminase IgA antibody in two clinical scenarios:

- Persistently high bone resorption markers [N-telopeptide (NTx) or C-telopeptide (CTx)] despite adherence to oral bisphosphonates
- Low (<50 mg/day) 24-hour urine calcium excretion in a patient consuming a recommended daily calcium intake

Urine calcium excretions that are consistently low, despite an adequate calcium intake, are strongly suggestive of poor calcium absorption and a high probability of celiac disease in patients with normal renal function. One of the more common conditions that lead to poor calcium absorption is celiac disease. Celiac disease may contribute to osteoporosis by preventing calcium or bisphosphonate absorption.

There are other gastrointestinal (GI) conditions in which oral bisphosphonates are probably not absorbed: gastrojejunostomy, small bowel resections, hemigastrectomies, and other clinical states in which upper-GI transit time is rapid, including gastric stapling—and all of these GI conditions may be related to bisphosphonate "treatment failure." The fundamental absorption characteristics of oral bisphosphonates are very erratic and fastidious in the first place, with less than 1% of an oral bisphosphonate formulation absorbed under the best circumstance. Hence, it does not take much of an alteration of GI tract function to abolish bisphosphonate absorption. If clinicians could measure a bisphosphonate blood level, clinical decisions regarding the uncertainty about bisphosphonate absorption could be resolved. Yet there are no clinically available bisphosphonate assays, so clinicians are often left in the dark about the bioavailability of oral bisphosphonates.

A high 24-hour urinary calcium excretion might also contribute to treatment failure. Hypercalciuria might be associated with bone loss because the high urinary calcium excretion might be related to a disease that directly contributes to bone loss (e.g., primary hyperparathyroidism, renal tubular acidosis), or the hypercalciuria might, per se, contribute to a negative calcium balance [15,16]. Hypercalciuria does not necessarily mean the patient is in negative calcium balance (calcium balance studies are not pragmatic to do in clinical practice) because hyperabsorption may be contributing to the hypercalciuria without the excess urinary calcium coming from the large bone reservoir of calcium. Nevertheless, a patient who is hypercalciuric and has a fracture or is losing BMD while on pharmacological treatment may benefit by lessening urine calcium excretion [17,18].

Hypercalciuria is best lowered by a thiazide diuretic, and this author prefers either a hydrochlorothiazide-amiloride combination or chlorthalidone (50 mg/day). After 6 to 8 weeks of the diuretic, the 24-hour urine calcium and serum calcium should be remeasured for two reasons: to see if (a) the thiazide is effective in normalizing the urinary calcium excretion (<300 mg/day) and (b) if hypercalcemia develops when normocalciuria is achieved. If hypercalcemia develops after achieving normocalciuria, then one may have unmasked primary hyperparathyroidism—the "thiazide-challenge test" [19]. Patients with mild primary hyperparathyroidism may be normocalcemic because they are hypercalciuric; for example, the kidney is protecting the blood (and brain) from hypercalcemia. Hence, if sustained hypercalcemia develops once normocalciuria is maintained, then additional testing for primary hyperparathyroidism may be indicated. If the patient does not develop hypercalcemia after becoming normocalciuric, then the clinician may continue the thiazide to see what effect normocalciuria has on the previous loss of BMD. If the BMD loss is reversed with a thiazide-induced normocalciuria, then the thiazide may be continued with or without combination therapy for the osteoporosis [20]. If there is no effect of normocalciuria on BMD, fractures, or kidney stone history (or if noncontrast CT of the kidneys has been done to rule out asymptomatic nephrocalcinosis), then the thiazide should be discontinued, because many of these hypercalciuric patients are so-called "healthy hypercalciurics"—they exhibit elevated urinary calcium excretion of no clinical relevance [21].

In those patients who are "treatment failures" defined by sustaining fractures or losing BMD while on therapy and who also have a persistently high bone resorption marker while on oral bisphosphonates where GI absorption may be the cause of treatment failure, the clinician has two options:

- Switching to an intravenous bisphosphonate to guarantee the delivery of the bisphosphonate to bone
- Switching therapy to subcutaneous teriparatide or calcitonin

If an intravenous bisphosphonate is chosen, there are three available. Two of these are currently being used off-label [i.e., they do not have a Food and Drug Administration (FDA) registration for an osteoporotic indication (pamidronate and zolendronic acid)], and the other is an intravenous bisphosphonate recently approved by the FDA for osteoporosis (ibandronate) [22–24]. The dose of pamidronate is usually 30 mg diluted in 250 mL D5W given over 2 hours, with an occasional patient requiring 60 mg every 3 months. The dose determination is decided by monitoring the bone resorption marker (NTx/CTx) between doses. This author measures the first marker 1 month after the first IV bisphosphonate infusion and the second marker 2 weeks before the second bisphosphonate infusion. The resorption marker should be maintained within a level consistent with sustained suppression of bone turnover levels. Urine NTx values in the 30s or lower [nm bone collagen equivalents (BCE)/nm creatinine], or serum CTx values between 0.5 and 3.2 pmol/L—the so-called "therapeutic" range—are seen in most treated patients in the clinical trials on the registered doses of bisphosphonates [25,26]. Sustained turnover marker suppression to some consistent level seems to be important to the improvement in bone strength, particularly with intermittent bisphosphonate dosing regimens [26,27]. In the early intermittent intravenous bisphosphonate studies (1 mg every 3 months of ibandronate), in which the spine BMD increased to levels seen in other bisphosphonate studies that did have fracture risk reduction, fracture risk reduction was not seen, probably because of inadequate and nonsustained suppression of bone turnover between dosing schedules at this dose [27]. The FDA-approved ibandronate dose of 3 mg every 3 months kept bone resorption markers more consistently suppressed between dosing intervals, which, in theory, should improve bone strength similarly to the fracture reduction–proven daily ibandronate dosing regimen [28].

If the 5 mg/year intravenous zolendronic acid becomes FDA-approved for osteoporosis, it may still be important to measure the postinfusion bone resorption markers (1 month and 11 month postinfusion), not necessarily to be secure in the maintenance of the suppression of bone turnover but to gauge when the next zolendronic acid dose is needed. There may be a heterogeneity in the duration of response to zolendronic acid–induced reduction in bone resorption, as may be the case with any intermittent bisphosphonate dosing regimen. Some patients may not have a rise from the nadir of resorption marker after zolendronic acid infusion until 18 to 24 months after infusion, so a standard infusion of zolendronic acid every 12 months might not be the correct dosing schedule for all patients. In theory, one might want to apply an intermittent bisphosphonate dosing regimen if the resorption marker between dosing schedules is still within a "therapeutic" range currently defined by observations of what may be adequate suppression of bone turnover as opposed to the theoretical concept of "oversuppression" of bone turnover—an untested hypothesis in human beings [29,30].

If teriparatide is chosen for "treatment failures," there is no reason to continue any prior therapy other than being certain the patient continues with vitamin D and calcium. In addition, there is no reason to give a patient a therapeutic "break" from a bisphosphonate before starting parathyroid hormone (PTH) [31,32]. After the teriparatide treatment period is complete (e.g., 2 years) the clinician must decide what to provide the patient in the context that the patient had previously "failed" an oral (usually bisphosphonate) therapy. If the treatment failure was related to the use of an oral bisphosphonate, then an IV bisphosphonate would be the best consideration after PTH administration. In the future, if oral bisphosphonate absorption or bisphosphonate long-term use is of any concern, alternative anabolic or antiresorptive agents may become a consideration for use in the sequential treatment of osteoporosis [33–35].

Determining the success or lack of success of treatments for post-menopausal osteoporosis is not an easy task. Yet fracturing during therapy despite good persistence with therapy or losing BMD or continual height loss due to progression of known prevalent vertebral compression fractures always raises questions in the minds of both physicians and patients about what else might be done to prevent the progression of osteoporosis clinical end points. To the extent that there are no evidence-based data that switching to an intravenous bisphosphonate or an anabolic agent has any better results with regard to fracture risk reduction than what the patient is already receiving or that "treatment failure" can be defined with certainty, this chapter offers some clinical advice on management of this difficult and not infrequently encountered medical problem.

REFERENCES

1. **Blake GM, Fogelman I.** Bone densitometry and fracture risk prediction. Eur J Nucl Med Mol Imaging 2004;31:785–786.
2. **Miller PD, Bonnick SL, Rosen C.** Guidelines for the clinical utilization of bone mass measurement in the adult population. Society for Clinical Densitometry. Calcif Tissue Int 1995;57:251–252.
3. **Miller PD.** Bone density and markers of bone turnover in predicting fracture risk and how changes in these measures predict fracture risk reduction. Curr Osteoporos Rep 2005;3:103–110.
   This article provides a review of the usefulness of surrogate markers such as bone mineral density (BMD) and bone turnover markers in assessing response to osteoporosis therapy.
4. **Miller PD, Hochberg MC, Wehren LE,** et al. How useful are measures of BMD and bone turnover? Curr Med Res Opin 2005;21:545–553.
   A review of the role of bone mineral density (BMD) and bone turnover markers in the management of osteoporosis.
5. **Weinstein RS.** True strength. J Bone Miner Res 2000;15:621–625.
6. **Bouxsein ML.** Determinants of skeletal fragility. Best Pract Res Clin Rheumatol 2005;19:897–911.
   This is a review of biomechanical aspects of age-related fractures, the mechanisms by which antiresorptive and anabolic therapies for osteoporosis may affect bone strength, and current and future methodologies for improving assessment of bone strength.

7. **Holick MF.** High prevalence of vitamin D inadequacy and implications for health. Mayo Clin Proc 2006;81:353–373.

   This article highlights the prevalence of vitamin D deficiency and the factors that lead to this condition. The prevalence of vitamin D inadequacy has been reported in approximately 36% of healthy young populations and up to 57% of general medicine inpatients in the United States. This prevalence is even higher in Europe. Factors that contribute to the development of this disease include low sunlight exposure, age-related decreases in cutaneous synthesis, and diets low in vitamin D. The paper also discusses prevention and effects on skeletal and extraskeletal systems.

8. **Heaney RP, Rafferty K.** Assessing nutritional quality. Am J Clin Nutr 2006;83: 722–723.

9. **Heaney RP.** Serum 25-hydroxyvitamin D and parathyroid hormone exhibit threshold behavior. J Endocrinol Invest 2005;28:180–182.

10. **Fasano A, Berti I, Gerarduzzi T,** et al. Prevalence of celiac disease in at-risk and not-at-risk groups in the United States: A large multicenter study. Arch Intern Med 2003;163:286–292.

    The aim of the study was to determine the prevalence of celiac disease (CD) in the United States. Serum antigliadin antibodies and antiendomysial antibodies (EMA) were measured. Patients who were found to be positive for EMA subsequently had human tissue transglutaminase IgA antibodies and CD-associated human leukocyte antigen DQ2/DQ8 haplotypes measured. Intestinal biopsy was recommended and performed whenever possible for all EMA-positive subjects. Of a total of 13,145 subjects screened, the prevalence of CD was 1:22 in first-degree relatives, 1:39 in second-degree relatives, and 1:56 in symptomatic patients. These first- and second-degree relatives were asymptomatic. The overall prevalence of CD in not-at-risk groups was 1:133. All the EMA-positive subjects who underwent intestinal biopsy had lesions consistent with CD.

11. **Fasano A, Catassi C.** Current approaches to diagnosis and treatment of celiac disease: an evolving spectrum. Gastroenterology 2001;121:1527–1528.

    This review discusses the pathophysiology, symptomatology, and current treatment algorithms for celiac disease.

12. **Molteni N, Caraceni MP, Bardella MT,** et al. Bone mineral density in adult celiac patients and the effect of gluten-free diet from childhood. Am J Gastroenterol 1990;85:51–53.

    Forearm bone mineral densities (BMDs) of 22 celiac patients on gluten-free diet from childhood (young men 14, young women 8, age 13–20) and 29 untreated adult celiac patients at diagnosis (men 5, women 24, age 18–56, 14 with subclinical disease) were measured and compared with healthy sex- and age-matched controls. BMD was similar in patients treated from childhood and their controls [668.4 ± 65.3 vs. 654.9 ± 69.6 mg/cm^2 (mean ± SD)], but significantly lower in untreated patients than in their controls (598.3 ± 83.1 vs. 673.2 ± 42.7 mg/cm^2; $p < 0.001$). It was also significantly lower in the 12 younger untreated celiac patients (18–28 y) versus controls (619.4 ± 68.5 vs. 669.1 ± 39.3 mg/cm^2; $p < 0.01$). In the untreated women, but not their controls, a negative correlation ($p < 0.05$) was observed between bone mineral density and age.

13. **Hoyt R.** Celiac disease and osteoporosis. Arch Intern Med 2005;165:1922–1923.

14. **Farrell RJ, Kelly CP.** Diagnosis of celiac sprue. Am J Gastroenterol 2001;96: 3237–3246.

    A review of the clinical manifestations and approach to diagnosis of celiac sprue.

15. **Liebman SE, Taylor JG, Bushinsky DA.** Idiopathic hypercalciuria. Curr Rheumatol Rep 2006;8:70–75.

    This paper discusses the pathophysiology, complications, and treatment of idiopathic hypercalciuria, the most common metabolic bone disorder found in patients with nephrolithiasis.

16. **Krieger NS, Bushinsky DA, Frik KK.** Cellular mechanisms of bone resorption induced by metabolic acidosis. Semin Dial 2003;16:463–466.

    An in-depth review of the effects of metabolic acidosis on bone loss.

17. **Friedman PA, Bushinsky DA.** Diuretic effects on calcium metabolism. Semin Nephrol 1999;19:551–556.

    This review discusses the basic mechanisms of renal calcium excretion and how these are altered by diuretics.

18. **Coe FL, Parks JH, Bushinsky DA,** et al. Chlorthalidone promotes mineral retention in patients with idiopathic hypercalciuria. Kidney Int 1988;33:1140–1146.

    Seven patients with severe idiopathic hypercalciuria (urinary calcium excretion >350 mg/day) and recurrent nephrolithiasis were treated with chlorthalidone or trichlormethiazide and followed. Although intestinal calcium absorption decreased, the reduction in urinary calcium loss was more marked. Phosphate retention increased, whereas calcitriol, parathyroid hormone (PTH), calcium, phosphates, and magnesium levels were unchanged.

19. **Mohamadi M, Bivens L, Becker KL.** Effect of thiazides on serum calcium. Clin Pharmacol Ther 1979;26:390–394.

    In a retrospective study of 22 hypertensive patients treated with thiazide diuretics, transient self-limited hypercalcemia (usually resolving in 2–4 weeks despite continuation of the thiazide) was noted in 36% of the population. A positive correlation with total protein, albumin, and globulin was seen, suggesting depletion of extracellular fluid.

20. **Rejnmark L, Vestergaard P, Mosekilde L.** Reduced fracture risk in users of thiazide diuretics. Calcif Tissue Int 2005;76:167–175.

    The aim of this study was to assess whether thiazide diuretics (TD) reduced fracture risk. The study was a nationwide population-based case-control study with fracture in year 2000 as outcome and use of TD during the previous 5 years as the exposure variable. Individual use of TD was derived from the Danish National Pharmacological Database and related to fracture data from the National Hospital Discharge Register. A total of 64,699 patients (age = 40 y) who sustained a fracture during the year 2000 were compared with 194,111 age- and gender-matched controls. After adjustment for potential confounders, current use of TD was associated with a 10% [95% confidence interval (CI), 7%–12%] reduced risk of any fracture and a 17% (95% CI, 11%–23%) reduced risk of forearm fractures. In former TD users, the risk reduction was slightly less pronounced. Similar results were found in men and women, and in subjects younger than or 65 years of age and older.

21. **Coe FL, Parks JH, Moore ES.** Familial idiopathic hypercalciuria. N Engl J Med 1979;300:337.

    The frequency of hypercalciuria was determined in the families (73 relatives) of nine patients with idiopathic hypercalciuria who formed recurrent calcium oxalate renal stones. Forty-three percent of the first-degree relatives and 29% of other relatives had the disease, and no relationships to age and sex were found. The authors concluded that there is a familial form of hypercalciuria, which appeared to be transmitted as an autosomal dominant trait.

22. **Papapoulos SE.** Bisphosphonates: Pharmacology and use in the treatment of osteoporosis. In: Marcus R, Feldman D, Kelsey J, eds. *Osteoporosis.* San Diego: Academic Press;1996:1209–1234.

23. **Reid IR, Brown JP, Burckhardt P,** et al. Intravenous zoledronic acid in postmenopausal women with low bone mineral density. N Engl J Med 2002;346:653–661.

    In this 1-year, randomized, double-blind, placebo-controlled trial, 351 postmenopausal women with low bone mineral density (BMD) were randomized to placebo or intravenous zoledronic acid 0.25, 0.5, or 1.0 mg at 3-month intervals. In addition, one group received a 4-mg single dose intravenously, and another received two doses of 2 mg each, 6 months apart. Similar increases in lumbar spine BMD, 4.3% to 5.1%, were seen in all zoledronic acid groups compared with placebo ($p < 0.001$). In addition, mean percentage change in femoral neck BMD was 3.1% to 3.5% higher ($p < 0.001$). Markers of bone resorption were significantly suppressed in all zoledronic acid groups. Side effects included myalgia and fever.

24. **Delmas PD, Adami S, Strugala C,** et al. Intravenous ibandronate injections in postmenopausal women with osteoporosis: One-year results from the dosing intravenous administration study. Arthritis Rheum 2006;54:1838–1846.

    This was a noninferiority study of two regimens of intermittent intravenous injections of ibandronate (2 mg every 2 months and 3 mg every 3 months) and 2.5 mg of oral ibandronate daily. The study enrolled 1,395 postmenopausal women (ages 55–80 years) with osteoporosis [lumbar spine (L2–L4) bone mineral density (BMD) T-score less than –2.5]. Participants also received daily calcium (500 mg) and vitamin D (400 IU). At 1 year, mean lumbar spine BMD increases were as follows: 5.1% among 353 patients receiving 2 mg of ibandronate every 2 months, 4.8% among 365 patients receiving 3 mg of ibandronate every 3 months, and 3.8% among 377 patients receiving 2.5 mg of oral ibandronate daily. The intravenous regimens were superior to the oral regimen ($p < 0.001$). Hip BMD increases (at all sites) were also greater in the intravenous groups than in the oral group. Robust decreases in the serum CTx level were observed in all arms of the study. Both of the intravenous regimens were well tolerated, and no adverse effects on renal function were noted.

25. **Chavassieux PM, Delmas PD.** Bone remodeling: biochemical markers or bone biopsy? J Bone Miner Res 2006;21:178–179.

26. **Eastell R, Delmas PD.** How to interpret surrogate markers of efficacy in osteoporosis. J Bone Miner Res 2005;20:1261–1262.

27. **Recker R, Stakkestad JA, Chesnut CH 3rd,** et al. Insufficiently dosed intravenous ibandronate injections are associated with suboptimal antifracture efficacy in postmenopausal osteoporosis. Bone 2004;34:890–901.

This was a double-blind, placebo-controlled, randomized phase III study that aimed to determine the 3-year antifracture efficacy and safety of 1- and 0.5-mg intravenous ibandronate injections, given once every 3 months, in 2,862 women (55–76 years) with postmenopausal osteoporosis. All participants received daily vitamin D (400 IU) and calcium (500 mg) supplementation. A consistent trend toward a reduction in the incidence of new morphometric vertebral fracture was observed in the active treatment arms compared with placebo (9.2% vs. 8.7% vs. 10.7% in the 1-mg, 0.5-mg, and placebo groups, respectively), as well as in the incidence of nonvertebral and hip fractures, but the numbers did not reach statistical significance. Small increases in lumbar spine bone mineral density (4.0% and 2.9%, respectively) and decreases in biochemical markers of bone resorption and formation, compared with placebo, were observed.

28. **Adami S, Felsenberg N, Christiansen C,** et al. Efficacy and safety of ibandronate given by intravenous injection once every 3 months. Bone 2004;34:881–889.

29. **Recker RR, Barger-Lux MJ.** Bone remodeling findings in osteoporosis. In Marcus R, Feldman D, Kelsey J, eds. *Osteoporosis,* 2nd ed. San Diego: Academic Press; 2001:59–70.

30. **Ott SM.** Long-term safety of bisphosphonates. J Clin Endocrinol Metab 2005;90: 1897–1899.

31. **Miller PD, Bilezikian JP, Deal C,** et al. Clinical use of teriparatide in the real world: Initial insights. Endocr Pract 2004;10:139–148.

A review of the clinical applications of teriparatide in the treatment of osteoporosis in men and postmenopausal women.

32. **Hodsman AB, Bauer DC, Dempster D,** et al. Parathyroid hormone and teriparatide for the treatment of osteoporosis: A review of the evidence and suggested guidelines for its use. Endocr Rev 2005;10:2004–2006.

33. **Meunier PJ, Roux C, Seeman E,** et al. The effects of strontium ranelate on the risk of vertebral fracture in women with postmenopausal osteoporosis. N Engl J Med 2004;350:459–468.

Strontium ranelate (SR) was studied for its effectiveness and safety in treating postmenopausal osteoporosis. In a randomized, multicenter, double-blind, placebo-controlled experiment, 353 osteoporotic women ($T < 2.4$) who had at least one fracture were given different dosages of SR for 2 years. The dosages were as follows: 0.5 g, 1 g, and 2 g SR per day. Also, some women were given placebo. To assess SR's effects, lumbar bone mineral density (BMD), femoral BMD, new vertebral deformities, and bone turnover were noted. It was found that after 2 years, lumbar BMD increased by 1.4% in women who received 0.5 g SR per day and 3.0% in women who received 2 g SR per day, as compared with placebo ($p < 0.01$). Also, women who took 2 g SR per day had decreased vertebral deformities (0.56 relative risk; 95% CI), and they increased their levels of bone alkaline phosphatase. These same women had decreased cross-linked N-telopeptides, as compared to women who received placebo. In conclusion, it was found that 2 g SR per day was the best dosage for effectiveness and safety; it increased vertebral BMD and decreased the incidence of fractures.

34. **Deal C, Omizo M, Schwartz EN,** et al. Combination teriparatide and raloxifene therapy for postmenopausal osteoporosis: Results from a 6-month double-blind placebo-controlled trial. J Bone Miner Res 2005;20:1905–1911.

35. **McClung MR, Lewiecki EM, Cohen SB,** et al. AMG 162 Bone Loss Study Group. Denosumab in postmenopausal women with low bone mineral density. N Engl J Med 2006;354:821–831.

In this 2-year randomized, double-blind study, the effectiveness of lasofoxifene and raloxifene in preserving bone mass and preventing osteoporosis in postmenopausal women was studied. A group of 410 postmenopausal women ranging from the ages of 47 to 74 received one of four different treatments: 0.25 mg/day of lasofoxifene, 1.0 mg/day of lasofoxifene, 6.0 mg/day of raloxifene, or placebo. The baseline bone mineral density of the lumbar spine and hip was noted. It was found that the bone mineral density of the lumbar spine increased ($p \leq 0.01$) as follows: 3.6% for 0.25 mg lasofoxifene, 3.9% for 1.0 mg lasofoxifene, and 1.7% for 6.0 mg/day of raloxifene. It was found that in all treatments, there was decreased bone turnover as compared with the placebo ($p \leq 0.05$). After 2 years, it was found that both dosage treatments of lasofoxifene decreased low-density lipoprotein cholesterol ($p \leq 0.05$) by the following amounts: 20.6% for 0.25 mg/day of lasofoxifene, 19.7% for 1.0 mg/day of lasofoxifene, 12.1% for 6.0 mg/day of ralofoxifene, and 3.2% for placebo. Thus, all trends point to lasofoxifene as the best treatment for osteoporosis in postmenopausal women.

11

Future Therapeutic Options

Paul D. Miller

Current osteoporosis therapies have been shown to reduce the risk of fragility fractures generally from 50% to 65% over a period of 3 years. No pharmacological intervention for any disease abolishes risk, but future therapeutic options for the treatment of osteoporosis are being designed with the hope of improving on the risk reduction that can be currently achieved.

However, there are additional considerations in designing future choices for the pharmacological treatment of osteoporosis besides improved efficacy: improved safety profiles and fewer side effects, better formulations that might encourage adherence and persistence, and therapies that might increase bone strength through different mechanisms of action other than just by bone mineral density and reducing bone turnover [1–5]. The osteoporosis-specific pharmacological agents that are potential future therapeutic options are listed in Table 11.1.

Very recently, intravenous ibandronate (3 mg intravenous injection every 3 months) was registered for postmenopausal osteoporosis (PMO) (Fig. 11.1) [6]. The approval for intravenous ibandronate was made in the same manner that weekly or monthly bisphosphonate formulations were Food and Drug Administration (FDA)–approved on the basis of noninferiority comparative studies. Noninferiority studies compare the effects of the fracture-proven daily dosing with the intermittent dosing schedule, and, if the increases in axial bone mineral density (BMD) by dual-energy x-ray absorptiometry (DXA) are noninferior to each other, FDA registration can be achieved. Hence, quarterly intravenous ibandronate has become the first intravenous bisphosphonate to be FDA-approved for the treatment of PMO.

The agents that are being considered for either registration for postmenopausal osteoporosis management or are in early clinical development are the newer intravenous bisphosphonates (zolendronic acid) [7]; newer selective estrogen receptor modulators [bazedoxifene (BZA), lasofoxifene, and arzoxifene] [8–13]; human monoclonal antibodies to the RANK-ligand system (denosumab) [14]; new parathyroid hormone (PTH) sequences and/or routes of administration (1-84 PTH subcutaneously, 1-31 PTH subcutaneously, 1-34 PTH nasal spray, 1-34 PTH inhaled) [15–19]; and newer non-PTH anabolic agents [20,21]. In even earlier developmental stages, bone agents that might be applicable to the management of PMO are cathepsin K inhibitors, calciolytic agents, agents that alter the *Src* tyrosine kinase or the sclerostin pathways, and pathways that modulate the WINT pathway

TABLE 11.1.   Newer therapeutic options in development or under FDA consideration

Zolendronic acid, 5 mg IV once a year
Denosumab (formerly AMG 162), a fully human monoclonal antibody to RANKL
PTH 1-84 (PREOS)
Strontium ranelate (Protelos)
Cathepsin K inhibitors
Other selective estrogen receptor modulators (SERMs)
Src tyrosine (STK) inhibitors
Sclerostin inhibitors

FDA, Food and Drug Administration; PTH, parathyroid hormone.

[22–26]. WINT is a membrane-bound osteoblast receptor. The WINT pathway is necessary for osteoblastogenesis.

In the initial dose-ranging studies of zolendronic acid, a single intravenous infusion of 4 mg over 15 minutes increased BMD and reduced biochemical markers of bone turnover [N-telopeptide (NTx)], results that were sustained for at least 12 months [7] (Figs. 11.2 and 11.3). Hence, in the FDA application for the treatment of PMO, the suggested dosing frequency will be every 12 months. In clinical practice there seems to be a large heterogeneity to the off-set of the long duration of zolendronic effect on bone turnover, as measured by bone resorption markers. In the unpublished offset of zolendronic acid in

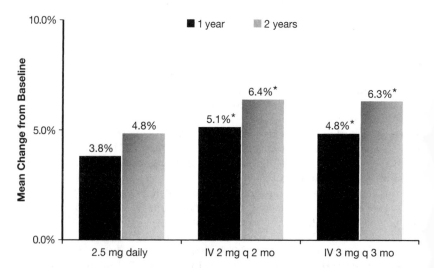

Figure 11.1.   Increases in lumbar spine bone mass density on oral versus intravenous ibandronate. Per-protocol population. Both intravenous doses were not inferior to daily doses at 1 year. Test for superiority: *p < 0.001 vs. daily. (Adapted from Delmas PD, Adami S, Strugala C, et al. Intravenous ibandronate injections in postmenopausal women with osteoporosis: One-year results from the dosing intravenous administration study. Arthritis Rheum 2006;54:1838–1846, with permission from GlaxoSmithKline & Roche Laboratories, Inc., Medical Affairs.)

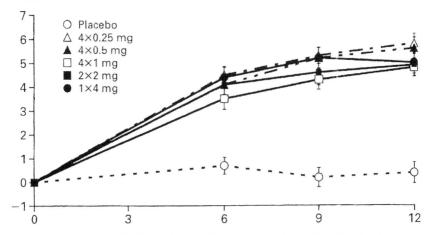

Figure 11.2   Effect of dosing regimens of intravenous zoledronic acid on lumbar spine bone mineral density in postmenopausal women with osteoporosis; p < 0.001 all doses versus placebo throughout the study. (From Reid IR, Brown JP, Burckhardt P, et al. Intravenous zoledronic acid in postmenopausal women with low bone mineral density. N Engl J Med 2002;346:653–661, with permission.)

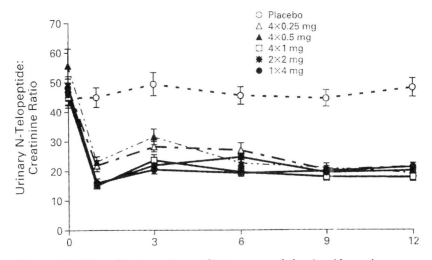

Figure 11.3.   Effect of dosing regimens of intravenous zoledronic acid on urinary N-telopeptide in postmenopausal women with osteoporosis; p < 0.01 all doses versus placebo throughout the study. (From Reid IR, Brown JP, Burckhardt P, et al. Intravenous zoledronic acid in postmenopausal women with low bone mineral density. N Engl J Med 2002;346:653–661, with permission.)

the PMO clinical trials, in which the dose will be 5 mg per day, some patients may have a persistent suppression of bone turnover markers far beyond 12 months. It is not known if the label will recommend measuring the urinary cross-linked NTx or serum C-telopeptide of type I collagen (CTx) in order to decide when a second dose of zolendronic acid may be required. Since it is unknown what level of bone turnover is ideal, or if there is a lower level of bone turnover that becomes harmful to bone strength, when the bone turnover is induced by antiresorptive treatment, it is also unclear if the dosing interval of zolendronic acid should be anything other than an every-12-months schedule. If the pending results of the yearly intravenous zolendronic acid clinical trials (HORIZON) show that zolendronic acid in a 5 mg/year dosing interval reduces the risk of fracture, then an annual dose will become the standard dosing interval.

The second-generation SERMs (selective estrogen selective modulators) are being designed with the purpose of having fewer side effects, especially hot flushes that limit to some degree the wide use of raloxifene. In addition, there is hope that the second-generation SERM agents might have a broader antifracture efficacy beyond reduction in vertebral fractures. Lasofoxifene received an approvable letter from the FDA in 2005 but has not gained FDA approval for PMO, pending additional uterine safety data.

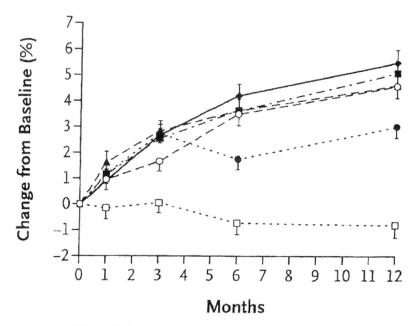

Figure 11.4.   Effect of dosing regimens of denosumab, given every 6 months, on lumbar spine bone density in postmenopausal women; p < 0.01 for 60 mg, 100 mg, 210 mg and alendronate versus placebo. □ Placebo (*n* = 46), ● 14 mg denosumab (*n* = 53), ▲ 60 mg denosumab (*n* = 46), ▶ 100 mg denosumab (*n* = 41), ■ 210 mg denosumab (*n* = 46), ○ 70 mg alendronate weekly (*n* = 46). (From McClung MR, Lewiecki EM, Cohen SB, et al., for the AMG 162 Bone Loss Study Group. Denosumab in postmenopausal women with low bone mineral density. N Engl J Med 2006;354:821–831, with permission.)

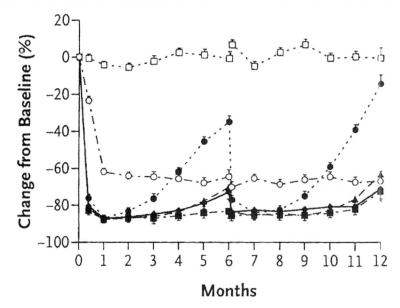

Figure 11.5.   **Effect of dosing regimens of denosumab, given every 6 months, on C-telopeptide in postmenopausal women; p < 0.0001 for 60 mg, 100 mg, 210 mg and alendronate versus placebo.** □ Placebo (n = 46), ● 14 mg denosumab (n = 53), ▲ 60 mg denosumab (n = 46), ▶ 100 mg denosumab (n = 41), ■ 210 mg denosumab (n = 46), ○ 70 mg alendronate weekly (n = 46). **(From McClung MR, Lewiecki EM, Cohen SB, et al., for the AMG 162 Bone Loss Study Group. Denosumab in postmenopausal women with low bone mineral density. N Engl J Med 2006;354:821–831, with permission.)**

Bazedoxifene has recently been filed for FDA registration. It remains to be seen if the second-generation SERMs will show a similar reduction in breast cancer risks as has been shown with raloxifene [27].

Anti-RANK-ligand antibody (denosumab) has recently been shown to increase BMD and reduce bone turnover markers in phase II clinical trials [14] (Figs. 11.4 and 11.5). The phase III fracture trial is using the dose of 60 mg of denosumab subcutaneously every 12 months for registration. The OPG-RANK ligand–RANK system is intimately involved in the coupling between osteoblastic and osteoclastic regulation. The preosteoblast produces competitive proteins: osteoprotogerin (OPG) and RANK ligand. Depending on which of these two osteoblastic-derived proteins gains access to the osteoclastic membrane receptor rank determines osteoclastic cell differentiation and activity [28]. The anti-RANK-ligand antibody binds to RANK ligand, inhibiting the latter to binding to the receptor rank. The net result is a decrease in bone resorption, a decrease in bone turnover, and an increase in BMD. Because this monoclonal antibody is not retained in bone (as are bisphosphonates), it may allow an alternative approach to the treatment of PMO that may not have the same concerns about long-term bone retention time that bisphosphonates may have.

The alternate PTH anabolic formulations are being designed to offer different routes of administration (nasal, inhaled, and oral), avoiding the daily subcutaneous injections of the current FDA-approved PTH (teriparatide). In Europe the subcutaneous injection formulation of the 1-84 PTH has been approved for the treatment of PMO. To date, the data from the 1-84 PTH clinical trial show its capacity to reduce the risk of incident vertebral compression fractures in postmenopausal women, both without as well as with a prevalent vertebral compression fracture [15] (Fig. 11.6). These data might lead to consideration of the earlier use of PTH in a lower-risk, postmenopausal population because a plausible hypothesis is to "make new bone" first, with PTH, then to maintain that newly formed bone with an antiresorptive agent.

Strontium ranelate has also been approved in Europe for the treatment of PMO. This agent, which is anabolic as well as possibly anticatabolic to bone cell lines, reduces the incidence of vertebral compression fractures (primary end point) [20] (Fig. 11.7) and nonvertebral fractures. There needs to be an adjustment in the measured increase in BMD in patients being monitored on strontium because about 50% of the increase in axial BMD is due to the strontium molecule effect of blocking the transmission of the DXA-derived photon [29]. The formulation of strontium ranelate is cumbersome. The formulation is a powder and must be diluted in a large volume of water for its daily usage.

The cathepsin K inhibitors and the calciolytic agents are the next in line for phase II clinical trials [22,25]. Cathepsin K resides in the osteoclast and must be released in order for bone resorption to take place. Inhibitors of cathepsin K result in inhibition of bone resorption [30]. Calcimimetic agents

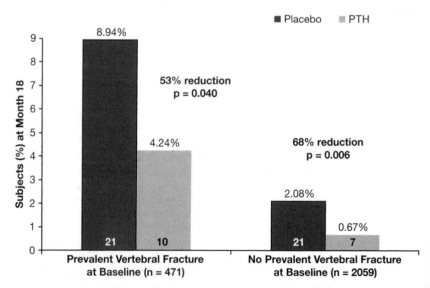

Figure 11.6.   (1-84) PTH in reducing new vertebral fractures in patients with or without fracture at baseline (intention to treat; ITT): results from the TOP (Treatment of Osteoporosis with PTH) trial. (Adapted from Greenspan SL, Bone HG, Marriott TB, et al. Preventing the first vertebral fracture in postmenopausal women with lost bone mass using PTH[1-84]: Results from the TOP study. J Bone Miner Res 2005;20:536, with permission.)

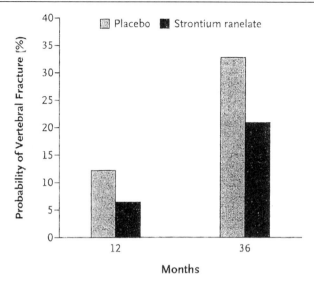

Figure 11.7.   **Vertebral fracture reduction by strontium ranelate: proportion of patients who had one or more new vertebral fracture(s). ■ Placebo, □ strontium ranelate. (From Meunier PJ, Slosman DO, Delmas PD, et al. Strontium ranelate: Dose-dependent effects in established postmenopausal vertebral osteoporosis—a 2-year randomized placebo controlled trial. J Clin Endocrinol Metab 2002;87:2060–2066, with permission.)**

are agents that "trick" the parathyroid hormone cell calcium receptor. Already FDA-approved for the treatment of severe secondary hyperparathyroidism in patients with end-stage renal disease is cinacalcet, which alters the calcium receptor to perceive that the serum calcium is higher than it truly is, with the suppression of endogenous PTH production [31]. On the other side of modulating the calcium receptor are the calciolytics, which alter the receptor to believe that the serum calcium is lower than it really is, with the result being the stimulation of endogenous PTH release. In the early pharmacokinetic (PK) studies of the calciolytic agents that are being considered for phase II clinical trials are doses that stimulate endogenous PTH production in a manner similar to the PK serum peaks and area under the curve observed with the subcutaneous administration of teriparatide. The calciolytic agents in development are an oral formulation that has the potential advantage of avoiding daily injections.

Finally, the discovery of the osteoblast-housed WINT pathway and the better clarification of its regulation by the tremendous basic science that has been devoted to understanding this pathway has also led to molecules to influence WINT (*Src* tyrosine kinase, sclerostin, and the LRP 5 gene [24,26,32] (Fig. 11.8). These developments may yield other means of altering bone remodeling and bone formation that may offer additional choices for the treatment of PMO.

The area of future therapeutics for the management of PMO is exciting—and may offer menus of choices for individualizing treatment according to

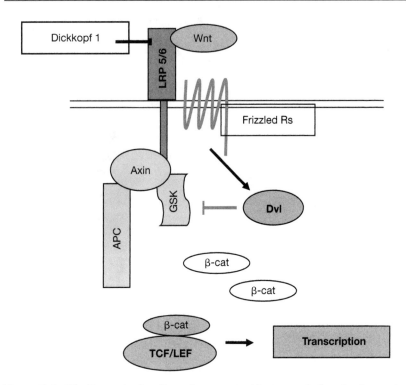

Figure 11.8. Wnt/β-catenin signaling enhances osteoblastogenesis. Inactivating mutations of Wnt co-receptor LRP-5 cause osteoporosis. Activating mutations of LRP 5/6 that do not bind Dkk-1 cause high bone mass. Dkk-1 binds LRP-5/6, preventing Wnt-Frizzled signal. Wnt/β-catenin signal is essential for osteogenesis. (Adapted from Ott SM. Sclerostin and Wnt signaling: The pathway to bone strength. J Clin Endocrinol Metab 2005;90:6741–6743.)

the needs and risk of the individual patient. Future therapies may also allow improved adherence and compliance and may be associated with fewer side effects or risks and easier routes of administration.

REFERENCES
Annotations by Leslie Dalaza

1. **Bouxsein, ML.** Determinants of skeletal fragility. Best Pract Res Clin Rheumatol 2005;19:897–911.

   This review article discusses the factors involved in declining bone strength. It is known that with older age, there is an increased occurrence of fractures. Thus, the topics of bone mineral density, age-related fractures, and resistance to fractures are reviewed. Also, therapies thought to improve bone strength, such as anticatabolic and anabolic therapies, are explored. In like manner, improved methods to evaluate bone strength in patients are examined.

2. **Weinstein RA.** True strength. J Bone Miner Res 2000;15:621–625.

   It is thought that with increased bone mineral density (BMD), mechanical strength will also increase. However, it was found that in the bone disease osteopetrosis, an increased mineral density correlates with a higher risk of bone fractures. It is hypothesized that in the presence of increased mineral density and skeletal mass, along with one or more of three mutations (incisors-absent, osteopetrosis, and/or toothless), the osteopetrotic rat will have weaker bones. The BMD of the tibial diaphysis, metaphysis, femoral diaphysis, and femoral neck was quantified using peripheral quantitative computed tomography (pQCT). Breaking tests were used to examine tibial and femoral midshafts, as well as strength of the femoral neck. It was found that osteopetrotic mutants showed equal or higher BMD and bone mineral content (BMC) than their normal litter mate (NLM) counterparts— while the mechanical breaking force of the bones was equal or lower. Osteopetrotic mutants were found to have a thin cortex and primary trabecular bone in their long bone shafts. Thus, osteopetrotic rats have increased bone density and decreased bone strength.

3. **Seeman E, Delmas PD.** Bone quality—the material and structural basis of bone strength and fragility. N Engl J Med 2006;354:2250–2261.

4. **Miller PD, Hochberg MC, Wehren LE,** et al. How useful are measures of BMD and bone turnover? Curr Med Res Opin 2005;21:545–553.

    Bone mineral density (BMD) and bone turnover are the current biochemical markers used to analyze preclinical and clinical studies of osteoporosis. BMD is thought to contribute to the majority of bone strength, and as a result is the current predictor for osteoporosis and fracture risk. However, both markers have caused confusion in the research world. Still, BMD and bone turnover are the best alternative biochemical markers as of yet.

5. **Miller PD.** Bone density and markers of bone turnover in predicting fracture risk and how changes in these measures predict fracture risk reduction. Curr Osteoporos Rep 2005;3:103–110.

    Bone mineral density (BMD) and bone turnover markers (BTMs) allow clinicians to assess their patients with osteoporosis. Typically, increases in BMD and/or reductions in BTMs correlate with decreased risk of vertebral and nonvertebral fractures. Knowing changes in BMD is particularly useful in allowing for early feedback to patients. Also, improvement in bone strength can be correlated to increased BMD after 12 or 24 months of therapy. Thus, BMD and BTM markers are both useful in managing patients' osteoporosis.

6. **Delmas PD, Adami S, Strugala C,** et al. Intravenous ibandronate injections in postmenopausal women with osteoporosis: One-year results from the dosing intravenous administration study. Arthritis Rheum 2006;54:1838–1846.

    Oral bisphosphonates are the usual treatments for postmenopausal women with osteoporosis. However, due to ineffectiveness of oral bisphosphonates, intravenous bisphosphonate (such as ibandronate) was studied as a possible suitable alternative. Thus, this study identified the best intravenous dosages for ibandronate in women affected with osteoporosis following menopause. A group of 1,395 women (between 55 and 80 years old) affected by osteoporosis [lumbar spine (L2-L4) bone mineral density (BMD) at a T-score < -2.5] and postmenopausal by at least 5 years comprised the population studied. Intravenous injections of ibandronate (2 mg every 2 months and 3 mg every 3 months) were compared. Also, 2.5 mg of oral ibandronate was given daily because it has already been proved to be effective in preventing fractures. After 1 year, the change of BMD of the lumbar spine was noted. Also, the hip BMD and level of C-telopeptide of type I collagen (CTx) were measured after 1 year. The intravenous regimens were found to be more effective ($p < 0.001$) than the oral form of ibandronate. After 1 year, the lumbar spine BMD increased by the following percentages: The 353 patients who received 2 mg of ibandronate every 2 months increased their mean lumbar spine BMD by 5.1%; the 365 patients who received 3 mg of ibandronate every 3 months increased their mean lumbar spine BMD by 4.8%; and the 377 patients who received a daily dose of 2.5 mg of oral ibandronate increased their mean lumbar spine BMD by 3.8%. Similar results were found with hip BMD; intravenous ibandronate proved more effective than oral ibandronate. Decreases in serum CTx level were noted. The intravenous ibandronate did not deleteriously affect renal function. Intravenous dosages of ibandronate (2 mg every 2 months or 3 mg every 3 months) were found as effective as the daily 2.5-mg oral dosage of ibandronate. Thus, all three regimens were effective in preventing fractures in women with postmenopausal osteoporosis.

7. **Reid IR, Brown JP, Burckhardt P,** et al. Intravenous zoledronic acid in postmenopausal women with low bone mineral density. N Engl J Med 2002;346:653–661.

    Bisphosphonates are the medicines of choice for osteoporosis. Their administration requires an empty stomach; it was found that this could reduce compliance in patients. Also, there are limits to maximal dosing due to the ability of the gastrointestinal tract to tolerate bisphosphonates. Thus, optimal intravenous dosages of bisphosphonates are being explored. A 1-year, randomized, double-blind, placebo-controlled experiment examined a group of 351 postmenopausal women with low bone mineral density (BMD). They were treated with five regimens of zoledronic acid (a bisphosphonate), and its effects on bone turnover and density in the lumbar spine were noted. The women either received placebo or intravenous zoledronic acid every 3 months, in doses of 0.25 mg, 0.5 mg, or 1 mg. Also, one group received a year dosage of 4 mg taken once, and another group received two dosages of intravenous zoledronic acid at 2 mg at a 6-month interval. BMD of zoledronic acid–treated patients increased for the lumbar spine (4.3%–5.1% higher than placebo, $p <$ 0.001) and the femoral neck (3.1%–3.5% higher than placebo, $p < 0.001$). Although the side effects included myalgia and pyrexia, the rates of patient dropout between those treated with zoledronic acid and placebo were found to be similar. Zoledronic acid was as effective as oral dosing of bisphosphonates for bone turnover and increasing bone density. Thus, it is suggested that annual infusion of zoledronic acid may prevent fractures in postmenopausal women with osteoporosis.

8. **Ronkin S, Northington R, Baracat E,** et al. Endometrial effects of bazedoxifene acetate, a novel selective estrogen receptor modulator, in postmenopausal women. Obstet Gynecol 2005;105:1397–1404.

   Healthy postmenopausal women were treated with bazedoxifene in order to see the drug's effect on the endometrium. A group of 497 postmenopausal women took part in a two-part, 6-month, double-blind, randomized study including placebos. In this study, the women were given 2.5, 5.0, 10, 20, 30, or 40 mg/day of bazedoxifene; 0.625 mg estrogen and 2.5 mg medroxyprogesterone acetate served as the control. The women kept daily diaries of any occurrence of amenorrhea, and at baseline and at 6 months, their endometrial thickness was assessed using transvaginal ultrasonography. Women who received 2.5 to 20 mg/day of bazedoxifene had no difference in endometrial thickness from baseline, as compared with those who took placebo. However, in the women who took 30 and 40 mg bazedoxifene the change of endometrial thickness from baseline was smaller than that of the placebo-treated women. None of the women exhibited endometrial hyperplasia. It was found that both groups experienced amenorrhea: The women who took 2.5 to 20 mg bazedoxifene had amenorrhea rates of 57% to 74%, whereas 90% of those women who took 30 and 40 mg bazedoxifene stopped menstruating by 6 months. It was found that 30 and 40 mg/day of bazedoxifene resulted in decreased thickness of the endometrium and increased amenorrhea, as compared with the placebo. Thus, bazedoxifene is thought to have endometrial antagonistic effects.

9. **Ke HZ, Qi H, Chidsey-Frink KL,** et al. Lasofoxifene (CP-336,156) protects against the age-related changes in bone mass, bone strength, and total serum cholesterol in intact aged male rats. J Bone Miner Res 2001;16:765–773.

   Lasofoxifene (LAS), a selective estrogen receptor modulator (SERM), was studied in male rats for its effects on bone mass and strength. Male Sprague-Dawley rats were used in this study, and 15 of them were necropsied as controls. Between the two groups, it was found that there was no change in body weight and prostate weight. For a period of 6 months, the male rats were given either 0.01 mg/kg/day ($n = 12$) or 0.1 mg/kg/day ($n = 11$) of LAS and compared with the controls. It was found that the controls increased in their fat body mass and decreased in their lean body mass. The LAS rats decreased in fat body weight and mass, and decreased in cholesterol, whereas their lean body mass remained unchanged. It was shown that LAS in these rats prevented an increase in serum osteocalcin and also prevented a decrease in total bone density and cortical thickness of the distal femoral metaphysis. In fact, there was a decrease in traveler bone volume (−46%). LAS was found to increase the prevention of decreased strength (−47%) and stiffness of the fifth lumbar vertebral body. In conclusion, LAS has been proven effective in preventing age-related changes in bone mass, structure, and turnover—as well as inhibiting bone resorption. Thus, this study supports the use of LAS in elderly men.

10. **Gennari L.** Lasofoxifene: A new type of selective estrogen receptor modulator for the treatment of osteoporosis. Drugs Today (Barc) 2006;42:355–367.

    For conditions such as aging and hormone-induced tumors, selective estrogen receptor modulators (SERMs) are used as estrogen antagonists and/or agonists. For instance, tamoxifen and toremifene are medications used in treating breast cancer; in addition, they are found to be good for bone mineral density. Also, raloxifene is used to prevent and treat postmenopausal osteoporosis and fractures. However, SERMs do not come without side effects. Because some SERMs are found to cause thromboembolic disorders and very rarely uterine cancer, there is widespread concern over their long-term use. The best alternative to be found was lasofoxifene (CP 336, 156) (LAS), for it is similar to estradiol and is found to have improved bioavailability. In phase II studies, it was proven that LAS at the minimal dosage of 0.25 mg/day was effective in preventing bone loss and decreasing cholesterol. Now, LAS is in phase III of development, so as to treat postmenopausal women with osteoporosis.

11. **Howell A.** Future use of selective estrogen receptor modulators and aromatase inhibitors. Clin Cancer Res 2001;7:4402–4412.

Depending on the cellular or tissue environment, selective estrogen receptor modulators (SERMs) act as estrogen agonists or antagonists. The first group of SERMs comprises triphenylethylene SERMs. They include tamoxifen, toremifene, and GW5638. With isomerization of triphenylethylene SERMs, fixed-ring SERMs such as benzothiophene arzoxiphene (LY353381), which is in phase III trials, are produced. Also, there are SERMs based on the estradiol molecule. They include ICI 182, 780, and SR16234, which has just begun trials. There are two types of aromatase inhibitors: those that inactivate aromatase (i.e., androstenedione and exemestane) and those that inhibit the prosthetic heme of the aromatase (i.e., triazole aromatase inhibitors). Of course, many combinations of these drugs exist and could be used to treat a patient. The decision rests on what works to prevent the progression of disease.

12. **Goldstein SR, Siddhanti S, Ciaccia AV, Plouffe L Jr.** A pharmacological review of selective oestrogen receptor modulators. Hum Reprod Update 2000;6:212–224.

Selective estrogen receptor modulators (SERMs) are nonsteroidal estrogen agonists or antagonists, depending on the tissue environment. They are molecules of interest for treatment of postmenopausal osteoporosis, hormone-dependent cancers, and cardiovascular disease. The first type of SERMs are triphenylethelenes. They include clomiphene (which increases ovulation), tamoxifen (which increases bone mineral density), and toremifen. Both tamoxifen and toremifen are used to treat breast cancer and do stimulate the endometrium. The second group of SERMs consists of benzothiophene, and that includes raloxifene, which treats postmenopausal women and decreases the instance of vertebral fractures. A major problem of SERMs is their ability to increase the risk of venous thromboembolism. Thus, many other selective estrogen receptor modulators are in clinical development.

13. **McClung MR, Siris E, Cummings SR,** et al. Prevention of bone loss in postmenopausal women treated with lasofoxifene compared with raloxifene. Menopause 2006;13:377–386.

In this 2-year randomized, double-blind study, the effectiveness of lasofoxifene and raloxifene in preserving bone mass and preventing osteoporosis in postmenopausal women was evaluated. A group of 410 postmenopausal women ranging from the ages of 47 to 74 received one of four different treatments: 0.25 mg/day of lasofoxifene, 1.0 mg/day of lasofoxifene, 6.0 mg/day of raloxifene, or placebo. The baseline bone mineral density of the lumbar spine and hip was noted. It was found that the bone mineral density of the lumbar spine increased ($p \leq 0.01$) as follows: 3.6% for 0.25 mg lasofoxifene, 3.9% for 1.0 mg lasofoxifene, and 1.7% for 6.0 mg per day of raloxifene. It was found that in all treatments, there was decreased bone turnover as compared with the placebo ($p \leq 0.05$). After 2 years, it was found that the treatments decreased low-density lipoprotein cholesterol ($p \leq 0.05$) by the following amounts: 20.6% for 0.25 mg/day of lasofoxifene, 19.7% for 1.0 mg/day of lasofoxifene, 12.1% for 6.0 mg/day ralofoxifene, and 3.2% for placebo. Thus, all trends point to lasofoxifene as the best treatment for osteoporosis in postmenopausal women.

14. **McClung MR, Lewiecki EM, Cohen SB,** et al., for the AMG 162 Bone Loss Study Group. Denosumab in postmenopausal women with low bone mineral density. N Engl J Med 2006;354:821–831.

In this study, the effects of the human antibody denosumab, known to inhibit RANKL (receptor activator of nuclear factor-kappaB ligand), were tested in 412 postmenopausal women with low bone mineral density (BMD) (T-score, −1.8 to −4.0 at lumbar spine, −1.8 to −3.5 at proximal femur). The treatment regimens were as follows: 14 mg, 60 mg, 100 mg, or 210 mg of denosumab every 3 months; 70 mg of oral alendronate weekly; or placebo. Also, the baseline levels of serum alkaline phosphatase and urine telopeptides were noted, for bone turnover comparison. It was found that the BMD of the lumbar spine increased by 3.0% to 6.7% in all levels of denosumab, and the hip BMD increased by 1.9% to 3.6% in all levels of denosumab. Likewise, the lumbar spine BMD increased by 4.6% and the hip BMD by 2.1% with 70 mg of oral alendronate. Both hip and lumbar spine BMD decreased by 0.6% with placebo. However, the radius BMD increased by 0.4% to 1.3% in all levels of denosumab, and decreased by 0.5% for 70 mg alendronate; there was a 2.0% decrease with placebo. Also, serum levels of C-telopeptides decreased. Thus, it was found that denosumab increased BMD and decreased resorption in postmenopausal women with low BMD. Denosumab is thought to be effective for the treatment of osteoporosis.

15. **Greenspan SL, Bone HG, Marriott TB,** et al. Preventing the first vertebral fracture in postmenopausal women with lost bone mass using PTH(1-84): Results from the TOP study. J Bone Miner Res 2005;20:536.

16. **Miles RR, Sulka JP, Halladay DL,** et al. Parathyroid hormone (hPTH 1–38) stimulates the expression of UBP41, an ubiquitin-specific protease, in bone. J Cell Biochem 2002;85:229–242.

Many different genes are thought to mediate the effects of parathyroid hormone (PTH), a hormone that induces bone formation. Differential display reverse transcriptase was used to screen for genes in osteoblasts of the femoral metaphyseal spongiosa of young rats. After an injection of 8 μg/100 g of human PTH (hPTH) (1–38) into the rats, a cDNA was cloned of a 348-amino-acid protein, and sequence analysis was performed. It was found that this protein coded for ubiquitin protease UBP41 (expressed in osteoblast UMR106, ROS17/2.8, and BALC), and was 98% homologous to the mouse UBP41, 93.7% homologous to the human UBP41, and 82.5% homologous to that of chickens. A Northern blot showed that after 1 hour of exposure to hPTH, a 3.8–4 kb of UBP41 increased: six- to eightfold in the metaphyseal region and threefold in the diaphyseal region. After 24 hours, however, the levels of UBP41 messenger ribonucleic acid (mRNA) expression returned to control levels. It was found that at continuous exposure to hPTH (1-38), there was a sustained elevation of PTH (131), which stimulated cyclic adenosine monophosphate (cAMP) and parathyroid hormone–related protein (PTHrP), thus resulting in UBP41 mRNA expression. In addition, it was found that with injection of prostaglandin E_2 (PGE2), expression of UBP41 mRNA increased as well, but returned to control levels within 6 to 24 hours. Overall, it was found that in PTH-treated primary osteoblasts and UMR106 cells, UPB41 mRNA expression increased 3.6- to 13-fold. When UMR106 cells were treated with PGE2, forskolin, and dibutryl cyclic adenosine monophosphate (cAMP), UBP41 mRNA expression increased 4-, 4.5-, and 2.4-fold, respectively. Such UPB41 mRNA expression was found in the brain, kidney, skeletal muscle, testis, and liver. Thus, it is thought that UBP41 upregulates osteotropic agents through the PKA/cAMP pathway.

17. **Condon SN, Darnbrough S, Burns CJ,** et al. Analogues of human parathyroid hormone (1-31)NH(2): Further evaluation of the effect of conformational constraint on biological activity. Bioorg Med Chem. 2002;10:731–736.

Analogs were constructed of human parathyroid hormone (hPTH) based on cyclo(Lys(18)-Asp(22))[Ala(1),Nle(8), Lys(18),Asp(22),Leu(27)]hPTH(1-31)NH(2) (2, EC(50) = 0.29 nM. It was found that by truncation by 2 at the N- or C-terminal end, agonist activity decreased, as measured by the adenylate cyclase activity in the ROS17/2.8 cell line. Scanning of alanine and glycine in the N-terminus of 2 was consistent with data obtained on linear hPTH (1-34). The primary sequence of hPTH (1-31)NH(2) was evaluated by placement of [i, i+4] lactam. Ring size and orientation at the 18 and 22 positions of lactam were studied as well.

18. **Chen SC, Eiting K, Cui K,** et al. Therapeutic utility of a novel tight junction modulating peptide for enhancing intranasal drug delivery. J Pharm Sci 2006;95:1364–1371.

In previous studies, it was found that tight junction modulating (TJM) peptides decreased transepithelial electrical resistance (TER) in *in vitro* nasal epithelial tissue. Now TJM peptides are being evaluated for use in transepithelial drug formations. It has been found that at neutral to acidic pH and at or below room temperature, TJM peptide is stable. With this knowledge, there is potential for TJM peptides to enhance low molecular weight drugs such as acetylcholinesterase inhibitors, salmon calcitonin, parathyroid hormone (1-34) [PTH (1-34)], and PYY (3-36). It was found that TJM peptides improved drug permeation across epithelial tissue. Also, the combination of PYY (3-36) and TJM peptide in rabbits resulted in increased bioavailability. Thus the TJM peptide can advance the development of intranasal formulations.

19. **Kronenberg H.** PTHrP and skeletal development. Ann N Y Acad Sci 2006;1068: 1–13.

Endochondral bone development necessitates parathyroid hormone–related protein (PTHrP), which is synthesized by perichondrial cells and chondrocytes. Chondrocytes have PTH/PTHrP receptors, which increase proliferation and delay differentiation. It is thought that PTHrP stimulates the G_s (which stimulates proliferation of chondrocytes, suppresses p57, phosphorylates transcription factor SOX9, and suppresses mRNA synthesis of RunX2) and G_q (which opposes proliferation) family of heterotrimeric proteins. Indian hedgehog (Ihh) is needed for synthesis of PTHrP and is synthesized when the chondrocytes stop proliferating. Thus, PTHrP regulates growth and differentiation of chondrocytes.

20. **Meunier PJ, Slosman DO, Delmas PD,** et al. Strontium ranelate: Dose-dependent effects in established postmenopausal vertebral osteoporosis—a 2-year randomized placebo controlled trial. J Clin Endocrinol Metab 2002;87:2060–2066.

Strontium ranelate (SR) was studied for its effectiveness and safety in treating postmenopausal osteoporosis. In a randomized, multicenter, double-blind, placebo-controlled experiment, 353 osteoporotic women ($T < 2.4$) who had at least 1 fracture were given different dosages of SR for 2 years. The dosages are as follows: 0.5 g, 1 g, and 2 g SR per day. Also, some women were given placebo. To assess SR's effects, lumbar bone mineral density (BMD), femoral BMD, new vertebral deformities, and bone turnover were noted. It was found that after 2 years, lumbar BMD increased by 1.4% in women who received 0.5 g SR per day and 3.0% for women who received 2 g SR per day, as compared with placebo ($p < 0.01$). Also, women who took 2 g SR per day had decreased vertebral deformities (0.56 relative risk; 95% CI) and increased bone alkaline phosphatase. These same women had decreased cross-linked N-telopeptides, as compared with women who received placebo. In conclusion, it was found that 2 g SR per day was the best dosage for effectiveness and safety; it increased vertebral BMD and decreased incidences of fractures.

21. **Delmas PD.** Clinical effects of strontium ranelate in women with postmenopausal osteoporosis. Osteoporos Int 2005;16 (Suppl 1):S16–19.

Treatments for osteoporosis are needed in order to better the quality of life of those with this disease. In this article, two separate trials investigated the safety and effectiveness of strontium ranelate (SR). The first trial, Spinal Osteoporosis Therapeutic Intervention (SOTI), produced results, whereas in the second trial, Treatment of Peripheral Osteoporosis Study (TROPOS), results are still pending. By including more than 6,700 postmenopausal women, it was found that after 3 years of analysis in SOTI, SR decreased new vertebral and clinical fractures as follows: at 1 year (RR 0.48, $p = 0.003$; RR = 0.51, $p < 0.001$) and at 3 years (RR = 0.62, $p < 0.001$; RR = 0.59, $p < 0.001$). In conclusion, it was found that SR decreased back pain and height loss (as compared with the placebo group) and was well tolerated in the gastrointestinal tract. Thus, SR is a significant medication in treating postmenopausal women with osteoporosis.

22. **Deaton DN, Tavares FX.** Design of cathepsin K inhibitors for osteoporosis. Curr Top Med Chem 2005;5:1639–1675.

This review article discusses the therapeutic approaches to treating osteoporosis. The treatment of choice discussed is that of the cathepsin K inhibitors, which are expressed in the osteoclasts and are important factors in degrading bone. Glaxo Wellcome researchers have been trying to develop improved molecular inhibitors, which include cyanamides, ketoheterocycles, and ketoamides. Exploration of S(3), S(2), S(1), and S(1') subsites with P(3), P(2), P(1), and P(1') probes suggests that ketoamide-based inhibitors given orally are the best in bioavailability.

23. **Martin TJ, Quinn JM, Gillespie MT,** et al. Mechanisms involved in skeletal anabolic therapies. Ann N Y Acad Sci 2006;1068:458–470.

Parathyroid hormone (PTH) is involved in anabolic activity for bone, when administered intermittently. However, if the levels of PTH are maintained, osteoclast formation occurs and bone resorption results. PTH-related protein (PTHrP) is thought to be a possible regulator of bone formation. In conjunction with bisphosphonates, it is thought that PTHrP stops the anabolic response to PTH and promotes the differentiation of osteoblast precursors. Perhaps there exists a coupling factor like receptor activator of nuclear factor-kappaB ligand (RANKL). It is found that a mutation in the LRP5 gene results in inheritance of a bone mass syndrome. However, inactivating mutations of LRP5 result in bone loss. Studies are in progress to explore the Wnt/frizzled/beta-catenin pathway in experimental models.

24. **Ott SM.** Sclerostin and Wnt signaling—the pathway to bone strength. J Clin Endocrinol Metab 2005;90:6741–6743.

25. **Ritz E.** Calcimimetics: Fooling the PTH receptor. Pediatr Nephrol 2005;20:15–18. Epub Oct 27, 2004.

The calcium sensory receptors from bovine parathyroid cells were studied, for increasing (calcimimetics) or decreasing (calciolytics) sensitivity to calcium—therefore, suppressing or stimulating parathyroid hormone (PTH) respectively. In primary and secondary hyperparathyroidism, calcimimetics decreased levels of PTH. And an advantage in secondary hyperparathyroidism is the lowering of calcium serum and phosphate concentration.

26. **Sawakami K, Robling AG, Ai M,** et al. The WNT co-receptor LRP5 is essential for skeletal mechanotransduction, but not for the anabolic bone response to parathyroid hormone treatment. J Biol Chem 2006;628:23698–23711; Epub June 20, 2006.

Low-density lipoprotein receptor-related protein 5 (LRP5) is a key regulator in bone mass. The introduction of loss-of-function mutations is known to result in the autosomal recessive osteoporosis-pseudoglioma disorder. This syndrome is characterized by decreased bone strength and mass. A study was performed on mice with loss-of-function mutations in the LRP5 gene, to understand the osteogenic response. It was found that in Lrp5-null (Lrp5 (−)/(−)) mice, there was a decrease in bone mineral density and bone strength, reduced mechanical loading by 88% to 99%, and inability of osteoblasts to produce osteopontin after mechanical stimulus. To further investigate these findings, 40 μg/kg/day of PTH was infused in Lrp5 (−)/(−) and Lrp5 (+)/(+) mice. Thus, it was found the Lrp5 was necessary for mechanotransduction in osteoblasts. Further, PTH may be an effective mode of treatment for increasing bone mass.

27. **Stearns V.** Raloxifene and tamoxifene had similar efficacy for preventing invasive breast cancer in women at increased risk. Evid Based Med 2006;11:177–178.

28. **Boyle WJ, Simonet WS, Lacey DL.** Osteoclast differentiation and activation. Nature 2003;423:337–342.

29. **Blake G, Fogelman I.** Long-term effect of strontium ranelate treatment on BMD. J Bone Miner Res 2005;20:1901.

30. **Block GA, Martin KJ, de Francisco AL,** et al. Cinacalcet for secondary hyperparathyroidism in patients receiving hemodialysis. N Engl J Med 2004;350: 1516–1525.

Dialysis patients with secondary hyperparathyroidism are usually treated with vitamin D and calcium. However, it is noted that hypercalcemia and hyperphosphatemia may occur, resulting in cardiovascular disease. To combat the effects of this, calcimimetics, such as cinacalcet hydrochloride, are being tested in two identical randomized, double-blind, placebo-controlled trials to target the calcium sensing receptors. Thus, for 26 weeks, hemodialysis patients with uncontrolled secondary hyperparathyroidism were treated either with cinacalcet (371 patients) or placebo (370 patients). Daily doses of 30 to 180 mg of cinacalcet were given to achieve parathyroid hormone (PTH) levels of 250 pg/mL or less, and the primary end point was defined as those stable at this level for 14 weeks. It was found that 43% of the patients taking cinacalcet reached the primary end point as compared with 5% ($p < 0.001$) of patients taking placebo. Also, the mean PTH level for patients taking cinacalcet decreased by 43% and increased by 9% ($p < 0.001$) for patients taking placebo. In addition, the serum levels of calcium and phosphorus decreased by 15% in patients taking cinacalcet, while the serum levels remained stable ($p < 0.001$) for patients taking placebo. In conclusion, cincacalcet is effective in decreasing levels of PTH and improving calcium and phosphorus homeostasis in dialysis patients with secondary hyperparathyroidism.

31. **Canalis E.** Novel treatments for osteoporosis. J Clin Invest 2000;106:177–179.

32. **Grey A, Reid IR.** Emerging and potential therapies for osteoporosis. Expert Opin Investig Drugs 2005;14:265–278.

Osteoporosis is a public health problem that is currently consuming society's resources; however, prevention of fractures is limited in scope and efficiency. Studies today are developing and refining therapies for osteoporosis. For instance, there are drugs that inhibit osteoclastic bone resorption, estrogenic compounds, bisphosphonates, and RANKL (receptor activator of nuclear factor-kappaB ligand), among many others. Also, parathyroid hormone (PTH) therapy (including its analogues) seems promising in preventing fractures in patients with osteoporosis.

12

Clinical Cases

Pauline M. Camacho and Paul D. Miller

CASE 1

History
A 61-year-old white woman had a dual-energy x-ray absorptiometry (DXA) scan ordered by her primary-care physician. Other than mild essential hypertension, she had no other known medical problems. She fractured her wrist after a fall 3 years earlier. She had lost 2 inches in height since her 30s. After the DXA results were given to her, she started taking Viactiv calcium chews 3 times a day. Her mother may have suffered from osteoporosis. She denied a history of kidney stones, smoking, or excessive alcohol intake.

Physical Examination
A grade 2 thoracic kyphosis was detected. The rest of the examination was unremarkable.

DXA Images

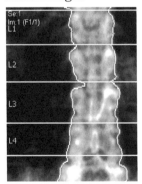 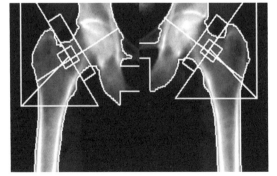

Region	BMD (g/cm²)	Young-Adult T-Score	Age-Matched Z-Score
L1	0.767	-3.0	-1.5
L2	0.767	-3.6	-2.0
L3	0.874	-2.7	-1.1
L4	0.821	-3.2	-1.6
L1-L2	0.767	-3.3	-1.8
L1-L3	0.807	-3.0	-1.5
L1-L4	0.811	-3.1	-1.5
L2-L3	0.825	-3.1	-1.6
L2-L4	0.823	-3.1	-1.6
L3-L4	0.848	-2.9	1.4

Region	BMD (g/cm²)	Young-Adult T-Score	Age-Matched Z-Score
Neck			
Left	0.619	-3.5	-1.8
Right	0.647	-3.3	-1.6
Mean	0.633	-3.4	-1.7
Difference	0.027	0.2	0.2

Laboratory Findings

Hemoglobin (12–15 mg/dL)	13 mg/dL
Serum creatinine (0.7–1.5 mg/dL)	0.8 mg/dL
ALT (7–35 IU/Ll)	23 IU/Ll
25-OHD (target >30 ng/mL)	24 ng/mL
Intact PTH (10–65 pg/mL)	72 pg/mL
Ionized calcium (1.10–1.30 mmol/L)	1.15 mmol/L
Total serum calcium (8.9–10.3 mg/dL)	9.0 mg/dL
Phosphorus	3.8 mg/dL
24-hour urine calcium (100–300 mg/24 h)	135 mg/24 h
Bone-specific alkaline phosphatase	21 μg/L
Premenopausal female: 4.5–16.9 μg/L	
Postmenopausal female: 7.0–22.4 μg/L	
Male 25 years and older: 6.5–20.1 μg/L	

ALT, alanine aminotransferase; PTH, parathyroid hormone.

Teaching Points

Dr. Camacho

- Patients frequently underestimate the significance of low trauma fractures. It is important to stress that fractures that result from a fall from a standing position are technically "fragility or osteoporotic fractures."
- This patient's DXA image shows that she is osteoporotic by World Health Organization (WHO) criteria. Lumbar spine T-score is -3.1, and femoral neck T-score is -3.5. However, looking closely at the Z-scores, they fall between -1.6 and -2.0.

This implies that the patient is close to two standard deviations below other women her age in terms of bone density, highly suggesting premature bone loss.

- A careful work-up for secondary causes of osteoporosis was warranted and subsequently revealed vitamin D deficiency and secondary hyperparathyroidism. Urinary calcium excretion is in the low-normal range.
- Vitamin D deficiency should be treated, in this case with vitamin D 50,000 IU once a week for 3 months, subsequently reduced to 50,000 IU once a month. Various treatment regimens are discussed in Chapter 7.
- Although vitamin D deficiency is frequently a result of poor nutritional intake and inadequate sun exposure in the elderly, the patient should be questioned about symptoms of malabsorption and a family history of celiac sprue. If clinically suggested, celiac antibodies must be obtained.
- It has not yet been studied whether an antiresorptive agent should be given to such patients with vitamin D deficiency as part of the initial therapy. Although rare, there are reports of hypocalcemia induced by bisphosphonates in this population. This patient's vitamin D levels were corrected to a current goal of greater than 30 ng/mL. One year after correction of her PTH levels to normal range, an antiresorptive agent was started.

CASE 2

History

A 49-year-old white woman was referred to the clinic because of her recent DXA results. Menopause was at age 40, and the patient was on estrogen replacement therapy (ERT) upon presentation to the clinic. She had taken alendronate for 3 months and Caltrate-D (elemental calcium 1,200 mg/day plus 800 IU vitamin D). Her sister, who is 2 years older, and her mother had osteoporotic fractures. She has not suffered from any fractures, but did report one episode of kidney stones 3 years earlier. She is a smoker (one half a pack per day). There was hyperthyroidism many years ago, but she is euthyroid on her current thyroid hormone replacement.

Physical Examination

Physical examination was significant only for a nonpalpable thyroid.

DXA Images

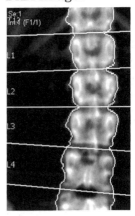
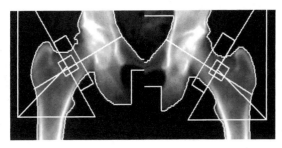

Region	BMD (g/cm²)	Young-Adult T-Score	Age-Matched Z-Score
L1	0.790	-2.8	-1.9
L2	0.903	-2.5	-1.5
L3	0.870	-2.7	-1.8
L4	0.799	-3.3	-2.4
L2-L4	0.852	-2.9	-1.9
Region	BMD (g/cm²)	Young-Adult T-Score	Age-Matched Z-Score
Neck			
Left	0.642	-2.8	-1.8
Right	0.607	-3.1	-2.1
Mean	0.625	-3.0	-2.0
Difference	0.034	0.3	0.3

Laboratory Findings

Hemoglobin (12–15 mg/dL)	13 mg/dL
Serum creatinine (0.7–1.5 mg/dL)	0.9 mg/dL
ALT (7–35 IU/L)	30 IU/L
25-OHD (target >30 ng/mL)	35 ng/mL
Intact PTH (10–65 pg/mL)	54 pg/mL
Ionized calcium (1.10–1.30 mmol/L)	1.15 mmol/L
Total serum calcium (8.9–10.3 mg/dL)	9.0 mg/dL
Phosphorus	3.6 mg/dL
24-hour urine calcium (100–300 mg/24 h)	435 mg/24 h
Bone-specific alkaline phosphatase	20 μg/L
Premenopausal female: 4.5–16.9 μg/L	
Postmenopausal female: 7.0–22.4 μg/L	
Male 25 years and older: 6.5–20.1 μg/L	
24-hour urine NTx/creatinine	18 nM/mM creatinine
Normal adult female	
Premenopausal: 17–94 nM BCE/mM creatinine	
Postmenopausal: 26–124 nM BCE/mM creatinine	
Normal adult male: 21–83 nM BCE/mM creatinine	
TSH (0.2–5 UU/L)	2.18 UU/L

ALT, alanine aminotransferase; PTH, parathyroid hormone; NTx, N-telopeptide; BCE, bone collagen equivalents; TSH, thyroid-stimulating hormone.

Teaching Points

Dr. Camacho

- The patient has osteoporosis based on WHO criteria.
- Similar to Case 1, this patient has low Z-scores and appears to have an inappropriate degree of bone loss for her age.
- Her metabolic bone work-up showed idiopathic hypercalciuria. Normal urinary calcium excretion is 1.5 to 3 mg/kg/24 hours or 100–300 mg/24 hours. Her vitamin D and parathyroid hormone (PTH) levels are normal, and there is no evidence of excessive intake of calcium. This is likely the reason why she has osteoporosis at a relatively young age. There is a familial tendency for this disease, and her sister and mother should be evaluated as well.
- Patients with idiopathic hypercalciuria respond very well to hydrochlorothiazide (HCTZ). She was started on 25 mg every day, and after 3 months her repeat urinary calcium had normalized at 280 mg/24 hours. Alendronate therapy was continued.
- Although HCTZ will correct the secondary cause, there is no strong evidence that this medication alone reduces fractures among patients with idiopathic hypercalciuria. Thus, bisphosphonate therapy should be used for these individuals together with the HCTZ.
- Urinary N-telopeptide (NTx) is suppressed to premenopausal range because of her prior intake of alendronate.

CASE 3

History
A 50-year-old woman was sent for osteoporosis management. She has no history of fractures or height loss. Menopause was at age 47. The patient is still suffering from menopausal symptoms, including hot flashes and vaginal dryness. She is in good general health, maintains an active lifestyle, and does not smoke. She drinks 2 glasses of skim milk per day and eats a few ounces of cheese.

Physical Examination
Physical examination was unremarkable.

DXA Images

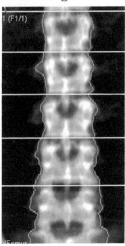
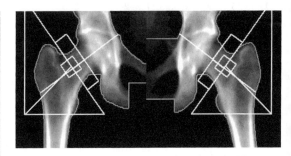

Region	BMD (g/cm²)	Young-Adult T-Score	Age-Matched Z-Score
L1	0.998	-1.1	-0.8
L2	1.017	-1.5	-1.2
L3	1.053	-1.2	-0.9
L4	1.066	-1.1	-0.8
L2-L4	1.048	-1.3	-0.9

Region	BMD (g/cm²)	Young-Adult T-Score	Age-Matched Z-Score
Neck			
Left	0.790	-2.1	-1.3
Right	0.862	-1.5	-0.7
Mean	0.826	-1.8	-1.0
Difference	0.072	0.6	0.6

Laboratory Findings

Hemoglobin (12–15 mg/dL)	13.5 mg/dL
Serum creatinine (0.7–1.5 mg/dL)	0.9 mg/dL
ALT (7–35 IU/L)	30 IU/L
25-OHD (target >30 ng/mL)	35 ng/mL
Intact PTH (10–65 pg/mL)	54 pg/mL
Ionized calcium (1.10–1.30 mmol/L)	1.15 mmol/L
Total serum calcium (8.9–10.3 mg/dL)	9.0 mg/dL
Phosphorus	3.6 mg/dL
24-hour urine calcium (100–300 mg/24 h)	165 mg/24 h
Bone-specific alkaline phosphatase	20 μg/L
Premenopausal female: 4.5–16.9 μg/L	
Postmenopausal female: 7.0–22.4 μg/L	
Male 25 years and older: 6.5–20.1 μg/L	
TSH (0.2–5 UU/L)	2.18 UU/L

ALT, alanine aminotransferase; PTH, parathyroid hormone; TSH, thyroid-stimulating hormone.

Teaching Points
Dr Miller

- This patient has osteopenia by WHO criteria, but the femoral neck T-score of -2.1 does not necessarily mean she has previously lost bone mass. This could easily be her peak adult bone mass acquired at the age of 20 years.
- The normal laboratory values have excluded most of the secondary conditions that may cause a loss of bone mineral density (BMD)—and two more should be added: a transglutaminase IgA antibody screening for asymptomatic celiac disease and a serum or urinary bone resorption marker [C-telopeptide (CTx) or NTx].
- Her absolute fracture risk is low. According to the soon-to-be-published WHO study, which validated 10-year absolute risk for all fractures in an untreated postmenopausal woman, her 10-year risk is less than 10%—not a high enough risk to justify any treatment beyond calcium, vitamin D, and exercise.
- She has menopausal symptoms, and national recommendations would be to use the lowest dose hormonal therapy that can control her menopausal symptoms and vaginal dryness; and at the same time would probably protect her skeleton from postmenopausal bone loss, which should be reassessed in 2 years by a repeat determination of BMD.
- If her NTx were elevated, and elevated bone resorption was not due to any other cause of high bone resorption, then a resorption marker could be rechecked within 3 months of initiating HT to see if it has declined at least 40% from baseline as an early feedback of efficacy and proper dose.

CASE 4

History

A 78-year-old white woman was referred for second opinion to the Bone Clinic. She was first diagnosed to have osteoporosis through a DXA scan in 1997. She was started on alendronate then. Calcitonin nasal spray was added after a few years, and she continued to take this for four years. She takes Tums (500 mg nonelemental calcium carbonate/pill) three times a day. Fracture history included foot fractures in 1994 and thoracic compression fractures in 2000, 2003, and 2004. She underwent vertebroplasty in 2003 and again in 2004. Menopause was at age 33, and she denied use of ERT. So far, she had lost 4 inches in height. She lives with chronic severe back pain. She had gastric ulcers in 1967 and a perforated ulcer in 1989. She admitted to occasional loose stools. Her sister is currently being treated with teriparatide and also has had two vertebroplasties.

Physical Examination

Physical examination showed an elderly, frail-looking woman. She has a grade 4 thoracic kyphosis. She walks without assist, but has a tentative gait. Noted was a grade 1 systolic ejection murmur at the base. The rest of the examination was unremarkable.

Follow-up

She was advised to increase her elemental calcium intake to 1,200 to 1,500 mg/day and 800 IU of vitamin D. Subsequent urinary calcium excretion increased to 155 mg/24 hours.

Both antiresorptive agents were discontinued, and the patient was started on teriparatide 20-μg sq every day for 2 years. Subsequent DXA showed a 9.4% improvement in lumbar spine BMD and 2% improvement in femoral neck BMD. The patient has not experienced any recurrent fractures.

DXA Images

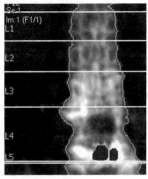
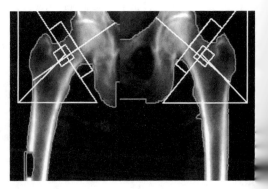

Region	BMD (g/cm²)	Young-Adult T-Score	Age-Matched Z-Score
L1	0.639	-4.1	-1.6
L2	0.796	-3.4	-0.9
L3	1.194	-0.1	2.5
L4	1.135	-0.5	2.0
L1-L2	0.723	-3.7	-1.2
L1-L3	0.919	-2.1	0.4
L1-L4	1.005	-1.5	1.0
L2-L3	1.024	-1.5	1.0
L2-L4	1.077	-1.0	1.5
L3-L4	1.158	-0.3	2.2

Region	BMD (g/cm²)	Young-Adult T-Score	Age-Matched Z-Score
Neck			
Left	0.730	-2.6	0.5
Right	0.633	-3.4	-0.4
Mean	0.682	-3.0	0.1
Difference	0.097	0.8	0.8

Laboratory Findings

Hemoglobin (12–15 mg/dL)	12.8 mg/dL
Serum creatinine (0.7–1.5 mg/dL)	1.3 mg/dL
ALT (7–35 IU/L)	32 IU/L
25-OHD (target >30 ng/mL)	35 ng/mL
Intact PTH (10–65 pg/mL)	62 pg/mL
Ionized calcium (1.10–1.30 mmol/L)	1.28 mmol/L
Total serum calcium (8.9–10.3 mg/dL)	9.0 mg/dL
Phosphorus (2.6–4.4 mg/dL)	3.6 mg/dL
24-hour urine calcium (100–300 mg/24 h)	120 mg/24 h
Bone-specific alkaline phosphatase	20 μg/L
Premenopausal female: 4.5–16.9 μg/L	
Postmenopausal female: 7.0–22.4 μg/L	
Male 25 years and older: 6.5–20.1 μg/L	
24-hour urine NTx/creatinine	8 nM BCE/mM
Normal adult female	
Premenopausal: 17–94 nM BCE/mM creatinine	
Postmenopausal: 26–124 nM BCE/mM creatinine	
Normal adult male: 21–83 nM BCE/mM creatinine	
1-25 OHD (15–75 ng/mL)	60 ng/mL
TSH (0.2–5 UU/L)	1.5 UU/L
SPEP/UPEP	Normal
Anti-endomysial and anti-gliadin Ab	Negative

ALT, alanine aminotransferase; PTH, parathyroid hormone; NTx, N-telopeptide; BCE, bone collagen equivalents; TSH, thyroid-stimulating hormone; SPEP/UPEP, serum/urine protein electrophoresis.

Teaching Points

Dr. Camacho

- The patient indeed has severe osteoporosis, as evidenced by recurrent fractures, significant height loss, and densitometric evidence of low BMD.
- She has multiple risk factors, including a strong family history of osteoporosis, previous fractures, and early menopause.
- Her DXA image revealed significant degenerative changes in L3, and the vertebroplasty in L5, both of which elevate her BMD. These need to be excluded in the analysis of lumbar spine BMD.
- Despite taking two antiresorptive agents for osteoporosis, she continued to have recurrent fractures. Compliance is likely not an issue because her urinary NTx is suppressed. This case speaks for failure of therapy, thus warranting a change in therapy and a thorough work-up for secondary causes of osteoporosis.
- Surprisingly, the patient is not vitamin D–deficient. Her urinary calcium is low to normal, which could be either from renal insufficiency, poor intake of calcium, or poor absorption of her calcium supplements.
- Teriparatide is indicated for persons with severe osteoporosis, patients with multiple compression fractures, and those who fail treatment with bisphosphonates. Given the development of fractures despite adequate suppression of bone resorption and numerous years of antiresorptive therapy, anabolic therapy was tried. The absence of fractures in 2 years is likely proof of fracture reduction from the drug.
- Teriparatide is currently indicated only for 2 years of use. Published studies support the use of antiresorptive agents after discontinuation of anabolic therapy.

CASE 5

History

A 73-year-old woman who was of Polish decent came to the clinic after her primary-care physician told her that she has severe osteoporosis based on her DXA scan. A recent lumbar compression fracture prompted the DXA scan. She developed the compression fracture as well as a wrist fracture after a fall. In addition, she also suffered from a spontaneous pubic bone fracture 4 years prior. She carries the diagnosis of irritable bowel syndrome and is lactose intolerant. Menopause was at age 40, and she denied ever using ERT. She takes Flovent for asthma, but was never on oral glucocorticoids for an extended period of time. She complains of constant pain in her pelvis and hips.

Physical Examination

Physical examination showed a thin, elderly woman with grade 1 thoracic kyphosis. Bone tenderness was elicited upon palpation of both tibias. She has hyperactive reflexes and Chvostek sign. The rest of the examination was unremarkable.

DXA Images

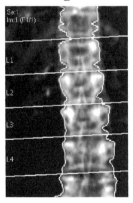
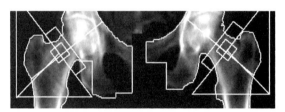

Region	BMD (g/cm²)	Young-Adult T-Score	Age-Matched Z-Score
L1	0.653	-4.0	-1.4
L2	0.747	-3.8	-1.2
L3	0.750	-3.7	-1.1
L4	0.708	-4.1	-1.5
L2-L4	0.732	-3.9	-1.3

Region	BMD (g/cm²)	Young-Adult T-Score	Age-Matched Z-Score
Neck			
Left	0.600	-3.7	-0.8
Right	0.648	-3.3	-0.4
Mean	0.624	-3.5	-0.6
Difference	0.048	0.4	0.4

Laboratory Findings

Hemoglobin (12–15 mg/dL)	11 mg/dL
Serum creatinine (0.7–1.5 mg/dL)	1.3 mg/dL
ALT (7–35 IU/L)	32 IU/L
25-OHD (target >30 ng/mL)	9 ng/mL
Intact PTH (10–65 pg/mL)	125 pg/mL
Ionized calcium (1.10–1.30 mmol/L)	1.10 mmol/L
Total serum calcium (8.9–10.3 mg/dL)	9.2 mg/dL
Phosphorus (2.6–4.4 mg/dL)	3.0 mg/dL
24-hour urine calcium (100–300 mg/24 h)	76 mg/24 h
Bone-specific alkaline phosphatase	63.8 μg/L
Premenopausal female: 4.5–16.9 μg/L	
Postmenopausal female: 7.0–22.4 μg/L	
Male 25 years and older: 6.5–20.1 μg/L	
24-hour urine NTx/creatinine	150 nM BCE/mM
Normal adult female	
Premenopausal: 17–94 nM BCE/mM creatinine	
Postmenopausal: 26–124 nM BCE/mM creatinine	
Normal adult male: 21–83 nM BCE/mM creatinine	
1-25 OHD (15–75 ng/mL)	60 ng/mL
TSH (0.2–5 UU/L)	1.5 UU/L
SPEP/UPEP	Normal
Anti-endomysial and anti-gliadin Ab	Antigliadin Ab-positive

ALT, alanine aminotransferase; PTH, parathyroid hormone; NTx, N-telopeptide; BCE, bone collagen equivalents; TSH, thyroid-stimulating hormone; SPEP/UPEP, serum/urine protein electrophoresis.

Teaching Points

Dr. Miller

- This patient has severe osteoporosis, and her fracture risk is very high, based on prior fragility fractures, and her increased age and low T-score.
- She has a low 25-hydroxyvitamin D level and an elevated parathyroid hormone and normal serum calcium concentration, making this most likely secondary hyperparathyroidism.
- The secondary hyperparathyroidism results from both her low vitamin D level and calcium malabsorption due to the probable presence of celiac disease, which leads to a selective calcium malabsorption (and at times, iron as well).
- Her elevated bone-specific alkaline phosphatase (BSAP) is most likely reflective of osteomalacia, due to severe vitamin D deficiency.

- Although she has a positive celiac antibody test, she still should have a small bowel biopsy because there are false-positive antibody tests and celiac disease is a histological diagnosis—and changes a patient's diet for life.
- She should have her vitamin D level normalized first with high-dose vitamin D before starting pharmacological therapy, which should suppress her BSAP and PTH.
- Once this is accomplished, she could either receive an intravenous bisphosphonate (oral bisphosphonates are not absorbed in the presence of celiac disease) or teriparatide.
- I would choose teriparatide first (once the BSAP is normal) and use for 2 years and then stop and follow with an intravenous bisphosphonate.

CASE 6

History

This patient is a 39-year-old premenopausal woman who had a DXA scan upon her request. She denies a personal or family history of fractures. She is generally healthy, exercises regularly, and drinks 2 glasses of skim milk per day. Menstrual cycles are regular. She read an article on osteoporosis and insisted that her primary care physician order a DXA scan.

Physical Examination

Physical examination was unremarkable.

DXA Images

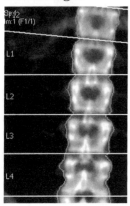
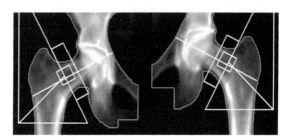

Region	BMD (g/cm²)	Young-Adult T-Score	Age-Matched Z-Score
L1	0.989	-1.2	-0.9
L2	1.032	-1.4	-1.1
L3	1.114	-0.7	-0.5
L4	1.044	-1.3	-1.0
L2-L4	1.063	-1.1	-0.9

Region	BMD (g/cm²)	Young-Adult T-Score	Age-Matched Z-Score
Neck			
Left	0.979	-0.5	0.3
Right	0.980	-0.5	0.3
Mean	0.980	-0.5	0.3
Difference	0.000	0.0	0.0

Laboratory Findings

Hemoglobin (12–15 mg/dL)	13 mg/dL
Serum creatinine (0.7–1.5 mg/dL)	0.8 mg/dL
ALT (7–35 IU/L)	25 IU/L
25-OHD (target >30 ng/mL)	35 ng/mL
Total serum calcium (8.9–10.3 mg/dL)	9.2 mg/dL
Phosphorus (2.6–4.4 mg/dL)	3.0 mg/dL
TSH (0.2–5 UU/L)	1.5 UU/L

ALT, alanine aminotransferase; TSH, thyroid-stimulating hormone.

Teaching Points
Dr. Camacho

- The patient is a premenopausal woman; it is important to know that the WHO criteria technically apply only to postmenopausal women. Thus, one must be careful in giving her the label of osteopenia or low bone mass.
- Her risk factor analysis shows that she is at low risk for fractures.
- This patient should be reassured and encouraged to continue with her healthy lifestyle.
- Her total elemental calcium intake should be 1,000 mg/day and vitamin D 400 IU/day.
- The patient will not need another DXA scan until after menopause unless she experiences fractures later on.

CASE 7

History

A 60-year-old frail-looking white woman has a history of two previous thoracic compression fractures. She has poorly controlled diabetes mellitus type 2 and end-stage renal disease (ESRD) and has been on hemodialysis for the past 3 years. The patient admitted to 3 inches of height loss. There is a maternal history of osteoporosis and diabetes mellitus. She does not smoke or drink.

Physical Examination

Physical examination revealed a small, thin woman with dorsal kyphosis. There was a soft systolic ejection murmur at the base and mild prominence of the thyroid gland.

DXA Images

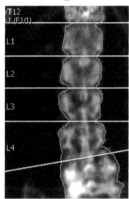
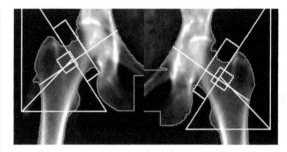

Region	BMD (g/cm²)	Young-Adult T-Score	Age-Matched Z-Score
L1	0.631	-4.2	-1.8
L2	0.693	-4.2	-1.9
L3	0.735	-3.9	-1.6
L4	0.737	-3.9	-1.5
L1-L2	0.662	-4.2	-1.9
L1-L3	0.687	-4.0	-1.7
L1-L4	0.703	-4.0	-1.7

Region	BMD (g/cm²)	Young-Adult T-Score	Age-Matched Z-Score
Neck			
Left	0.689	-2.9	-0.2
Right	0.644	-3.3	-0.5
Mean	0.667	-3.1	-0.3
Difference	0.044	0.4	0.4

Laboratory Findings

Hemoglobin (12–15 mg/dL)	10 mg/dL
Serum creatinine (0.7–1.5 mg/dL)	5.6 mg/dL
ALT (7–35 IU/L)	32 IU/L
25-OHD (target >30 ng/mL)	9 ng/mL
Intact PTH (10–65 pg/mL)	325 pg/mL
Ionized calcium (1.10–1.30 mmol/L)	1.10 mmol/L
Total serum calcium (8.9–10.3 mg/dL)	8.9 mg/dL
Phosphorus (2.6–4.4 mg/dL)	5.0 mg/dL
Bone-specific alkaline phosphatase	63.8 μg/L
Premenopausal female: 4.5–16.9 μg/L	
Postmenopausal female: 7.0–22.4 μg/L	
Male 25 years and older: 6.5–20.1 μg/L	
1-25 OHD (15–75 ng/dL)	12 ng/mL
TSH (0.2–5 UU/L)	0.45 UU/L

ALT, alanine aminotransferase; PTH, parathyroid hormone; TSH, thyroid-stimulating hormone.

Teaching Points

Dr. Miller

- Patients with low T-scores or fragility fractures who are on dialysis (stage 5 chronic kidney disease) need double tetracycline-labeled quantitative bone histomorphometry to make the correct diagnosis of the etiology of bone fragility.
- This requirement is because patients with renal osteodystrophy (all forms—adynamic bone disease, hyperparathyroid bone disease, osteomalacia) all have low T-scores and are subject to fracture. Hence neither the WHO criteria nor the presence of fractures can be used to diagnose osteoporosis in patients with ESRD. These patients can also get osteoporosis for many reasons and may be candidates for treatment with bisphosphonates, which are contraindicated in patients with adynamic bone disease or osteomalacia.
- Biochemical profiling can discriminate among the various forms of renal bone disease in groups of patients but not in individual patients—hence a biopsy is needed to make the exact diagnosis.
- Her elevated PTH and BSAP levels are more consistent with hyperparathyroid bone disease but not diagnostic—her PTH level would need to be greater than 600 pg/mL before there can be a greater degree of certainty that she has pure hyperparathyroid bone disease.
- Her 25-hydroxyvitamin D is low (as it often is in this population, like many other older or unhealthy people) and should be corrected first.
- If the bone biopsy shows hyperparathyroidism (osteitis fibrosa cystica), then she should be treated with either cinacalcet or a vitamin D analogue to suppress her PTH level to about 200 pg/mL.

- If the bone biopsy shows no evidence of severe hyperparathyroid bone disease or adynamic/osteomalacia bone disease, she would be a candidate for a bisphosphonate because she has osteoporosis by exclusion.
- Even though by Food and Drug Administration (FDA) label bisphosphonates are contraindicated in patients with glomerular filtration rates (GFRs) less than 30 mL/min, the clinician must do something to treat these osteoporotic high-risk patients.
- If bisphosphonates are used, this author would use half the usual dosing regimen and restrict the use to no more than 3 years because the bone retention of bisphosphonates may be greater in patients with severe reductions in GFR.

INDEX

Page numbers followed by "f" indicate figures; page numbers followed by "t" indicate tables.

A

Age-related bone loss
pathophysiology of, 17, 18f
Age-related fracture risk, 28
Alendronate, 128–129, 133, 135, 150, 158
Amenorrhhea, 83
Anabolic therapy, 132–133
Androgen deprivation therapy, 82, 83
Annotated references
biochemical evaluation, 70–80
bone densitometry using dual-energy x-ray absorptiometry for monitoring, 52–61
diagnosis, 11–14
fracture risk, 32–47
future treatment options, 194–201
pathogenesis, 19–24
secondary causes, 92–114
tailoring treatment to individual patients, 162–175
treatment options, 135–147
treatment success, 180–185
vitamin D deficiency, 121–126
Anorexia, 83, 84
fractures in, 161
Anticonvulsants, 85
Anti-RANK-ligand antibody
lumbar spine bone mass and, 190f, 191f, 191
Antiresorptive-induced changes
in spinal bone mineral density, 49, 50f
Antiresorptive therapy, 127–130
Arizoxifene, 187

B

Bazedoxifene, 187
Biochemical evaluation, 63–80, 64t
annotated references on, 70–80
tests for, 63–67
vitamin D deficiency and, 119
Biochemical markers of bone turnover, 68, 68t
fracture risk baseline determination, 69
fracture risk reduction prediction and, 69
limitation of, 69–70
monitoring effectiveness of, 68–69

postmenopausal bone loss and, 69
selection of, 70
Bisphosphonates, 127–130, 158–159, 160, 161, 181
intravenous, 180
oral
bioavailability of, 179
side effects and clinical issues with, 130–131
Bone
effects of glucocorticoids on, 18–19, 19f
Bone biopsy
double tetracycline-labeled, 161
Bone densitometry
using dual-energy x-ray absorptiometry for monitoring, 49–61, 50f
annotated references on, 52–61
value of, 50–51
Bone density
fracture risk versus, 3, 4f
Bone formation
and bone resorption
balance between, 192–193
Bone loss
age-related
pathophysiology of, 17, 18f
glucocorticoid-induced, 160
hormonal therapy to prevent, 158
osteoporotic
factors in, 16t
period of, 17
post-solid-organ transplantation, 160
Bone mass
lumbar spine
anti-RANK-ligand antibody and, 190f, 191f, 191
denosumab and, 190f, 191f, 191
intravenous zoledronic acid and, 188, 189f
oral versus intravenous ibandronate and, 187, 188f
peak, 16, 17f
Bone mineral density, 177
areal versus volumetric measurement of
anabolic therapy and, 51–52
bone turnover markers and, 157
dual-energy x-ray absorptiometry to measure, 32

Bone mineral density *(continued)*
fracture risk and, 25, 26f
increases in
pharmacologically-induced, 49, 50t
low
future fracture risk and, 27, 27t
in hip
teriparatide in, 159
with prior fracture, 152
medications and, 84–85
Bone remodeling cycle, 15–16, 16f
Bone resorption
and bone formation
balance between, 192–193
markers of, 156–157
Bone turnover markers, 156–157, 177
biochemical. *See* Biochemical markers
of bone turnover

C
Calciolytic agents, 187, 192–193
Calcitonin, 131, 150
Calcitriol
in vitamin D deficiency, 120
Calcium
serum total or ionized, 64t, 64–65
Calcium absorption
in celiac disease, 178
inadequate, 178
Calcium and creatinine test
24-hour urine, 66
Calcium homeostasis
vitamin D deficiency and, 117
Calcium therapy, 133–134
Cathepsin K inhibitors, 187, 192–193
Causes
secondary, 81–114, 82t
annotated references, 92–114
Celiac antibodies, 67
Celiac sprue, 90, 178
Cinacalcet, 193
Clinical cases
39-year-old woman with healthy
lifestyle, 216–217
49-year-old woman with idiopathic
hypercalciuria and osteoporosis,
206–207
61-year-old woman with low trauma
fractures and osteoporosis,
203–205
50-year-old woman with osteoporosis,
208–209
60-year-old woman with previous
compression fractures, 218–220

73-year-old woman with thoracic
kyphosis, 213–215
78-year-old woman with thoracic
kyphosis and osteoporosis,
210–212
Clinical picture, 1–3
Complete blood count, 63, 91
Crohn disease, 89
Cushing disease
screening for, 67
Cushing syndrome, 90
Cyclosporine, 85–86

D
Denosumab
lumbar spine bone mass and, 190f,
191f, 191
Depo-Provera
bone mass density and, 160
Diagnosis, 11–14
among males, 6–7
among nonwhite population, 3t,
3–11
annotated references on, 11–14
using peripheral devices, 7
Disease
burden of, 1
Dorsal kyphosis, 2
Dual-energy x-ray absorptiometry, 3,
49
of anteroposterior lumbar spine, 8f
femoral neck markers for, 9f
least significant change and, 51
to measure bone mineral density, 32
misinterpretations of, 7–11, 8f, 9f,
10f
multiple compression fractures on, 9f
in osteomalacia, 120
Paget disease and, 10f
showing sclerotic facet changes, 8f
vertebral fractures and, 30–32, 156

E
End-organ failure, 89
Endometriosis
bone mass density and, 160
Estrogen
hypogonadism and, 82
Estrogen receptor modulators
selective, 190–191
Etidronate, 150
Exercises
weight-bearing, 134

F

Fall(s)
    hip fracture and, 157–158
    prevention of, 134
        strategies for, 157–158
Femoral neck marker
    on dual-energy x-ray absorptiometry
        scans, 11
Femur Strength Index, 157
Fluoride, 149
Food and Drug Administration (FDA)
        registered therapies, 149, 150,
        150t
Forearm
    fractures of, 26
Fracture(s)
    compression
        on dual-energy x-ray
            absorptiometry scan, 9f
        vertebral, 26, 27, 27f
    of forearm, 26
    fragility. See Fragility fracture(s)
    of hip, 26
    humeral/shoulder, 26
    individual risk factors for, 154, 155t,
        157
    and normal or osteopenic T-scores,
        5–6, 6f
    osteoporotic
        in women, 2, 2f
    predictive risk of
        for future fractures, 26, 26t
    reduction of
        assessment of, 177–178
    of ribs, 26
    risk of
        age and, 28
        in women, 3, 4f
        annotated references on, 32–47
        assessment of, 25–47
        versus bone density, 3, 4f
        bone mineral density and, 25, 26f
        combined effect of risk factors on,
            28–29
    risk score for, 153, 154f, 155f, 155t
    specific types of
        treatment to reduce risk of, 158–159
    vertebral. See Vertebral fracture(s)
    vitamin D deficiency and, 118–119
Fragility fracture(s), 2–3
    definition of, 25
    and future fractures, 151–152
    history of, 25–28
    in hypogonadism, 161
    predictors of, 151, 151t
        risk of, 187
        treatment of, 154–155
        in younger patients, 161
Frailty scores, 157

G

Gastrointestinal diseases, 89–90
Glomerular filtration rate, 63
Glucocorticoid-induced osteoporosis,
        18–19, 134–135
Glucocorticoids
    effects on bone, 18–19, 19f
    inhaled, 84–85
    oral, 84
    vitamin D deficiency and, 118

H

Height loss, 1–2
Hematologic diseases, 90
Heparin, 85
Hip
    fractures of, 26
        falls and, 157–158
        low bone mineral density in
            teriparatide in, 159
    rotation of
        on dual-energy x-ray
            absorptiometry scans, 11
Hip protectors, 134
Hip structural analysis, 157
Hormonal therapy
    to prevent bone loss, 158
Hormone replacement therapy, 131–132,
        133, 149
Humerus/shoulder
    fractures of, 26
25-Hydroxyvitamin D, 65, 91
    measurement of, 119
Hypercalcemia
    due to calcitriol treatment, 120–121
Hypercalciuria, 66, 179
    idiopathic, 90–91
Hyperparathyroidism
    primary, 65, 88–89, 179
    secondary, 86
Hyperthyroidism, 86
Hypocalcemia
    signs of, 119–120
Hypocalciuria, 66
Hypoestrogenism, 83
Hypogonadism, 18, 82–84
    conditions producing, 82
    fragility fractures in, 161

I

Ibandronate, 130, 150, 158, 180
  intravenous, 187
    versus oral
      lumbar spine bone mass and, 187,
        188f
Immunosuppressants, 84, 85–86
Insulin-like growth factor 1
  decreased, 83
International Society for Clinical
        Densitometry (ISCD), 51
  guidelines for vertebral fracture
        assessment, 31

K

Kidney disease
  chronic
    parathyroid hormone goals in, 63,
      64t
Kidney function
  decrease in
    vitamin D deficiency and, 118
  estimation of
    tests for, 63
Kyphoplasty, 134
Kyphosis
  dorsal, 2

L

Lasofoxifene, 187
Liver function tests, 64
Long hip axis length, 157

M

Malabsorption
  vitamin D and, 117–118
Medications. *See* Pharmacological
        agents
Men
  osteoporosis in, 18, 82, 135
  younger
    tailoring therapy to, 160–162

N

N-teleopeptide
  urinary
    zoledronic acid and, 188, 189f
National Osteoporosis Risk Assessment
        (NORA), 6, 26

O

Osteoblastogenesis
  osteoblast-housed WINT pathway
        and, 193, 194f
Osteoblasts, 15
Osteoclasts, 15
Osteocytes, 15
Osteogenesis imperfecta, 160
Osteomalacia, 86–87
  calcium deficiency in, 120
  definition of, 119
  dual-energy x-ray absorptiometry in,
        120
  symptoms of, 119
Osteopenia
  fragility fractures and, 152f, 152–153,
        153f

P

Paget disease
  on dual-energy x-ray absorptiometry
        scan, 10f
Pamidronate, 150, 180
Parathyroid hormone, 1–84, 150
  goals
    in chronic kidney disease, 63, 64t
  increase in secretion of, 117
  intact
    levels of, 66
  synthetic human. *See* Teriparatide
Pathogenesis
  annotated references on, 19–24
Pharmacologic therapy, 127
  recommendations on, 128t
Pharmacological agents
  bone mineral density and, 84–85
  in development or under
        consideration, 187, 188t
  in future therapies, 187
  for prevention and treatment, 149,
        150t
  vitamin D deficiency and, 118
Phosphorus
  serum, 65
Postmenopausal osteoporosis, 16–17,
        18f, 127–134
Premenopausal women
  tailoring therapy to, 160–162
Prevention
  pharmacological agents for, 149,
        150t
Protein electrophoresis
  serum, 67
  urine, 67

R

Raloxifene, 131, 133, 150, 158
  and teriparatide, 160
Rib fractures, 26
Risedronate, 129–130, 150, 158

S

Sclerotic facet changes
  on dual-energy x-ray absorptiometry
    scan, 8f
Screening, 91
Selective estrogen receptor modulators,
    190–191
Serum creatinine, 63
Serum protein electrophoresis, 67
Spinal bone mineral density
  antiresorptive-induced changes in, 49,
    50f
Spine
  anteroposterior lumbar
    on dual-energy x-ray
      absorptiometry scan, 8f
  lumbar
    bone mass
      anti-RANK-ligand antibody and,
        190f, 191f, 191
      denosumab and, 190f, 191f,
        191
      oral versus intravenous
        ibandronate and, 187, 188f
Spine artifacts
  on dual-energy x-ray absorptiometry
    scans, 7–11
Strontium ranelate, 150, 192

T

T-scores, 5
Tacrolimus, 85–86
Teriparatide, 51, 132–133, 135, 150, 160,
    192, 193
  fracture risk and, 160
  in low hip bone mineral density, 159
  for nonunion of fractures, 161–162
  populations targeted for use of,
    159–160
  and raloxifene, 160
  in treatment failures, 181
Testosterone
  hypogonadism and, 82
Testosterone panel
  free, 67
Therapy. *See* Treatment

Thiazide diuretics
  in hypercalciurea, 179
Thyroid-stimulating hormones, 67
Transplantation, 89
Treatment
  failure of
    examination of laboratory tests of,
      178
    measures following, 177–185
  pharmacological agents for, 149, 150t
  success of, 177–185
    annotated references on, 180–185
    measurement of, 177
  tailoring to individual patients,
    149–175
    annotated references on, 162–175
Treatment options, 127–147
  annotated references on, 135–147
  future, 187–202
    annotated references on, 194–201
Triamcinolone, 84–85

U

Urine calcium and creatinine test
  24-hour, 66
Urine creatinine clearance
  24-hour, 63
Urine protein electrophoresis, 67

V

Vertebral compression fracture(s), 26,
    27, 27f
Vertebral fracture(s)
  assessment of, 31–32
    risk determined by, 30–32
  dual-energy x-ray absorptimetry and,
    156
  reduction by strontium ranelate, 192
Vertebral markers
  on dual-energy x-ray absorptiometry
    scans, 11
Vertebroplasty, 134
Vitamin D
  levels of
    in celiac disease, 178
  metabolism of, 116f, 116–117
  pleotropic effects of, 117
Vitamin D deficiency, 65, 86–88
  acquired, 115–126
  annotated references on, 121–126
  biochemical evaluation for, 119
  clinical conditions causing, 117–118
  definition of, 115–116

Vitamin D deficiency *(continued)*
    effects on calcium homeostasis, 117
    epidemiology of, 115
    and fractures, 118–119
    medications and, 118
    treatment of, 120
        monitoring of, 121
Vitamin D insufficiency, 178
Vitamin D supplementation, 133, 134

W
Weight-bearing exercises, 134
WINT pathway
    osteoblast-housed
        and osteoblastogenesis, 193, 194f
World Health Organization (WHO)
    absolute risk project, 29–30, 30f, 31t

criteria for assessment of severity, 5,
    5t
criteria use and misuse, 5–6
fracture risk and, 152f, 152–154, 153f,
    155f

X
X-ray absorptiometry scans
    dual-energy. *See* Dual-energy x-ray
        absorptiometry

Z
Z-scores, 5
Zolendronic acid, 150, 180, 187,
    188–189, 190
    urinary N-telopeptide and, 188, 189f